OFFICE ANDROLOGY

CONTEMPORARY ENDOCRINOLOGY

P. Michael Conn, SERIES EDITOR

Office Andrology, edited by *PHILLIP E. PATTON AND DAVID E. BATTAGLIA*, 2005
Stem Cells in Endocrinology, edited by *LINDA B. LESTER*, 2005
Male Hypogonadism: *Basic, Clinical, and Therapeutic Principles,* edited by *STEPHEN J. WINTERS*, 2004
Androgens in Health and Disease, edited by *CARRIE J. BAGATELL AND WILLIAM J. BREMNER*, 2003
Endocrine Replacement Therapy in Clinical Practice, edited by *A. WAYNE MEIKLE*, 2003
Early Diagnosis of Endocrine Diseases, edited by *ROBERT S. BAR*, 2003
Type I Diabetes: *Etiology and Treatment,* edited by *MARK A. SPERLING*, 2003
Handbook of Diagnostic Endocrinology, edited by *JANET E. HALL AND LYNNETTE K. NIEMAN*, 2003
Pediatric Endocrinology: *A Practical Clinical Guide,* edited by *SALLY RADOVICK AND MARGARET H. MACGILLIVRAY*, 2003
Diseases of the Thyroid, 2nd ed., edited by *LEWIS E. BRAVERMAN*, 2003
Developmental Endocrinology: *From Research to Clinical Practice,* edited by *ERICA A. EUGSTER AND ORA HIRSCH PESCOVITZ*, 2002
Osteoporosis: *Pathophysiology and Clinical Management,* edited by *ERIC S. ORWOLL AND MICHAEL BLIZIOTES*, 2002
Challenging Cases in Endocrinology, edited by *MARK E. MOLITCH*, 2002
Selective Estrogen Receptor Modulators: *Research and Clinical Applications,* edited by *ANDREA MANNI AND MICHAEL F. VERDERAME*, 2002
Transgenics in Endocrinology, edited by *MARTIN MATZUK, CHESTER W. BROWN, AND T. RAJENDRA KUMAR*, 2001
Sports Endocrinology, edited by *MICHELLE P. WARREN AND NAAMA W. CONSTANTINI*, 2000
Gene Engineering in Endocrinology, edited by *MARGARET A. SHUPNIK*, 2000
Endocrinology of Aging, edited by *JOHN E. MORLEY AND LUCRETIA VAN DEN BERG*, 2000
Human Growth Hormone: *Research and Clinical Practice,* edited by *ROY G. SMITH AND MICHAEL O. THORNER*, 2000
Hormones and the Heart in Health and Disease, edited by *LEONARD SHARE*, 1999
Menopause: *Endocrinology and Management,* edited by *DAVID B. SEIFER AND ELIZABETH A. KENNARD*, 1999
The IGF System: *Molecular Biology, Physiology, and Clinical Applications,* edited by *RON G. ROSENFELD AND CHARLES T. ROBERTS, JR.*, 1999
Neurosteroids: *A New Regulatory Function in the Nervous System,* edited by *ETIENNE-EMILE BAULIEU, MICHAEL SCHUMACHER, AND PAUL ROBEL*, 1999
Autoimmune Endocrinopathies, edited by *ROBERT VOLPÉ*, 1999
Hormone Resistance Syndromes, edited by *J. LARRY JAMESON*, 1999
Hormone Replacement Therapy, edited by *A. WAYNE MEIKLE*, 1999
Insulin Resistance: *The Metabolic Syndrome X,* edited by *GERALD M. REAVEN AND AMI LAWS*, 1999
Endocrinology of Breast Cancer, edited by *ANDREA MANNI*, 1999
Molecular and Cellular Pediatric Endocrinology, edited by *STUART HANDWERGER*, 1999
Gastrointestinal Endocrinology, edited by *GEORGE H. GREELEY, JR.*, 1999
The Endocrinology of Pregnancy, edited by *FULLER W. BAZER*, 1998

OFFICE ANDROLOGY

Edited by

PHILLIP E. PATTON, MD

and

DAVID E. BATTAGLIA, PhD

Department of Obstetrics and Gynecology,
Oregon Health and Science University,
University Fertility Consultants, Portland, OR

HUMANA PRESS
TOTOWA, NEW JERSEY

999 Riverview Drive, Suite 208
Totowa, New Jersey 07512

www.humanapress.com

For additional copies, pricing for bulk purchases, and/or information about other Humana titles, contact Humana at the above address or at any of the following numbers: Tel: 973-256-1699;Fax: 973-256-8341; E-mail: orders@humanapr.com.com or visit our website at humanapress.com

This publication is printed on acid-free paper. ∞
ANSI Z39.48-1984 (American National Standards Institute)
Permanence of Paper for Printed Library Materials.

Production Editor: C. Tirpak
Cover Design: Patricia Cleary

Cover Illustration: From Fig. 4, Chapter 4, "Specialized Sperm Testing: Pros and Cons," by Kirk C. Lo, Aron Johnson, Larry I. Lipshultz, and Dolores J. Lamb.

Printed in the United States of America. 10 9 8 7 6 5 4 3 2 1
eISBN: 1-59259-876-5

Library of Congress Cataloging-in-Publication Data

Office andrology / edited by Phillip E. Patton, and David E.Battaglia.
p. ; cm. -- (Contemporary endocrinology)
Includes bibliographical references and index. ISBN 1-58829-318-1 (alk. paper)
1. Andrology. 2. Infertility, Male. I. Patton, Phillip E. II. Battaglia, David Edward.
III. Series: Contemporary endocrinology (Totowa, N.J.)
[DNLM: 1. Infertility, Male--diagnosis. 2. Genital Diseases, Male. 3. Infertility, Male--therapy.
4. Insemination, Artificial. WJ 709 O32 2005]
RC875.O35 2005
612.6'1--dc22

2004027128

Preface

The investigation and management of male infertility can be a formidable diagnostic challenge to family physicians, urologists, and reproductive specialists alike. For the first time, health care providers can access a comprehensive resource that covers a broad spectrum of relevant clinical issues related to male infertility disorders.

In *Office Andrology*, a variety of topics including basic sperm biology, male reproductive endocrinology, immunology, specialized sperm testing, and genetic issues of male infertility are reviewed by recognized experts in the field. In addition, this book features a pragmatic review of the investigation, diagnostic testing, and management of the infertile male. Controversial medical and surgical treatment options are focus areas that should assist the practicing clinician. For the reproductive specialist, the text covers timely topics, including gender selection, HIV discordance couples, and posthumous reproduction in a thoughtful and comprehensive manner.

The goal of *Office Andrology* is to provide a practical guide for those requiring concise answers to both the urbane and complex scenarios attendant on male infertility. Practitioners wishing a greater understanding of the available diagnostic and treatment options will find *Office Andrology* especially useful in their clinical practice.

Phillip E. Patton, MD
David E. Battaglia, PhD

Contents

Contributors

Karen E. Adams, MD, FACOG, *Department of Obstetrics and Gynecology, Oregon Health and Science University, Portland, OR*
David E. Battaglia, PhD, *Department of Obstetrics and Gynecology, Oregon Health and Science University, University Fertility Consultants, Portland, OR*
Keith L. Blauer, MD, *Reproductive Care Center, Salt Lake City, UT*
Emmett F. Branigan, MD, *Bellingham IVF and Infertility Center, Bellingham, WA*
Lisa V. Brock, *Attorney General's Office, State of Washington, Olympia, WA*
William Byrd, PhD, HCLD, *Department of Obstetrics and Gynecology, University of Texas Southwestern Medical Center, Dallas, TX*
Grace M. Centola, PhD, HCLD(ABB), *Offices for Fertility and Reproductive Medicine, New York, NY; Professional ReproLab Consulting, Macedon, NY*
Eugene F. Fuchs, MD, *Department of Surgery, Division of Urology, Oregon Health and Science University, Portland, OR*
Wayne J.G. Hellstrom, MD, *Department of Urology, Tulane University School of Medicine, New Orleans, LA*
Aron Johnson, *Department of Obstetrics and Gynecology, Oregon Health and Science University, University Fertility Consultants, Portland, OR*
David S. Karabinus, PhD, *Genetics and IVF Institute, Fairfax, VA*
Dolores J. Lamb, PhD, HCLD, *Scott Department of Urology, Department of Molecular and Cellular Biology, Baylor College of Medicine, Houston, TX*
Larry I. Lipshultz, MD, *Scott Department of Urology, Baylor College of Medicine, Houston, TX*
Kirk C. Lo, MD, *Scott Department of Urology, Baylor College of Medicine, Houston, TX*
Anna C. Mastroianni, *Attorney General's Office, State of Washington, Olympia, WA.*
R. Dale McClure, MD, FRCS(C) *Section of Urology, Virginia Mason Medical Center, Seattle, WA*
Sharon T. Mortimer, PhD, *Oozoa Biomedical Inc., West Vancouver, BC, Canada*
Kinloch Nelson, MD, *Virginia Urology, Hanover Medical Park, Mechanicsville, VA*
Robert D. Oates, MD, *Department of Urology, Boston University School of Medicine, Boston, MA*
Darius A. Paduch, MD, *Department of Urology, Weill Medical College of Cornell University, New York, NY*

PHILLIP E. PATTON, MD, *Department of Obstetrics and Gynecology, Oregon Health and Science University, University Fertility Consultants, Portland, OR*
JOSEPH E. PEÑA, MD, *Department of Obstetrics and Gynecology, Columbia Presbyterian Medical Center, New York, NY*
MARK V. SAUER, MD, *Department of Obstetrics and Gynecology, Columbia Presbyterian Medical Center, New York, NY*
PETER SCHLEGEL, MD, *Department of Urology, Weill Medical College of Cornell University, New York, NY*
SHERMAN J. SILBER, MD, *Infertility Center of St. Louis, St. Luke's Hospital, St. Louis, MO and Department of OB-GYN Infertility Center, New York, NY*
PAUL TUREK, MD, *Department of Urology, University of California San Francisco, San Francisco, CA*
MUSTAFA F. USTA, MD, *Department of Urology, Tulane University School of Medicine, New Orleans, LA*
ULRIKE ZENKE, MD, *Department of Urology, University of California San Francisco, San Francisco, CA*

1 Essentials of Sperm Biology

Sharon T. Mortimer, PhD

CONTENTS

INTRODUCTION

That the spermatozoon has a role in reproduction has been known for centuries, but the specifics of its contribution have only come to be understood in relatively recent times. Antoni van Leeuwenhoek was the first to describe "semen animals" (spermatozoa) in an ejaculate in 1677, and in 1679, he discovered the presence of spermatozoa in the *vas deferens* and testicular tissue, leading him to conclude that sperm production was the sole purpose of the testis *(1)*. In 1683, he wrote that he was certain "that man comes not from an egg but from an animalcule in the masculine seed," and in 1685, he concluded that each spermatozoon contained both a person in miniature and a persistent and living soul. This argument was in contradiction to Harvey's and de Graaf's hypotheses that it was the egg that contained the miniature and entire human, and the semen was merely the vehicle of a stimulating spirit that started the growth of the egg into the embryo.

Acceptance of the equal role of the spermatozoon and oocyte in reproduction began in the latter part of the 19th century, and the understanding of the structure and function of spermatozoon was developed during the 20th century, following improvements in the technology of microscopy and the identification of DNA as genetic material.

From: *Contemporary Endocrinology: Office Andrology*
Edited by: P. E. Patton and D. E. Battaglia

This chapter aims to provide an overview of the biology of the spermatozoon, including its role in fertilization.

SPERM PRODUCTION

Spermatozoa are highly specialized haploid cells produced in the testes of adult males. Each testis is comprised largely of convoluted seminiferous tubules, which are packed loosely into lobes separated by bands of fibrous tissue. Each seminiferous tubule is a loop, with its ends draining into the rete testis, and then into the efferent ducts and epididymis. Within each lobe, the seminiferous tubule is enclosed by loose connective tissue containing blood vessels, nerves, and lymph vessels, as well as the Leydig cells, which produce testosterone in response to luteinizing hormone.

Seminiferous tubules of adult men have a stratified epithelium of several layers and a central lumen. The basal compartment is the outermost part of the tubule contents and contains the resting spermatogonia (the basic self-renewing stem cell of the male germline) and Sertoli cells, which act to regulate the development of the germinal cells along with the maturation and release of spermatozoa into the central lumen of the seminiferous tubule. Each Sertoli cell is joined to its neighbors by tight junctions, forming the blood–testis barrier, which prevents the passage of molecules between the basal and luminal compartment of the seminiferous tubules. Another effect of the blood–testis barrier is to prevent the initiation of an immune response to spermatozoa by the man's immune system, because these antigenically "foreign" cells are not produced until puberty.

Spermatozoa are produced from their progenitor spermatogonia in a series of processes termed "spermatogenesis," "spermiogenesis," and "spermiation." Spermatogenesis begins with six cycles of mitotic proliferation of a diploid spermatogonium, resulting in the production of a clone of daughter cells—the primary spermatocytes. The primary spermatocytes then leave the basal compartment and push into the adluminal compartment of the seminiferous epithelium, where they enter the meiotic prophase. At the completion of prophase, each primary spermatocyte produces two sondary spermatocytes, each of which then divides to produce two haploid spermatids. Because all of these cell divisions are not complete, the 64 spermatids created from each spermatogonium form a syncytium; i.e., they are all interconnected by cellular bridges of cytoplasm. Spermatids are still round cells at this stage, and they differentiate into mature spermatids or testicular spermatozoa in the process of spermiogenesis.

Spermiogenesis is a complex series of maturational and transformational processes that occur in the adluminal compartment of the seminiferous tubules. In this process, the nuclear histones are replaced by protamines, which then become crosslinked by disulphide bonds, making the chromatin highly condensed and resulting in a much smaller nucleus. The nucleus then moves into an eccentric position, closer to the cell membrane. The acrosome is generated by the Golgi complex, and this is applied to the part of the nucleus in contact with the cell membrane. One of the centrioles attaches to the opposite side of the nucleus and produces the axial filament, around which the axonemal structures develop to form the axial filament complex. Cytoplasmic reduction occurs, and the mitochondria become arranged around the proximal portion of the developing tail.

At the completion of spermiogenesis, spermatozoa are released, tail-first, into the lumen of the seminiferous tubule. The residual cytoplasm is pinched off at the neck region of the mature spermatid as it leaves the seminiferous epithelium in a process termed "spermiation." Following spermiation, the mature spermatids are transported to the rete testis and then to the epididymis where they undergo posttesticular sperm maturation, a series of morphological, biochemical, biophysical, and metabolic changes. The epididymis can be divided into three functional regions: the caput (head), corpus (body), and cauda (tail), with the general functions of sperm concentration, maturation, and storage, respectively. At the end of their transport through the epididymis, spermatozoa have acquired the ability to become motile when they come into contact with seminal fluid at ejaculation.

By definition, spermatozoa are not functionally mature until ejaculation, but there is a developing conflict between physiology and technology. The clinical procedure of injecting testicular or epididymal spermatozoa into oocytes in the process of intracytoplasmic sperm injection (ICSI) has resulted in the births of many babies worldwide in the past decade, suggesting that these immature spermatozoa are "fertile." Furthermore, recent reports of the successful use of epididymal spermatozoa for intrauterine insemination suggest that in the human, functional maturity of spermatozoa may be attained at an earlier developmental stage than in other species. However, it must be noted that for the vast majority of couples, the surgical retrieval of spermatozoa is unnecessary for fertility. Therefore, the remainder of this chapter reviews the biology of ejaculated spermatozoa.

SPERM STRUCTURE

A normal human spermatozoon is 55 to 70 μm in length and has three main structural regions: the head, midpiece, and tail (flagellum). The principal function of the sperm head is the contribution of its haploid set of chromosomes to the oocyte at fertilization, whereas the midpiece and tail provide the motility necessary for the spermatozoon to reach the site of fertilization (Fig. 1). The sperm head contains the cell's nuclear DNA, but the chromatin is heavily con-

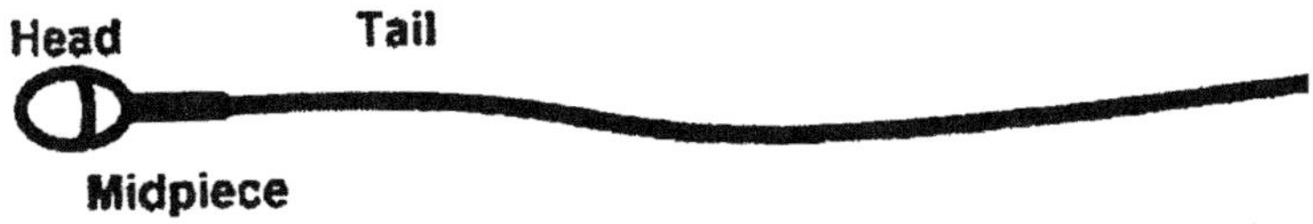

Fig. 1. Diagram of a human spermatozoon. The acrosome is shown covering the anterior portion of the head.

densed, and its protamines are highly crosslinked so that the sperm nucleus is stabilized and effectively inactivated until after fertilization. This makes the head of the spermatozoon inflexible, which assists in penetration of the oocyte's zona pellucida during fertilization. The anterior half to two-thirds of the sperm head is covered by the acrosome, the membrane-bound structure that originated from the Golgi complex during spermiogenesis. The acrosome contains hydrolytic enzymes that are released during the acrosome reaction. For the fertilizing spermatozoon, this occurs on or near the surface of the oocyte's zona pellucida.

The sperm midpiece contains the mitochondria that generate energy via oxidative phosphorylation; the centriole, used by the fertilized oocyte in its first cell division; and the beginnings of axoneme, the motility apparatus. The mitochondria are arranged helically around the proximal part of the axoneme, and they supply the adenosine triphosphate (ATP) necessary for flagellar motility.

The axoneme is a highly complex structure composed of microtubules and dynein that extends along most of the flagellum (Fig. 2). The central portion of the axoneme contains a pair of microtubules, which are connected to each other by linkages. These are surrounded by nine microtubule doublets, each consisting of an A subunit (a complete microtubule) and a B subunit (a C-shaped microtubule structure whose ends are attached to the A subunit). A pair of dynein arms are attached to each of the A subunits. Dynein is an ATPase, and it is thought that when the ATP generated by mitochondria reaches the dynein arms, their conformation changes, allowing them to reach out and attach to the B subunit adjacent microtubule. This attachment allows the first microtubule doublet to rachet forward relative to the second doublet. When this movement is completed, the dynein arms return to their normal conformation and release the second microtubule doublet. In turn, the dynein arms of the second microtubule doublet then reach out and attach to the B subunit of the third microtubule doublet, and the cycle continues around the nine pairs. This movement of microtubule doublets relative to each other generates and propagates the flagellar beat and confers motility.

Therefore, an absence of dynein arms in the axoneme, as occurs in Kartagener syndrome, renders the spermatozoa immotile and is a cause of infertility. However, in recent years, spermatozoa from men with Kartagener syndrome have

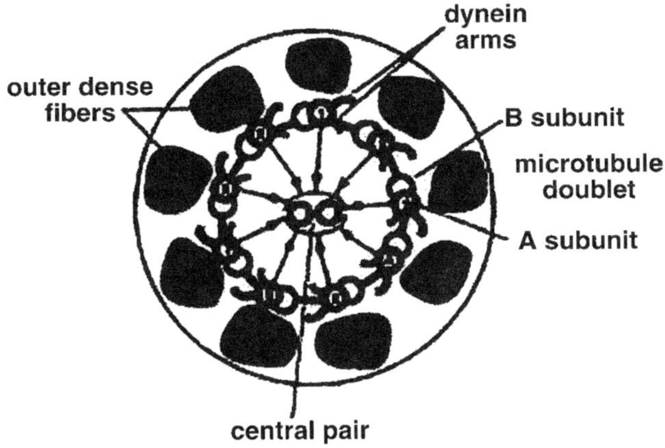

Fig. 2. Diagram of a cross-section of the sperm axoneme. (Adapted from ref. *2*.)

been used successfully in ICSI, because this technique removes the requirement of sperm motility for fertilization, resulting in the births of some normal children.

A set of nine outer dense fibers is arranged outside the microtubule doublets. The exact role for these fibers is unclear, but it is thought that they act to stiffen the proximal portion of the flagellum and also cause an elastic recoil of the axoneme after microtubule doublet sliding.

SPERM FUNCTION AND PHYSIOLOGY

Following their production in the testis, spermatozoa are transported through the caput and corpus regions of the epididymis, then stored in the proximal cauda epididymis. The spermatozoa mature during epididymal transit and storage and acquire functional competence. The most obvious maturational change in spermatozoa is the acquisition of the ability to move when in contact with seminal plasma or physiological culture media—a process referred to as "activation." Other changes during epididymal maturation of spermatozoa are alterations to the plasma membrane, chromatin condensation and stabilization, and possibly some final modifications to the shape of the acrosome.

At ejaculation, sperm are transported from their storage site and are mixed with prostatic fluid and seminal vesicle fluid before passage along the penile urethra. The first fraction of the ejaculate contains most of the spermatozoa, suspended in epididymal and prostatic fluid, whereas subsequent fractions contain both prostatic and vesicular fluid. During intercourse, the spermatozoa are deposited into the vagina, near the cervical os, and must swim through the cervical mucus, traverse the uterus, enter the oviduct, and reach the oocyte in its ampullary portion for fertilization to occur.

Mammalian spermatozoa cannot fertilize oocytes immediately upon ejaculation nor upon retrieval from the epididymis. A series of metabolic and physiological changes collectively termed "capacitation" must happen before spermatozoa acquire the ability to penetrate the zona pellucida and bind to the oocyte. In nature, these changes occur during transit through the female reproductive tract, but it is possible to induce capacitation in vitro using appropriate culture media and conditions; consequently, this is an integral step for successful in vitro fertilization.

It is indicated that modifications to the sperm plasma membrane, occuring during epididymal transit, act to stabilize the spermatozoon and prevent it from capacitating in the male reproductive tract, as the completion of capacitation marks the beginning of membrane destabilization events, which eventually lead to cell death. One function of capacitation is the removal of these stabilizing residues, such as cholesterol—the removal of which renders the plasma membrane more fusogenic, being critical for successful sperm–egg interaction. It is not possible to visualize the capacitation-related changes in the sperm plasma membrane, making it impossible to assay for capacitation alone, but it may be monitored through changes in chlortetracycline-binding patterns on the sperm head or by changes in lectin-binding sites. In the human, capacitation may begin with the removal of some sperm surface components during passage through cervical mucus owing to the high-shear forces to which the spermatozoa are exposed.

The cervix acts as a barrier to sperm penetration, resulting in the less-competent spermatozoa being excluded from reaching the uterus and oviduct. Generally, motility determines whether a spermatozoon will penetrate the cervical mucus, but passage of motile spermatozoa with antibodies bound to their surface is inhibited. As described previously, motility is dependent on the function of both the sperm midpiece (for energy generation) and tail (for beat development and propagation). If there are one or more defects in the midpiece or tail, a spermatozoon's motility will be impaired. Cervical mucus is receptive to spermatozoa only in the periovulatory period, as its secretion is under endocrine control, but even at this time, spermatozoa experience high-shear forces during penetration. Therefore, for successful passage through the cervical mucus, spermatozoa must be highly progressively motile with significant lateral head movement, reflecting the amplitude of the flagellar beat. The morphology of the spermatozoon does not necessarily equate with mucus-penetrating ability, but because immotile (or poorly motile) spermatozoa cannot pass the cervix, those spermatozoa with midpiece and/or tail abnormalities are excluded. Also, considering the observation that spermatozoa with head defects are at least twice as likely to have coexisting midpiece and/or tail defects, many spermatozoa with head abnormalities will not penetrate the cervix because of co-existing abnormal motility. However, if the only morphological abnormality of a spermatozoon is in its head shape, then the cervical mucus will not inhibit its passage.

Once past the internal os, the spermatozoa swim through the uterus and enter the oviduct via the uterotubal junction. The sperm movement pattern is likely still linear and progressive at this stage, but it is difficult to confirm this experimentally. Once spermatozoa enter the isthmus of the oviduct, it is thought that they bind to its epithelial cells, forming a "reservoir" where they are held in a quiescent "semicapacitated" state until ovulation.

Following ovulation, contractile movement of the oviduct, beating of the epithelial cilia, and sperm motility all contribute to sperm transport in the oviduct. The ampullary ciliary movements direct the fluid in the oviductal lumen from the ampulla toward the isthmus. Spermatozoa are constrained to swim against currents; hence, the directed current toward the isthmus forces the spermatozoa to swim in the opposite direction toward the ampulla, which is the site of fertilization. In accordance with careful studies only possible in experimental animals, it is postulated that small numbers of spermatozoa are released from the isthmus sequentially, resulting in relatively few spermatozoa in the ampulla at once.

Movement patterns (kinematics) of spermatozoa change concomitantly with capacitation with the development of a nondirected whiplash-style of movement referred to as "hyperactivated motility." In animal models, this hyperactivated motility has been observed in the ampulla, the site of fertilization, and has led to the development of several theories as to its physiological relevance. These include concepts of hyperactivation:

- Provides a mechanism to reduce the chance of entrapment of spermatozoa in the crypts of the oviduct.
- Maintains spermatozoa in the ampulla, thereby setting them up in a search pattern for the oocyte.
- Encourages stirring of ampullary fluid to maintain a homogeneous mixture of metabolites in the region where fertilization will occur.
- Confers upon the spermatozoon the ability to traverse the cumulus matrix, because hyperactivated spermatozoa have a tenfold higher efficiency at penetrating highly viscous media than nonhyperactivated spermatozoa.
- Provides power generation for zona pellucida penetration. (It has been estimated that the sperm–zona bonds that form in fertilization have a strength of about 4×10^{-4} μ*N*, whereas the force generated by the hyperactivated beat pattern is 2.7×10^{-2} μ*N*, two orders of greater magnitude. The force generated by nonhyperactivated spermatozoa is $<3 \times 10^{-4}$ μ*N*—not enough to disrupt the sperm–zona bond.)

It is likely that hyperactivation is an integral part of more than just one of the processes involved in sperm transport through the female reproductive tract and in sperm–egg interactions, and experimental animal studies predict that failure of hyperactivation would be associated with fertilization failure, both in vivo and in vitro.

When the spermatozoon encounters the cumulus–oocyte-complex, it traverses the cumulus matrix and binds to the zona pellucida, where it undergoes the acrosome reaction, a prerequisite for sperm–egg fusion. The acrosome reaction involves localized fusions of the plasma membrane and outer acrosomal membrane over the anterior portion of the sperm head. Vesicles composed of the plasma membrane and outer acrosomal membrane form, allowing the release of acrosomal contents, including hyaluronidase and acrosin, leaving the anterior portion of the head covered by the inner acrosomal membrane. Following completion of this reaction, the spermatozoon penetrates the zona pellucida. Although it has been taught for many years that zona penetration is a purely chemical process with the acrosomal enzymes digesting the glycoproteins of the zona pellucida, more recent work considering the role of hyperactivated motility suggests that it is more likely to be a combination of chemical softening and mechanical propulsion factors.

After successful penetration of the zona pellucida, the spermatozoon enters the perivitelline space, comes into contact with the microvilli of the oocyte plasma membrane (oolemma), and the postacrosomal region of the sperm head binds to the oolemma. Flagellar motility ceases at this time, and fusion is initiated between the oolemma and the equatorial segment of the spermatozoon. The whole spermatozoon is then engulfed by the oocyte. The nucleus of the sperm head decondenses to form the male pronucleus with a new nuclear envelope derived from components in the ooplasm. This can then fuse with the female pronucleus that was formed following the resumption of oocyte meiosis triggered by sperm-oolemma contact. The fertilized oocyte is referred to as a zygote, then subsequently as an embryo, after the first cleavage.

RELATIONSHIP BETWEEN SPERM PHYSIOLOGY AND INFERTILITY

The complexity of sperm structure and function means that it can be difficult to determine the pathophysiological reason(s) a man's infertility. If the developmental or maturational processes are perturbed, this could result in problems, such as:

- Low sperm concentration (from inefficient spermatogenesis)
- Poor sperm motility (caused by midpiece or axonemal abnormalities)
- Abnormal sperm morphology (owing to errors in spermiogenesis)

This list is clearly only illustrative—it could be extended to take in every step of each process, from the activation of spermatogonium to fertilization, and even further, because embryo development is affected by the quality of the nuclear DNA of fertilizing spermatozoon.

REFERENCES

1. Leeuwenhoek's perception of the spermatozoa. Adapted from Ruestow EG. J History Biol 1983;16:185–224. Available from: www.zygote.swarthmore.edu/fert1a. Accessed May 2003.
2. Mortimer ST. A critical review of the physiological importance and analysis of sperm movement in mammals. Hum Reprod Update 1997;3:403–439.

2 Endocrinology of Male Infertility

R. Dale McClure, MD, FRCS(C)

CONTENTS

INTRODUCTION

Understanding reproductive physiology is pivotal in the evaluation and therapy of endocrine abnormalities. Although an endocrinological cause of male infertility is uncommon (less than 2%) *(1)* identification is important, as specific hormonal therapy is often successful. The human testis is an organ of dual function: spermatogenesis, occuring in the seminiferous tubules, and secretion of steroid hormones (androgens) by the Leydig cells, present in the interstitial tissue. These testicular functions are intimately related, because testosterone synthesis is required not only for sperm production, but also for the development of secondary sexual characteristics and normal sexual behavior. The anterior

From: *Contemporary Endocrinology: Office Andrology*
Edited by: P. E. Patton and D. E. Battaglia © Humana Press Inc., Totowa, NJ

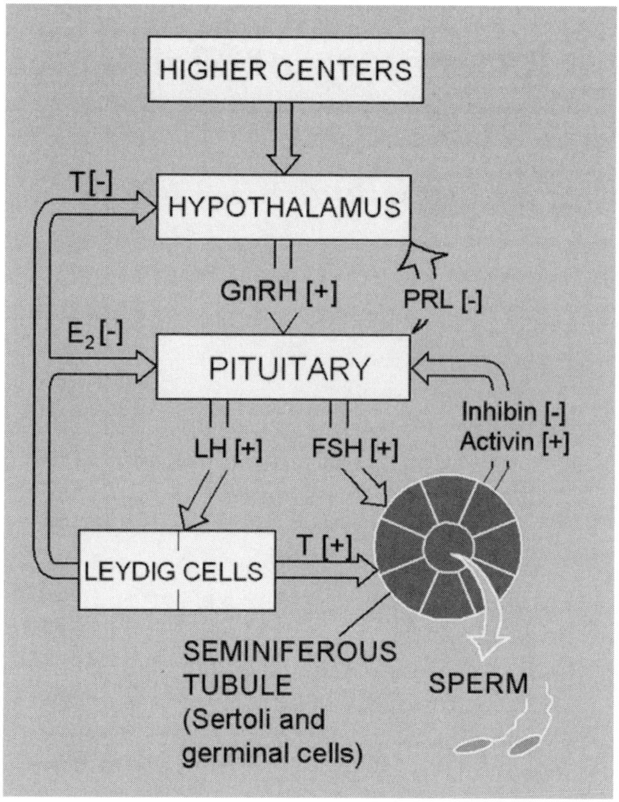

Fig. 1. Hypothalamic-pituitary-gonadal axis. LH, luteinizing hormone; FSH, follicle stimulating hormone; T, testosterone; DHT, dihydrotestosterone; E2, estradiol; GnRH, gonadotropin-releasing hormone; PR, prolactin; +, positive influence; –, negative influence.

pituitary controls both these functions through the secretion of gonadotropins, luteinizing hormone (LH), and follicle-stimulating hormone (FSH). In turn, the anterior pituitary is regulated by the hypothalamic secretion of gonadotropin-releasing hormone (GnRH). The extrahypothalamic central nervous system then influences the hypothalamus. The hypothalamic-pituitary-gonadal axis consists of a closed-loop feedback control mechanism directed at maintaining normal reproductive function (Fig. 1) *(2–5)*.

REPRODUCTIVE PHYSIOLOGY

The Hypothalamus

The hypothalamus—the integrative center of the reproductive axis—receives neural input from many brain centers and is the *pulse generator* for the cyclical secretion of pituitary and gonadal hormones *(4,5)*. The function and anatomical association of the pituitary gland with the hypothalamus is accomplished by the hypophyseal portal microvascular system. This portal vascular system provides a direct route for the delivery of hypothalamic-releasing hormones to the anterior pituitary gland. In contrast, reverse flow through this vascular route may allow pituitary hormones direct access to the hypothalamus, e.g., men with pituitary hyperprolactinemia often have problems both with impotence and libido *(5)*. The excess prolactin in these individuals has direct access to, and may affect, higher brain centers.

The single hypothalamic decapeptide, GnRH, has stimulatory effects on the pituitary gland, resulting in the synthesis and release of both gonadotropic hormones, LH and FSH. GnRH is released to the portal circulation in pulses occurring on the average basis of 1 pulse every 70 to 90 min and has a very short half-life in the blood of approx 2 to 5 min. The pulsatile secretion of GnRH appears to be essential for the stimulatory effects on LH and FSH release *(3,4)*. Alternatively, constant exposure of the gonadotropins to GnRH results in paradoxic inhibitory effects on LH and FSH, and the pituitary becomes desensitized through the continuous exposure of GnRH by the downregulation of pituitary receptors.

A variety of influences, including age, diet, stress, and exercise, may affect GnRH secretion *(4)*. Neurotransmitters (norepinephrine, dopamine, serotonin, and acetylcholine) and neuropeptides (endogenous opioid peptides) have both inhibitory and stimulatory effects on the hypothalamus *(4,5)*. Pituitary gonadotropins and gonadal steroids also modulate the pulse frequency and amplitude of GnRH secretion.

ANTERIOR PITUITARY

Binding to high-affinity receptors on pituitary cells (gonadotrophs), GnRH influences the release of the two primary pituitary hormones (LH and FSH) that regulate testicular function. These pituitary hormones are both glycoproteins composed of two polypeptide-chain subunits. The protein component of the α-subunits are identical and similar to other pituitary hormones (thyroid-stimulating hormone [TSH] and human chorionic gonadotropin [hCG]), but biological and immunological activity are conferred by the unique β-subunit *(2)*. Although both hormones are secreted in an episodic manner by the pituitary gland, the longer half-life of FSH in circulation is reflected by a more constant serum level than that of the more rapidly metabolized LH. The peak and trough pattern of blood levels of gonadotropins, particularly LH, is clinically important because a single measurement of circulating LH may be as much as 50% above or below the mean integrated hormone concentrations *(6)*.

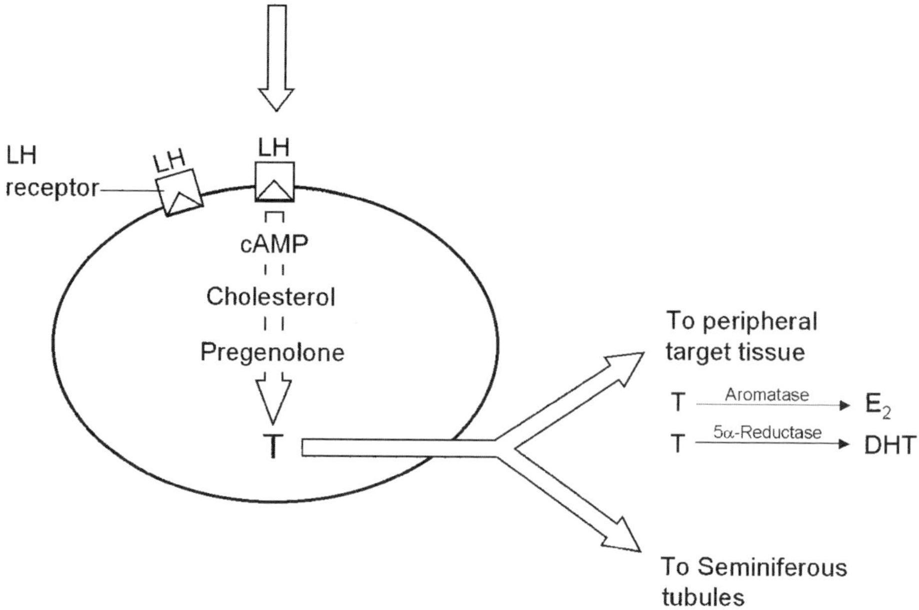

Fig. 2. Testosterone production and metabolism. cAMP, cyclic adenosine monophosphate; T, testosterone; E2, estradiol; DHT, dihydrotestosterone.

TESTES

LH interacts with specific high-affinity cell surface receptors on the plasma membrane of Leydig cells. Ligand binding stimulates a membrane-bound adenylate cyclase to enhance the formation of cyclic adenosine monophosphate (cAMP), which binds to the regulatory subunits of protein kinase. This, in turn, causes dissociation of regulatory subunit and activation of the catalytic subunit of the enzyme. The activated Leydig cell protein kinase operates through several steps to stimulate the enzyme synthesis of testosterone synthesis (Fig. 2) *(2,3)*.

FSH targets the epithelium of the seminiferous tubule and binds to membrane receptors on the Sertoli's cells. The second messenger is the cAMP, and activation of adenylate cyclase stimulates cAMP-dependent protein kinase and RNA and protein synthesis, including synthesis of the androgen-binding protein and aromatase enzyme that converts testosterone to estradiol (Fig. 3) *(2,3)*.

FEEDBACK CONTROL OF GONADOTROPINS

The hypothalamic-pituitary-gonadal system is a closed-loop feedback system directed at maintaining normal reproductive function *(2–5)*. Gonadal hormones have inhibitory effects on the secretion of LH and FSH. Although testosterone—

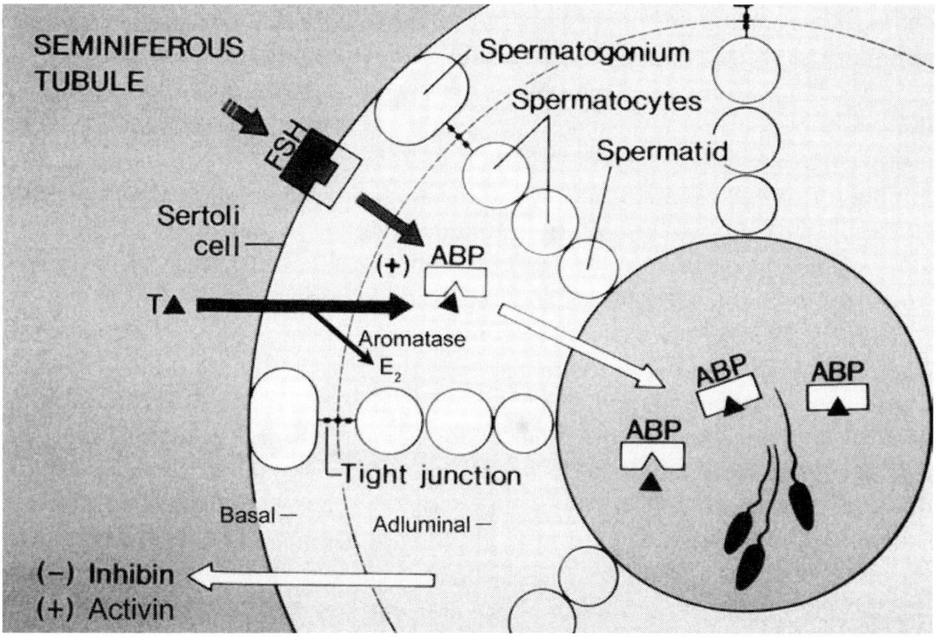

Fig. 3. Schematic representation of the seminiferous tubule. Follicle-stimulating hormone (FSH) and testosterone (T) act on the Sertoli cells to produce androgen-binding protein (ABP), inhibin, activin, as well as estradiol (E2).

the major secretory product of the testes—is a primary inhibitor of LH secretion in men, other testes products, including estrogens and other androgens, also inhibit LH secretion. Testosterone is metabolized in peripheral tissues to the potent androgen dihydrotestosterone (DHT) or potent estrogen, estradiol.

Both androgens and estrogens *independently* appear to modulate LH secretion. Estradiol is produced both by the testes and from peripheral conversion of androgenic precursors and is a more potent inhibitor of LH and FSH secretion. Infusions of gonadal steroids in amounts that accumulate physiological concentrations of the hormones in the blood demonstrate suppression of LH levels for testosterone and estradiol, suggesting that *both* hormones may have an important role in LH regulation. Gonadal sex steroids influence the *frequency* and/or *amplitude* of LH secretory pulses in men by acting at the level of the GnRH pulse generator in the hypothalamus and partly at the level of GnRH-stimulated LH secretion *(2–5)*.

The mechanism for the feedback control of FSH secretion is even more controversial than that of LH. After castration, FSH increases the indication of a negative feedback from testicular products. Like LH, both testosterone and estradiol are capable of suppressing FSH serum levels, but the influence of these two gonadal steroids in physiological function is still undefined *(2,4)*.

A nonsteroidal tubular factor may also be significant in the feedback regulation of FSH. *Inhibin* has been isolated and characterized in follicular fluid and is produced by the Sertoli cells of the testes. Inhibin has two subunits: α and β. Two inhibin forms have been isolated—inhibin A (α and β A subunits) and inhibin B (α and β B subunits)—both of which have been shown to cause selective suppression of FSH release in vitro *(4)*. The combination of the two β-subunits led to the formation of *activins*, which increase FSH secretion in vitro. In addition to inhibin, numberous gonadal peptides and growth factors, such as follistatin and transforming growth factor B, are also modulators of FSH secretion *(4)*. Reductions in spermatogenesis are accompanied by decreased production of inhibin, and this decline in negative feedback is associated with reciprocal elevation of FSH levels. Isolated levels of FSH constitute an important and sensitive marker of the status of the germinal epithelium *(2)*.

Even in pathological conditions with marked damage to the germinal tissue, serum FSH is not elevated to castrate levels unless Leydig cell function is also impaired. It appears that *both* gonadal steroids and peptides are important to maintain normal serum FSH concentrations.

PROLACTIN AND GONADOTROPINS

Hyperprolactinemia is linked with disturbed reproductive function reflected by a variety of symptoms and signs of hypogonadism. LH levels are inappropriately low relative to low-serum testosterone levels, indicating that the hypothalamic-pituitary axis fails to respond to reduced testicular testosterone production *(4,5)*. Prolactin may inhibit GnRH secretion either directly or through modulation of the dopaminergic pathways. Although the pituitary responds normally to GnRH administration, the pulse frequency of LH secretion is diminished in hyperprolactinemic individuals. Bromocriptine, a dopamine agonist with prolactin-lowering activities, improves sexual function *(7)*. Excessive prolactin may affect sexual functions by having a direct effect on the central nervous system and also from inhibition of androgen secretion. In individuals with elevated prolactin, libido does not return to normal as long as the prolactin levels remain elevated despite use of androgen therapy *(5)*.

ANDROGEN PHYSIOLOGY

Androgens regulate gonadotropin secretion, initiation and maintenance of spermatogenesis, formation of male phenotype during sexual differentiation, promotion of sexual maturation at puberty, and controlling sexual drive and potency *(2)*.

Testosterone is synthesized from pregnenolone within the Leydig cells. Testosterone production in men approximates 5 mg per day and the secretion occurs in an irregular pulsatile manner. There is a diurnal pattern: the peak level is in the early morning, and the nadir is in the evening *(8)*. Inside androgen target cells, testosterone can be converted to DHT by 5α-reductase. Both these androgens bind to the same high-affinity-androgen receptor protein; subsequently, the hormone receptor complex is attached to acceptor sites in the nuclei to affect the biologic response *(3–5)*.

Estrogens may either be secreted directly by the testes or formed in peripheral tissues. Like other steroid hormones, androgens and estrogens initiate their effect at the cellular level by interacting with high-affinity receptor proteins and are present in the highest concentration in androgen target tissues, e.g., the accessory organs of male reproduction. In the testes, androgen receptors are present both in Sertoli cells and Leydig cells.

In normal males, 2% of testosterone is *free* (unbound), and 44% is bound to a high-affinity sex hormone-binding globulin (SHBG), and the remainder is bound to albumin and other proteins. Free- and albumin-bound portions make up the measure known as *bioavailable testosterone (2–4)*. It was formerly believed that the physiologic active androgen moiety was the nonprotein-bound free testosterone. Now it appears that the cellular transfer of steroid hormones is more complicated and can involve hormone dissociation from the binding proteins, such as albumin-bound testosterone, within the microcirculation of the brain and liver *(9)*. SHBG has a higher affinity for testosterone than for estradiol, and changes in SHBG concentration can alter the hormonal milieu. Elevated estrogens, thyroid hormone, and healthy aging increases plasma SHBG and therefore decreases the free testosterone fraction *(10)*. Alternatively, androgens, growth hormone, and obesity depress SHBG levels and increase the active androgen fraction (Fig. 4) *(10,11)*.

HORMONAL CONTROL OF SPERMATOGENESIS

Spermatogenesis is primarily controlled by the gonadotropins—FSH and LH. LH indirectly affects spermatogenesis by stimulating endogenous testosterone production. The Sertoli cells possess specific high-affinity FSH receptors and produce androgen-binding protein, which carries androgens intracellularly, serves as an androgen reservoir within the seminiferous tubule, and transports testosterone from the testes into the epididymal tubule. The physical proximity of the Leydig cells to the seminiferous tubules, and the elaboration by the Sertoli cells of ABP, maintain an extremely high level of androgen concentration within the microenvironment of the developing spermatozoa *(2,3,5)*.

Hormonal requirements for the initiation and maintenance of spermatogenesis appear to be different. The maintenance immediately after hypophysectomy

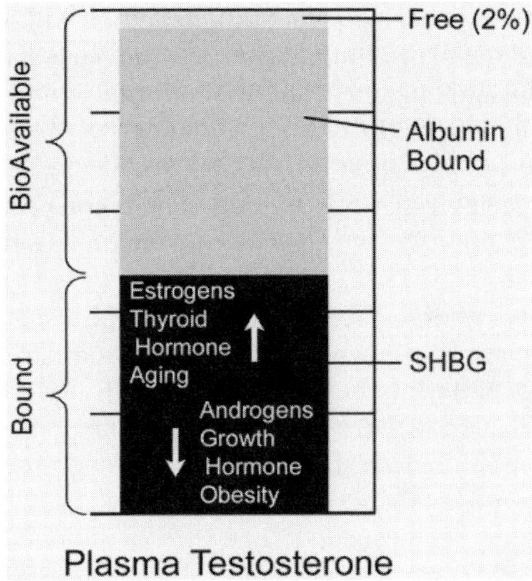

Fig. 4. Plasma testosterone distribution. SHBG, sex hormone-binding globulin.

(pituitary obliteration) requires testosterone alone; however, when the germinal epithelium regresses completely, both FSH and testosterone treatment are required. Qualitatively, testosterone will initiate and maintain spermatogenesis in humans, but quantitative restoration will not be achieved *(12)*. In humans, FSH is necessary for the maintenance of quantitatively normal sperm production *(13)* and is particularly important for initiating spermatogenesis in pubertal males and reinitiating spermatogenesis in men whose germinal epithelium has regressed after hypophysectomy. *Qualitative* sperm production can be achieved by replacement of either FSH or LH alone. However, both FSH and LH are necessary to maintain *quantitative* normal spermatogenesis in humans *(12)*.

DIAGNOSING ENDOCRINE ABNORMALITIES: CLINICAL FINDINGS

History

Specific childhood illnesses should be sought, including cryptorchidism, postpubertal mumps, orchitis, testicular trauma or pain (torsion), as well as the timing of puberty *(14)*. Precocious puberty may indicate the adrenal genital syndrome *(15)*. A detailed history of exposure to occupational and environmental toxins, excessive heat, and radiation should be elucidated *(16,17)*. Cancer chemotherapy has a dose-dependent, potentially devastating effect on the testicular germinal epithelium and may compromise Leydig cell function *(18)*.

Drug history should be reviewed; anabolic steroids, cimetidine, ketoconazole, and spironolactone may affect the reproductive cycle *(1,4,19)*. Unfortunately, the use of anabolic steroids is very common among potential athletes. Exogenous androgens exert their deleterious effects on the feedback level of the pituitary and hypothalamus by inhibiting gonadotropin release. Chronic use has also been shown to inhibit gonadotropin secretion and lower testosterone levels. Additionally, alcohol, marijuana, and cocaine have been implicated as reversible gonadotoxic agents *(14,19,20)*.

Decreased libido and impotence are the earliest symptoms of low testosterone. Loss of libido that is associated with headaches, visual abnormalities, and galactorrhea may suggest a pituitary tumor. Anosmia may be a symptom in individuals with hypothalamic hypogonadism. Other medical problems associated with infertility include thyroid disease and liver disease *(21,22)*. Chronic systemic diseases (e.g., renal, sickle cell, celiac, and HIV disease) are also related to abnormal reproductive hormonal axis *(14,23–25)*.

Physical Examination

When germ cell failure occurs before puberty, patients have obvious features of eunuchoidism (Table 1). When failure occurs after puberty, the diagnosis is more difficult unless it is linked with adrenal failure, because the regression of secondary sexual characteristics may take years.

Careful examination of the testes is essential in the examination. The seminiferous tubules account for approx 95% of testicular volume. The prepubertal testis measures approx 2 cm in length (2 mL-volume, as assessed by Prader orchidometer) and gradually increases in size with puberty. The normal adult testis is an average of 4.6 cm long (3.6–5.5-cm range) and 2.6 cm wide (2.1–3.2-cm range) with a mean volume of 18.6 ± 4.8 mL standard deviation (SD) (Fig. 5) *(2,26)*. When the seminiferous tubules are damaged before puberty, the testes are small and firm but characteristically small and soft with postpubertal damage.

Gynecomastia is a consistent feature of a feminizing state. Men with congenital hypogonadism may have related midline defects, such as anosmia, color blindness, cerebellar ataxia, hare lip, and cleft palate *(2,3,19)*. Hepatomegaly may be associated with problems of hormone metabolism. Proper neck examination may help rule out thyromegaly, a bruit, or nodularity linked with thyroid disease. The neurologic examination should test the visual field and reflexes.

SEMEN ANALYSIS

Examination of the seminal fluid provides important information concerning the integrity of the reproductive hormonal network, spermatogenesis, and patency of the reproductive tract. A normal microscopic examination eliminates the need for any further diagnostic studies.

Table 1
Features of Eunuchoidism

Eunuchoid skeletal proportions
Upper body:lower body ratio < 1
Arm span > 2 inches than height
Lack of adult male hair distribution
Sparse axillary, pubic, facial, and body hair
Lack of recession of hair on temporal lobe
Infantile genitalia
Small penis, testes, and prostate
Underdeveloped scrotum
Diminished muscular development and mass

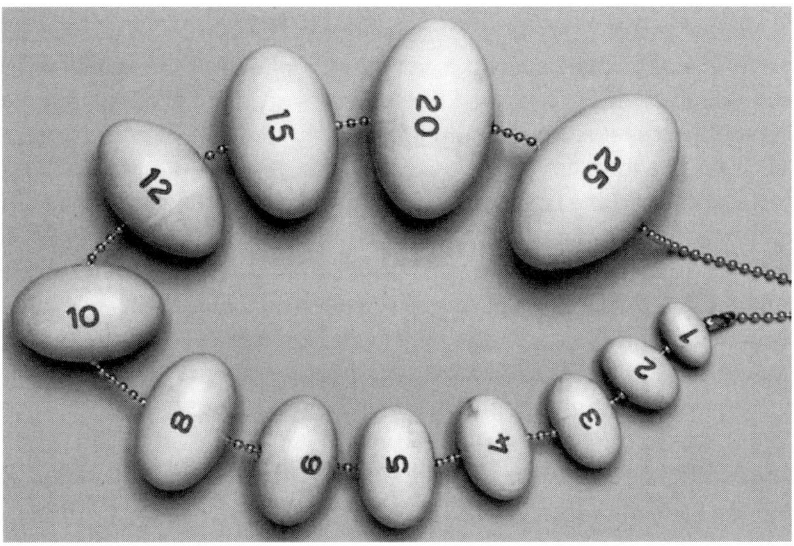

Fig. 5. A Prader orchidometer for measuring testicular volume.

BASELINE HORMONE EVALUATION

The classic hormone evaluation includes a serum testosterone and serum gonadotropins (LH and FSH). An algorithm for diagnosing endocrine causes of male infertility is illustrated in Fig. 6. A low-serum testosterone with inappropriately low LH levels usually warrants the investigation of serum prolactin levels *(14)*. A more recent study showed that obtaining serum FSH and testosterone

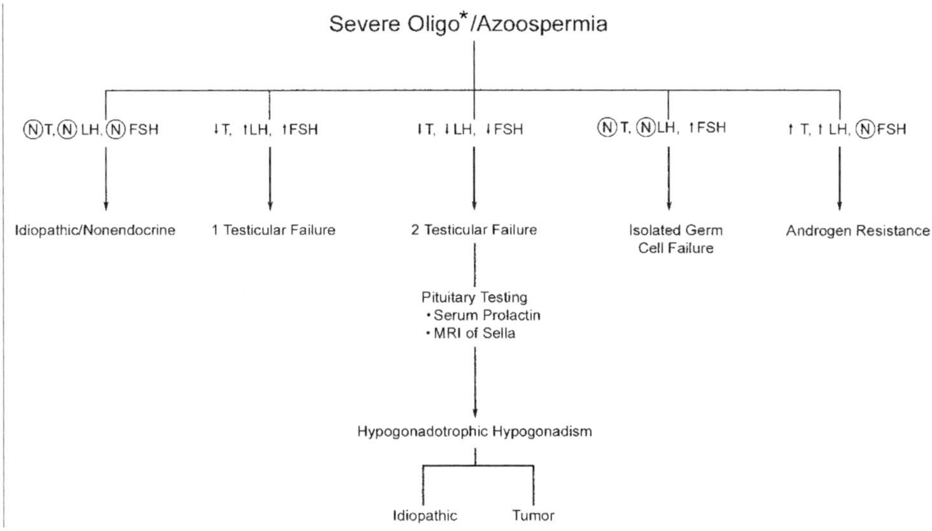

Fig. 6. Algorithm for the diagnosis of endocrine causes of male infertility. *, sperm counts < 5×10^6/mL.

only in men with sperm densities less than 10 million sperm/mL and soft testes will detect virtually all (99%) endocrine abnormalities *(27)*.

A single LH determination has limited prognostic accuracy (± 50%) because of the episodic nature of LH secretion and its short half-life *(6)*. In contrast, serum FSH has a longer half-life, and fluctuations in serum levels are less obvious. If an abnormal LH value is obtained in a single sample, then three serum samples can be collected over a 20-min interval and the samples pooled *(28)*. Estradiol levels are measured in patients presenting with gynecomastia, testicular masses, or history compatible with excessive exogenous estrogen exposure.

Testosterone secretion follows a diurnal cycle with an early morning peak around 8:00 AM followed by evening trough at 8:00 PM when the concentration falls to about 70% of the morning peak *(4,8,19)*. Testosterone values should therefore be drawn in the morning. The measurement of total (bound) testosterone usually provides a correct assessment of bioavailable testosterone. Free (unbound) testosterone is a more accurate marker of bioavailable testosterone, particularly when conditions of altered SHBG concentrations exist *(10)*. Elevated estrogens, thyroid hormone, and aging increase plasma SHBG and thus decrease levels of free testosterone. Alternatively, androgens, growth hormone, and obesity depress SHBG levels and increase the active androgen fraction. Measurement of the free-testosterone fraction should be made by equilibrium dialysis. Ultrafiltration or analog immunoassays are currently very unreliable *(29)*.

A low-serum testosterone level is one of the best indicators of hypogonadism of hypothalamic or pituitary origin. Mean serum LH and FSH concentrations are significantly lower in hypogonadotropic patients than in normal men, but they can overlap with the lower limits of normal in some individuals. In patients with hypogonadotropic hypogonadism, the pituitary hormones other than LH and FSH should also be assessed (adrenocorticotropic hormone, TSH, and growth hormone) to exclude the possibility of hypopituitorism. Thyroid dysfunction is such a rare cause of infertility that routine screening is discouraged.

Elevated serum FSH and LH values help to distinguish primary testicular failure (hypergonadotropic hypogonadism) from secondary testicular failure (hypogonadotropic hypogonadism).

Decreases in spermatogenesis are generally accompanied by reductions in inhibin production, and this decline in negative feedback is associated with a reciprocal elevation of FSH levels. Elevated FSH is usually a reliable indicator of severe germinal epithelial damage and is usually associated with azoospermia or severe oligospermia ($<5 \times 10^6$/mL). In azoospermic and severely oligospermic patients with normal FSH levels, primary spermatogenic defects cannot be distinguished from obstructive lesions by hormonal investigation alone. Therefore, scrotal exploration and testicular biopsy should be considered. Elevated serum FSH levels related to small atrophic testes implies severe infertility; biopsy is not warranted.

Hyperprolactinemia is reported to cause oligospermia, but the diagnostic value of routine prolactin measurements is extremely low in men with semen abnormalities unless decreased libido, impotence, and evidence of hypogonadism also exist. Prolactin measurement is warranted in patients with low-serum testosterone without an associated increase in serum LH. Individuals with gynecomastia or suspected androgen resistance (high-serum testosterone and LH with undermasculinization) should have a serum estradiol determination.

Individuals with a rapid loss of secondary sex characteristics, implying both testicular and adrenal failure, should undergo investigation of adrenal function. In men with a history of precocious puberty, congenital adrenal hyperplasia should be considered. In the common variant (21-hydroxylase deficiency), serum levels of 17-hydroxyprogesterone are elevated, as is urinary pregnanetriol. In the 11-hydroxylase deficiency, serum 11-deoxycortisol is elevated *(15)*.

DYNAMIC HORMONAL TESTING

Dynamic tests to determine the physiologic state of the hypothalamic-pituitary axis include stimulation tests with GnRH and hCG. The GnRH test evaluates the functional capacity of pituitary gonadotropins to release LH and FSH. Often, a single GnRH test is nondiagnostic, and chronic testing with GnRH is necessary. The ability of the testes to secrete testosterone is tested with the administration of hCG, which has a biologic activity similar to that of LH. The stimulation tests are usually in the realm of endocrinology and are used mainly in a research setting *(2,14)*.

CLASSIFICATION OF ENDOCRINE CAUSES OF INFERTILITY

The results of hormone testing can classify patients into primary and secondary hypogonadism. The primary type (hypergonadotropic hypogonadism) where the defect is at the testicular level with elevated serum LH or FSH or both. The secondary type (hypogonadotropic hypogonadism) where the defect is at the hypothalamic or pituitary level with inappropriately low-serum LH and FSH levels. Occasionally, there is selective involvement of LH but rarely of FSH by itself. Most infertile men with seminiferous tubule abnormalities have no detectable endocrinopathy and have normal serum LH, FSH, and testosterone levels. These characteristics typify eugonadotropic hypogonadism (Table 2).

PRIMARY HYPOGONADISM

Chromosomal Abnormalities

Somatic

Various somatic chromosomal abnormalities are associated with male infertility, and incidence increases as the sperm count decreases. In a study of 1263 barren couples, Kjessler found the overall incidence of male chromosomal abnormalities to be 6.2%. In a subgroup in which the male partner's sperm count was less than 10 million, the incidence rose to 11%. In the azoospermic subjects, 21% had significant chromosomal abnormalities *(30)*.

Y Chromosome

Approximately 7% of men with severe oligospermia and 13% of men with azoospermia harber structural alterations in the long arm of the Y chromosome (Yq) *(31,32)*, and gene defects (microdeletions) in this region may lead to defective spermatogenesis. There appears to be a specific region designated as azoospermic factor (AZF), and its absence or mutation accounts for azoospermia. Three nonoverlapping regions with *AZF* designated as *AZFa*, *AZFb*, and *AZFc (33)* can also be identified. Deletion of the *DAZ* (deleted in azoospermia) gene in the *AZFc* region is the most commonly observed microdeletion in infertile men. In addition to azospermia, men with abnormalities in testicular development, e.g., cryptorchidism, may also have Y chromosome microdeletions *(34)*. Testicular sperm extraction in conjunction with assisted reproductive techniques can result in pregnancies in these previously infertile men. Similar genetic defects are likely present in male offspring, and vertical transmission is described *(35)*. Prior to undergoing any

Table 2
Male Hypogonadism

Primary hypogonadism (hypergonadotropic hypogonadism)
Chromosomal abnormalities
Myotonic dystrophy
Bilateral anorchia (vanishing testes syndrome)
Sertoli-cell-only syndrome
Gonadal toxins (drugs and radiation)
Orchitis
Systemic diseases (hepatic, renal, sickle cell disease, and HIV)
Secondary hypogonadism (hypogonadotropic hypogonadism)
Hypogonadotropic eunuchoidism (Kallmann's hypogonadism)
Isolated LH or FSH deficiency
Multiorgan genetic disorders (congenital hypogonadotropic syndromes)
Pituitary disease
Androgens, estrogens, glucocorticoids (endogenous/exogenous excess)
Hyperprolactinemia
Hemochromatosis
Hypothyroidism or hyperthyroidism
Defective androgen synthesis or action
Reifenstein's syndrome
5-α reductase deficiency
Celiac disease
Eugonadotropic syndromes
Adult seminiferous tubule failure

LH, luteinizing hormone; FSH, follicle-stimulating hormone.

assisted reproductive techniques, appropriate genetic testing should be offered to these individuals.

Klinefelter's Syndrome

Klinefelter's syndrome is the most common cause of primary hypogonadism. It occurs in approx 1 in every 500 men and is a genetic disorder resulting from the presence of an extra X chromosome in the male *(2,19,36)*. In classic Klinefelter's syndrome, the karyotype of all cells is XXY as a result of either maternal or paternal meiotic nondisjunction during gametogenesis *(2)*.

Characteristically, these individuals have small firm testes, decreased androgenicity (delayed sexual maturation), azoospermia, and gynecomastia. As features of hypogonadism are often not evident until puberty, diagnosis is usually delayed. The reduction in testicular mass is usually owing to sclerosis and hyalinization of the seminiferous tubules; although the Leydig cells may appear hyperplastic, their total number per testis is normal. The testes are characteristically less than 2 cm long and always less than 3.5 cm (corresponding to volumes of 2 and 12 mL, respectively). These individuals have increased mean body height secondary to a longer lower body segment that is not secondary to the androgen deficiency but caused by the underlying chromosome abnormality *(2,3,19)*.

Gonadotropin levels are characteristically elevated, particularly FSH. Plasma testosterone can range from normal to low, but decreases with age. Serum estradiol levels are often increased secondary to elevated LH levels, and increased serum estradiol levels promote an increase in SHBG. Elevated SHBG results in higher levels of bound testosterone and lower levels of free testosterone, which explains the inconsistency between total serum testosterone levels and degree of androgenicity. Higher estrogen levels relative to testosterone cause the feminized appearance and gynecomastia. As these men have abnormal testosterone to estradiol ratio, aromatase inhibitors have been known to decrease the conversion of testosterone to estradiol, thereby increasing serum testosterone levels *(40)*. In the majority of these men, they will later require androgen replacement for optimal virilization and normal sexual function.

Several medical disorders occur at a greater frequency than normal in Klinefelter syndrome, including chronic pulmonary disease, varicose veins, cerebrovascular disease, glucose intolerance, and primary hypothyroidism *(37)*. There is also a 20-fold increase of breast cancer and these individuals may have mild mental deficiency and/or be socially maladjusted *(38)*. There are also variant syndromes characterized by more than two X chromosomes (Poly X syndrome) associated with more severe abnormalities than classical Klinefelter syndrome.

Approximately 10% of these patients have a chromosomal mosaicism (XXY/XY), which is the result of mitotic nondisjunction that occurs after fertilization. They have less severe features of Klinefelter syndrome and may be fertile when a normal (46,XY) clone of cells exists within the testes *(2,3,14,19)*. In the past, infertility was irreversible in classic Klinefelter syndrome. Presently, techniques using testicular microdissection have identified viable sperm allowing in vitro fertilization and intracytoplasmic sperm injection with resulting pregnancies *(39)*.

XX Disorder (Sex Reversal)

This is a rare (1/9000) variant of Klinefelter syndrome *(2,14,19)*. The signs are similar, except that the average height is less than normal, hypospadias is common, and the incidence of mental impairment is not increased. Although these patients have a 46,XX chromosome complement, this paradox is explained by the translocation of the testes determining factor normally found in the Y chromosome to the X chromosome. This is a result of frequent XY recombination that occurs during normal male meiosis.

Noonan's Syndrome (Male Turner's Syndrome)

This disorder occurs when genotypic XY males manifest features similar to those of Turner's syndrome *(41)*. Men typically have dysmorphic features like web neck, short stature, low-set ears, wideset eyes, and cardiovascular abnormalities. Most cases are sporadic, but affected families have been described in which inheritance is autosomal-dominant. Of these individuals, 75% have cryptorchidism at birth that may limit their future fertility. However, if testes are fully descended, fertility is possible and likely. FSH and LH levels depend on the degree of testicular function *(14,19)*.

Myotonic Dystrophy

Myotonic dystrophy is an autosomal-dominant disorder characterized by prolonged contraction of skeletal muscles (myotonica). Aside from the progressive muscle atrophy and weakness, associated abnormalities include lenticular opacities, frontal baldness, and impaired spermatogenesis (testicular atrophy) *(42)*. Pubertal development is usually normal, and testicular failure occurs in approx 80% of affected men between the ages of 30 and 40. Leydig cell function remains normal, and there is no gynecomastia. The serum FSH level is elevated proportionate to the degree of testicular atrophy. There is no therapy for the infertility; because testosterone levels are normal, androgen replacement is not required *(14)*.

Bilateral Anorchia (Vanishing Testes Syndrome)

This extremely rare disorder occurs in approximately 1 of every 20,000 males, presenting with nonpalpable testes and sexual immaturity owing to the absence of testicular androgens. The karyotype is normal, but serum LH and FSH levels are elevated, and serum levels of testosterone are extremely low. The absent testes can be from testicular torsion, trauma, vascular injury, or infection *(43)*. These patients have eunuchoid proportions but no gynecomastia, and therapy is directed at treating the underlying androgen deficiency.

These patients usually present with suspected bilateral cryptorchidism before puberty or with sexual infantilism during adulthood. To differentiate between anorchia and bilateral undescended testes, the testosterone response to human chorionic gonadotropin is extremely useful. Men with anorchia do not respond to hCG, whereas those with functioning testes do *(14)*.

Sertoli-Cell-Only Syndrome (Germinal Cell Aplasia)

This disorder is indicated by the absence of germ cells and presence of only Sertoli cells on testicular biopsy. The most likely cause of the syndrome is congenital absence or early neonatal loss of germ cells, but it may also be secondary to genetic defects or androgen resistance. Clinical findings include azoospermia associated with normal virilization, testes of normal consistency but slightly smaller size, and no gynecomastia *(14)*. Serum testosterone and serum LH levels are normal, but serum FSH is usually elevated *(44)*. With other testicular disorders (mumps, cryptorchidism, damage from radiation or toxins, and adult seminiferous tubule failure), the seminiferous tubules may also only contain Sertoli cells, but in these men, the testes are small, the histological pattern is not as uniform, and severe sclerosis and hyalinization are prominent features.

Gonadotoxins

Drugs

The germinal epithelium, a rapidly dividing tissue, is susceptible to agents that interfere with cell division. Cancer chemotherapy causes a dose-dependent, potentially devastating effect on the testicular germinal epithelium and may damage the Leydig cells. Effects vary with drug class and age of the patient *(18,45)*.

Drugs may cause infertility by directly inhibiting testosterone synthesis, blocking peripheral androgen action, inhibiting pituitary gonadotropin secretion, or enhancing estrogen levels. Cyproterone, ketoconazole, spironolactone, and alcohol all interfere with testosterone synthesis *(19)*. The most commonly administered drug known to be an androgen antagonist is cimetidine *(46)*. Men treated with cimetidine present with gynecomastia and may have decreased sperm density. Recreational drugs (marijuana, heroin, and methadone) are associated with lower serum testosterone levels without a concomitant elevation in plasma LH, suggesting a central abnormality as well as a testicular defect *(19,20)*.

Radiation

Germ cells are particularly sensitive to radiation, whereas Leydig cells are relatively resistant. A single exposure below 600 rad to germ cell damage is reversible, but above this level, permanent damage is likely *(2,17)*. Spermatogenesis may recover in some men, but it may take 2 to 3 yr. Elevated serum FSH levels reflect impaired spermatogenesis, which may return to normal with the recovery of spermatogenesis.

Environmental Toxins

A variety of chemical agents are toxic to spermatogenesis, including pesticides (e.g., dibromochloropropane), industrial solvents (e.g., carbon disulfide), and metals (lead, cadmium, and mercury) *(19,48)*. Other toxins are cigaret smoke, and it is likely that as yet unidentified toxins may contribute significantly to male factor infertility.

Orchitis

Approximately 15 to 25% of adult men who contract mumps (epidemic parotiditis) develop orchitis, which is commonly unilateral. Bilateral involvement occurs in only 10% of affected men and less than one-third of men with bilateral orchitis recover normal semen parameters *(47)*. Testicular atrophy can develop within 1 to 6 mo or can take years. With the advent of the mumps vaccine, the incidence of mumps and associated orchitis is becoming increasingly rare.

Systemic Disease

Chronic Renal Failure

Uremia is associated with decreased libido, impotence, altered spermatogenesis, and gynecomastia. Serum testosterone is decreased, and serum LH and FSH levels are increased. The cause of this dysfunction is multifactorial, with contributions from nutrition deficiency, estrogen excess, hyperprolactinemia, and nondialyzable uremic toxins *(23)*. In patients who have undergone successful renal transplantation, uremic hypogonadism improves.

Cirrhosis of the Liver

A large percentage of men with liver cirrhosis have testicular atrophy, impotence, and gynecomastia *(22)*. Serum testosterone levels and metabolic clearance rates are reduced, and testosterone binding to plasma proteins is increased secondary to increased SHBG. Serum estradiol rises because of decreased hepatic extraction of androgens and increased peripheral conversion of androgens to estrogen, resulting in gynecomastia. Independent of its effect on the liver, ethanol also acutely reduces testicular testosterone synthesis *(19,22)*.

Sickle Cell Disease

Many men with sickle cell disease have evidence of hypogonadism (delayed sexual maturation, impaired skeletal growth, reduced testicular size, and, in some, reduced sperm density). Serum testosterone is low, but studies have shown basal serum LH and FSH levels to be normal, elevated, or reduced. These discrepancies make it impossible to state definitively whether the hypogonadism of sickle cell disease is primary (testicular), secondary (pituitary-hypothalamic), or a mixture of both *(14,19)*.

Androgen Resistance Syndromes

Congenital androgen insensitivity results from either an androgen receptor abnormality or a defect in the enzyme responsible for peripheral androgen conversion (5-α reductase) *(49)*. These men are nearly always infertile.

Androgen-resistant syndromes constitute a category of phenotypic disorders in which 46,XY males with bilateral testes fail to develop as completely normal men. The clinical spectrum extends from infertility alone to pseudo-hermaphrodism. These patients have elevated rates of testosterone production and therefore high-baseline testosterone secondary to high-serum LH. The elevated LH levels are a consequence of the lack of feedback regulation from the resistance or absence of androgen receptors at the hypothalamic pituitary level to the androgen action. Diagnosis of androgen resistance is made by genital skin fibroblast culture and measurement of androgen receptor function.

Individuals with 5-α-reductase deficiency at birth have ambiguous genitalia, but at puberty, increased testosterone secretion from the testes results in incomplete virilization. Spermatogenesis is impaired because the testes are usually undescended, and these men are infertile *(14)*.

Celiac Disease

Individuals with celiac disease have been shown to have infertility (abnormalities in sperm motility and morphology) associated with a biochemical picture of androgen resistance *(24)*; that is, high-serum testosterone and high-LH concentrations. Dietary modification led to the normalization of biochemical abnormalities.

SECONDARY HYPOGONADISM (HYPOGONADOTROPIC SYNDROMES)

Isolated Gonadotropin Deficiency (Kallmann's Syndrome)

Although uncommon (1:10,000 men), this is second to Klinefelter's syndrome as a cause of hypogonadism *(2,3,19)*. The original report described the familial form associated with anosmia, but the eponym now refers to both variants, with and without anosmia. This syndrome may be associated with other congenital anomalies (congenital deafness, hare lip, cleft palate, craniofacial asymmetry, renal abnormalities, and color blindness) *(50)*. The hypothalamic hormone, GnRH, appears to be absent, as exogenous GnRH administration stimulates the release of both LH and FSH from the pituitary *(51,52)*. Except for the gonadotropin deficiency, anterior pituitary function is intact. Congenital GnRH deficiency can be inherited as autosomal-dominant, autosomal-recessive, or an X-linked condition. More than two-thirds of cases, however, are sporadic *(19)*.

During childhood, patients may present with a microphallus, cryptorchidism, or both, but a delay in sexual maturation is the usual presentation. The differential diagnosis includes constitutionally delayed puberty, but anosmia, somatic midline defects, or a positive family history may imply that sexual maturation may not proceed normally. Other distinguishing features of Kallmann's syndrome include a normal growth curve, a height age greater than bone age, and testes that are almost invariably less than 2 cm in diameter. Although basal serum testosterone levels are low, baseline serum LH and FSH in prepubertal patients may be within the lower limits of normal for their age group and thus will not aid the diagnosis. The GnRH stimulation test results in a rise of both serum gonadotropins. With severe deficiency, GnRH may have to be administered chronically to elicit a response.

Isolated Leutinizing Hormone Deficiency ("Fertile Eunuch")

These individuals have eunuchoid proportions with variable degrees of virilization and often gynecomastia. They also characteristically have large testes with an ejaculate that may contain a few sperm *(53)*. Serum FSH levels are normal, but both serum LH and serum testosterone concentrations are low normal. Serum testosterone increases after hCG administration indicating hypogonadotropic hypogonadism. The cause appears to be partial gonadotropin deficiency with adequate LH to stimulate high-intratesticular testosterone and resultant spermatogenesis but insufficient testosterone to promote virilization. These patients may be treated with hCG for virilization and full spermatogenesis *(14)*.

Isolated Follicle-Stimulating Hormone Deficiency

In this rare disorder, patients are normally virilized and have normal testicular size and baseline levels of LH and testosterone. Sperm counts range from azoospermic to severely oligospermic. Serum FSH levels are low and do not respond to GnRH. The use of gonadotropins may improve spermatogenesis and fertility *(2,14)*.

Congenital Hypogonadotropic Syndromes

These syndromes are associated with secondary hypogonadism and a multitude of other associated somatic findings *(54)*. The Prader-Willi Syndrome is characterized by hypogonadism, hypomentia, hypotonia at birth, and obesity. The Laurence-Moon-Bardet-Biedle Syndrome is characterized by mental retardation, retinitis pigmentosa, polydactyly, and hypogonadism. Other congenital hypogonadotropic syndromes are Lowe's Syndrome and congenital oculofacial paralysis (Möbius' Syndrome).

Pituitary Disease

Pituitary insufficiency may result from tumors, infarction, iatrogenic damage (surgery or radiation), or one of several infiltrative and granulomatous processes. If pituitary insufficiency occurs before puberty, growth retardation associated with adrenal and thyroid deficiency is a major clinical presentation.

Hypogonadism occuring in a sexually mature man usually has its origin in a pituitary tumor. The symptoms of decreasing libido, impotence, and infertility may be present years before the appearance of other signs of an expanding tumor, such as headache, visual field abnormalities, and deficiency of thyroid or adrenal hormones *(19,55)*. Once an individual has passed through normal puberty, it takes a long time for the secondary sexual characteristics to disappear unless adrenal insufficiency exists. Physical examination demonstrates small and soft testes, and the diagnosis is based on the finding of low-serum testosterone levels with low or normal plasma gonadotropin concentrations. Depending on the degree of panhypopituitarism, serum corticosteroids are reduced, as will serum TSH and growth hormone levels.

Estrogen Excess

Adrenal cortical, Sertoli cell, or interstitial cell tumors of the testes all may at times produce estrogen *(56)*. Similarly, hepatic cirrhosis has been associated with increased endogenous estrogen. Excessive estrogen acts primarily by suppressing pituitary gonadotropin secretion, resulting in secondary testicular failure.

Androgen Excess

Like estrogens, excessive androgen levels also suppress pituitary gonadotropins, leading to secondary testicular failure. The current use of exogenous androgens (anabolic steroids) by professional and nonprofessional athletes may cause temporary sterility *(57)*. Elevated endogenous androgen secretion may occur in men with testosterone-secreting tumors (e.g., Leydig cell tumors) or in individuals with congenital adrenal hyperplasia (e.g., 21-hydroxylase or 11β-hydroxylase deficiency) *(15)*.

Hyperprolactinemia

Excessive serum prolactin levels cause both reproductive and sexual dysfunction *(58,59)*. Prolactin-secreting tumors of the pituitary gland, whether from a microadenoma (< 10 mm) or macroadenoma, result in loss of libido, impotence, galactorrhea, gynecomastia, and altered spermatogenesis. Patients with a macroadenoma first present with visual field abnormalities and headaches, should undergo magnetic resonance imaging of the pituitary and laboratory assessment of anterior pituitary, thyroid, and adrenal function *(55)*.

Men with pituitary adenomas have low-serum testosterone levels, but basal serum levels of LH and FSH are either low or low normal and reflect an inadequate pituitary response to depressed testosterone, implicating impaired GnRH secretion. Signs and symptoms of other derangements in pituitary trophic hormones (hypothyroidism and hypoadrenalism) should be sought, particularly in individuals with a macroadenoma.

Other causes of elevated serum prolactin include central nervous system (CNS)-active drugs (antipsychotics, opiates, sedative hypnotics, and antidepressants) *(60)*. Antihypertensive drugs, such as α-methyldopa, reserpine, and verapamil, may also stimulate prolactin levels. Strenuous exercise, stress, nipple stimulation, and high-protein meals may also elevate serum prolactin. A slightly high prolactin level (21–40 ng/mL) warrants reconfirmation.

Because prolactin release by the pituitary lactotrophs is under tonic inhibition by the catecholamine dopamine, the dopamine agonist, bromocriptine, will lower prolactin concentration and can restore gonadotropin secretion and normal gonadal function in patients with prolactin-producing tumors. The usual dose is 5 to 10 mg per day. Side effects are dizziness, hypertension, headaches, nausea, and vomiting. Cabergoline, another dopamine agonist, can be administered once or twice a week and has less tendency toward nausea than bromocriptine. In certain individuals, surgical ablation may be required *(7)*. In the rare patient in whom infertility is the sole manifestation of elevated prolactin, treatment has resulted in normalization of sperm counts.

Glucocorticoid Excess

Whether glucocorticoid excess is exogenous (e.g., from treatment of ulcerative colitis, asthma, or rheumatoid arthritis) or endogenous (Cushing's syndrome), the result is decreased spermatogenesis *(19,61)*. Elevated plasma cortisol levels depress LH secretion and cause secondary testicular dysfunction. Even short-term therapy may result in lower serum testosterone levels. Correction of the glucocorticoid excess results in improvement of spermatogenesis.

Hyperthyroidism and Hypothyroidism

Both elevated and depressed levels of serum thyroid hormone alter spermatogenesis *(14,19,21)*. Hyperthyroid men may develop gynecomastia, a depressed sperm count and/or motility, and sexual dysfunction. Hyperthyroidism is evidenced by effects at both the pituitary and testicular levels with alterations in the secretion of releasing hormones and increased conversion of androgens to estrogens. Men with hypothyroidism may experience a decreased libido as well as other CNS effects. Decreased SHBG levels and lower total testosterone in these patients may indicate testicular failure. Either hypothyroidism or hyperthyroidism are extremely rare causes of infertility.

Hemochromatosis

Approximately 80% of men with this disease have testicular dysfunction. Their hypogonadism may be secondary to iron deposition in the liver or may be primarily testicular because of iron deposition in the testes *(62)*. Recently, iron deposits have been identified in the pituitary, implicating this gland as the major site of abnormality.

CASE PRESENTATION

Medical Treatment of Hypogonadotropic Hypogonadism

GS was a 32-yr-old gentleman with a known diagnosis of Kallman's syndrome presenting for treatment of infertility. At birth, he was found to have a small phallus and was bilaterally cryptorchid. Orchidopexy was performed and he subsequently received exogenous testosterone therapy to stimulate penile growth and for virilization. The diagnosis of Kallmann's syndrome had been made with the clinical findings of anosmia, color blindness, and the response of GnRH stimulation with a rise in both serum LH and FSH from previously undetected levels as well as an increase in serum testosterone.

Previous androgen therapy will not affect the testicular responsiveness to gonadotropins. The androgens, however, must be withdrawn for at least 2 mo prior to gonadotropin stimulation. Human gonadotropin has the biological activity of LH and stimulates Leydig cells to synthesize and secrete testosterone. Human chorionic gonadotropins (Pregnyl, Profasi, APL; 2000 IU intramuscularly 3 times/wk) were given to stimulate testosterone and obtain full androgenization (Fig. 7). Over a 4-mo period, hCG increased the testicular volume from 3 to 8 cc, but for full testicular growth, FSH needed to be added *(63)*. Serum testosterone was measured every month and kept between 300 and 600 ng/dL. The hCG dose was changed accordingly. Higher testosterone levels should be avoided as they may elevate serum estrogen levels and cause gynecomastia. If plasma testosterone concentration fails to respond to hCG, antibodies to hCG should be suspected *(64)*.

After 4 mo, the patient was well-virilized, but the testicular volume had only increased to 8 cc, and monthly semen analysis still revealed azoospermia. At this time, FSH was initiated *(14)*. FSH is available as human menopausal gonadotropin. The commercial preparation of Pergonal contains 75 IU of FSH and 75 IU of LH per vial. The initial dose was one vial intramuscularly three times per week given with hCG. Both solutions are compatible, and the same syringe may be used.

As it may take months for sperm to appear in the ejaculate after FSH administration, monthly semen analyses were performed *(65,66)*. After 5 mo of hCG and FSH, the patient achieved a volume of 12 cc and had a sperm count of 6 million per cc. At 12 mo, his testicular volume had increased to 14 cc, and his sperm count had risen to 12 million per cc. Pregnancy occurred 4 mo later. The sperm counts in most individuals receiving gonadotropin therapy are usually less

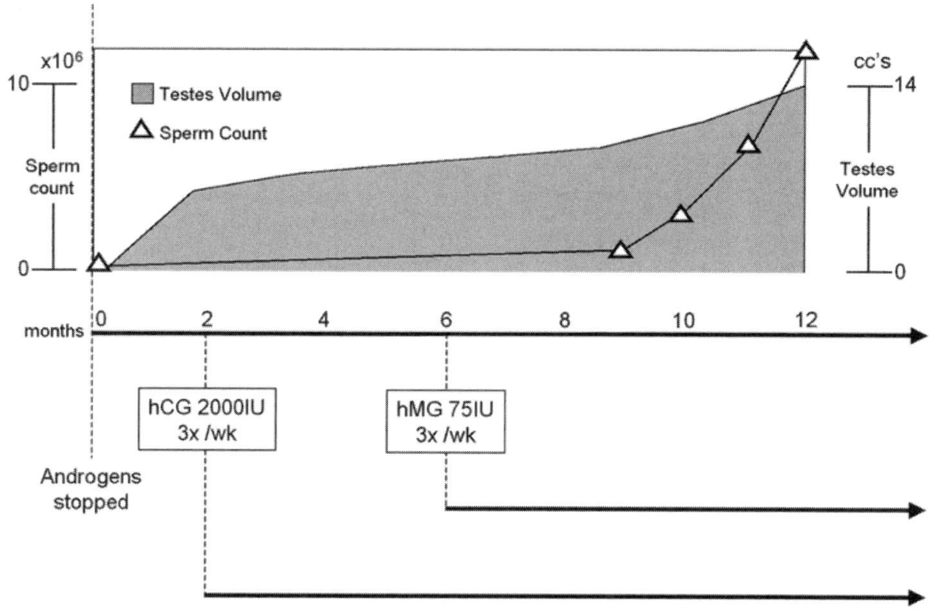

Fig. 7. Course of treatment of an individual with hypogonadotropic hypogonadism.

than 20 million. Burris found that 71% of 22 individuals who initiated a pregnancy had sperm counts less than 20 million per milliliter, indicating the quality of spermatogenesis as well as sperm function in these males are relatively normal *(67)*.

Once pregnancy occurs, if the patient wants further children, FSH can be stopped and spermatogenesis can be maintained on hCG therapy alone *(65)*. An alternative therapy would be to give GnRH subcutaneously in a pulsatile manner *(68)*. Unfortunately, this requires an infusion pump, which is expensive and is not proven to be superior to the combined hCG/FSH therapy. It is also not approved by the FDA. Therapy is monitored by its effect on gonadotropins, testosterone, and eventually on spermatogenesis.

REFERENCES

1. Baker HWG, Baker HG, deKretser DM, et al. Relative incidence of etiological disorders in male infertility. In: Santen RJ, Swerdloff RS, eds. Male Reproductive Dysfunction. Marcel Dekker, New York, NY, 1986, pp. 341–372.
2. Bardin CW, Paulsen CA. The testes. In: Williams RH, ed. Textbook of Endocrinology, 6th ed. Saunders, Philadelphia, PA, 1981.
3. Griffin JE, Wilson JD. Disorders of the testes and the male reproductive tract. In: Wilson JD, ed. Williams Textbook of Endocrinology, 9th ed. Saunders, Philadelphia, PA, 1998, pp. 819–875.

4. Veldhuis JD. Male hypothalamic-pituitary-gonadal axis. In: Lipshultz LI, Howards SS, eds. Infertility in the male, 3rd ed. Mosby-Year Book, St. Louis, MO, 1997, pp. 23–58.
5. Swerdloff RS, Wang C. Physiology of hypothalamic-pituitary function. In:Walsh PC, ed. Campbell's Urology, 7th ed., vol. 3. Saunders, Philadelphia, PA, 1998, p. 1239.
6. Santen RJ, Bardin CW. Episodic luteinizing hormone secretion in man: pulse analysis, clinical interpretation, physiologic mechanisms. J Clin Invest 1973;52:2617.
7. Moltich ME. Advances in pituitary tumor therapy: medical treatment of prolactinomas. Endocrinol Metab Clin North Am 1984;28:143.
8. Bremner WJ, Vitiello MV, Prinz PN. Loss of circadian rhythmicity in blood testosterone levels with aging in normal men. J Clin Endocrinol Metab 1983;56:1278.
9. Pardridge WM, Landaw EM. Testosterone transport in brain: primary role of plasma protein-bound hormone. Am J Physiol 1985;249:E534.
10. McClure RD. Androgen deficiency and the aging male: New urologic perspectives. Current Urology Reports 2001;2:453–459.
11. Giagulli VA, Kaufman JM, Vermeulen A. Pathogenesis of the decreased androgen levels in obese men. J Clin Endocrinol Metab 1994;79:997.
12. Matsumoto AM. Hormonal control of human spermatogenesis. In: Burger H, deKretser D, eds. The Testis. Raven Press, New York, NY, 1989:181–196.
13. Matsumoto AM, Karpas AE, Bremner WJ. Chronic human chorionic gonadotropin administration in normal men: Evidence that follicle-stimulating hormone is necessary for the maintenance of quanitatively normal spermatogenesis in man. J Clin Endocrinol Metab 1986;62:1184–1192.
14. McClure RD. Endocrine investigation and therapy. Urol Clin North Am 1987;14:471–488.
15. Bonaccorsi AC, Adler I, Figueiredo JF. Male infertility due to congenital adrenal hyperplasia: testicular biopsy findings, hormonal evaluation, and therapeutic results in three patients. Fertil Steril 1987;47:664–670.
16. Schrag SD, Dixon RL. Occupational exposures associated with male reproductive dysfunction. Ann Rev Pharmacol Toxicol 1985;25:567–592.
17. Shapiro E, Kinsella TJ, Makuch RW, et al. Effects of fractionated irradiation on endocrine aspects of testicular function. J Clin Oncol 1985;3:1232.
18. Byrne J, Mulvihill JJ, Myers MH, et al. Effects of treatment on fertility in long-term survivors of childhood or adolescent cancer. N Engl J Med 1987;317:1315–1321.
19. Winters SJ. Clinical disorders of the testis. In: DeGroot LJ, Jameson JL, eds. Endocrinology, 4th ed. Saunders, Philadelphia, PA, 2001, pp. 2269–2290.
20. Kolodny RC, Masters WH, Kolodner RM, Toro G. Depression of plasma testosterone levels after chronic intesive marijuana use. N Engl J Med 1974;290:872–874.
21. Kidd GS, Glass AR, Virgersky RA: The hypothalamic-pituitary-testicular axis in thyrotoxicosis. J Clin Endrocrinol Metab 1979;48:798.
22. Van Thiel DH, Galaver JS. Hypothalamic-pituitary-gonadal function in liver disease with particular attention to the endocrine effects of chronic alcohol abuse. Prog Liver Dis 1986;8:273–282.
23. Handelsman DJ. Hypothalamic-pituitary gonadal dysfunction in renal failure, dialysis and renal transplantation. Endocr Rev 1985;6:151–182.
24. Farthing MJG, Edwards CRW, Rees LH, Dawson Am. Male gonadal function in coeliac disease. 1. Sexual dysfunction, infertility, and semen quality. Gut 1982;23:608–614.
25. Poretsky L, Can S, Zumoff B. Testicular dysfunction in human immunodeficiency virus-infected men. Metabolism 1995;44:946.
26. Zachman M, Prader A, Kind HP, et al. Testicular volume during adolescence: Cross-sectional and longitudinal studies. Helv Paediatr Acta 1974;29:61.

27. Sigman M, Jarow JP. Endocrine evaluation of infertile men. Urol 1997;50:659–664.
28. Goldzieher JW, Dozier TS, Smith KD, et al. Improving the diagnostic reliability of rapidly fluctuating plasma hormone levels by optimized multiple-sampling techniques. J Clin Endocrinol Metab 1976;43:824.
29. Klee GC, Heser DW. Techniques to measure testosterone in the elderly. Mayo Clin Proc 2000;75(Suppl):S19–S25.
30. Kjessler B: Fracteurs genetiques dans la subfertile male humaine. In: Fecondite et Sterilite du Male: Acquisitions Recentes. Masson et Cie, Paris, 1972.
31. Najmabadi H, Huang V, Yen P, et al. Substantial prevalence of microdeletions of the Y chromosome in infertile men with idiopathic azoospermia and oligospermia detected using a sequence-tagged sitbased mapping strategy. J Clin Endocrinol Metab 1996;81:1347.
32. Pryor JL, Kent-First M, Muallem A, et al. Microdeletions in the Y chromosome of infertile men. N Engl J Med 1997;336:534–539.
33. Reijo R, Lee TY, Salo P, et al. Diverse spermatogenic effects in humans caused by Y chromosome deletions encompassing a novel RNA-binding protein gene. Nat genet 1995;10:383.
34. Foresta C, Moro E, Garolla A, et al. Y chromosome microdeletions in cryptorchidism and idiopathic infertility. J Clin Endrocrinol Metab 1999;84:3660.
35. Chang PL, Sauer MV, Brown S. Y chromosome microdeletion in a father and his four infertile sons. Hum Preprod 1999;14:2689–2694.
36. Bojesen A, Juul S, Gravholt CH. Prenatal and postnatel prevalence of Klinefelter syndrome: a national registry study. J Clin Endocrinol Metab 2003;88:622.
37. Schwartz D, Root AW. The Klinefelter syndrome of testicular dysgenesis. Endrocrinol Metab Clin North Am 1991;20:153.
38. Bender BG, Linden MG, Robinson A. Neuropsychological impairment in 42 adolescents with sex chromosome abnormalities. Am J Med Genet 1993;48:169.
39. Tournaye H, Staessen C, Liebaers I, et al. Testicular sperm recovery in nine 47, XXY Klinefelter patients. Hum Reprod 1996;11:1644.
40. Raman JD, Schlegel PN. Aromatase inhibitors for male infertility. J Urol 2002;167:624–629.
41. Mendez HMM, Opitz JM. Opitz JM. Noonan syndrome: a review. Am J Med Genet 1985;21:493–506.
42. Takeda R, Ueda M. Pituitary-gondal function in male patients with myotonic dystrophy: Serum leteinizing hormone, follicle stimulating hormone and testosterone levels and histological damage of the testis. Acta Endocrinol (Copenh) 1977;84:382–389.
43. Aynsley-Green A, Zachmann M, Illig R, et al. Congenital bilateral anorchia in childhood: A clinical, endocrine and therapeutic evaluation of twenty-one cases. Clin Endocrinol (Oxf) 1976;5:381–391.
44. Micic S, Ilic V, Micic M, et al. Endocrine profile of 45 patients with sertoli cell only syndrome. Andrologia 1983;15:228–232.
45. Schilsky RL, Lewis BL, Sherins RJ. Gonadal dysfunction in patients receiving chemotherapy for cancer. Ann Intern Med 1980;93:109–114.
46. Carlson HE, Ippoliti AF, Swerdloff RS. Endocrine effects of an acute and chronic cimetidine administrations. Dig Dis Sci 1981;26:428.
47. Beard CM, Benson RC Jr., Kelalis PP, et al. The incidence and outcome of mumps orchitis in Rochester, Minnesota 1935–1974. Mayo Clin Proc 1977;52:3.
48. Lipshultz LI, Ross CE, Whorton D, et al. Dibromochloropropane and its effect on testicular function in man. J Urol 1980;124:464.
49. Griffin JE, McPhaul MJ, Russell DW, Wilson JD. The androgen resistance syndromes: Steroid 5-alpha-reductase 2 deficiency, testicular feminization, and related disorders. In: Scriver

CR, Beaudet AL, Sly WS, Valle D, eds. The Metbolic and Molecular Bases of Inherited Disease, 8th edition. McGraw-Hill, New York, NY, 2001, p. 4117.
50. Christensen RB, Matsumoto AM, Bremner WJ. Idiopathic hypogonadotropic hypogonadism with anosmia (Kallmann's syndrome). Endocrinologist 1992;2:332–340.
51. de Roux N, Young J, Brailly-Tabard S, et al. The same molecular defects of the gonadotropin-releasing hormone receptor determine a variable degree of hypogonadism in affected kindred. J Clin Endocrinol Metab 1999;84:567.
52. Spratt DI, Carr DB, Merriam GR, et al. The spectrum of abnormal patterns of gonadotropin releasing hormone secretion in men with idiopathic hypogonadotropic hypogondism: clinical and laboratory correlations. J Clin Endocrinol Metab 1987;64:283–291.
53. Faiman C, Hoffman DL, Ryan RJ, Albert A. The "fertile eunuch" syndrome: Demonstration of isolated luteinizing hormone defieciency by radioimmunoassay technique. Mayo Clin Proc 1968;43:661.
54. Castro-Magana M, Bronsther B, Angulo MA. Genetic forms of male hypogonadism. Urology 1990;35:195–204.
55. Molitch ME. Pathologic hyperprolactinemia. Endocrinol Metab Clin North Am 1992;21:877–901.
56. Freeman DA. Steroid hormone-producing tumors of the adrenal, ovary, and testes. Endocrinol Metab Clin North Am 1991;20:751.
57. Knuth UA, Maiera H, Nieschlag E. Anabolic steroids and semen parameters in bodybuilders. Fertil Steril 1989;52:1041.
58. Carter JN, Tyson JE, Tolis G, et al. Prolactin-secreting tumors and hypogonadism in 22 men. N Engl J Med 1978;299:847.
59. Segal S, Yaffe H, Laufer N, Ben-David M. Male hyperprolactinemia: effects on fertility. Fertil Steril 1979;32:556.
60. Hell K, Wernze H. Drug-induced changes in prolactin secretion: clinical implications. Med Toxicol 1988;3:463–498.
61. MacAdams MR, White RH, Chipps BE. Reduction of serum testosterone levels during chronic glucocorticoid therapy. Ann Intern Med 1986;104:648.
62. Charbonnel B, Chupin M, Le Grand A, Buillon J. Pituitary function in idiopathic haemochromatosis: hormonal study in 36 male patients. Acta Endocrinol (Copenh) 1981;98:178.
63. Burris AS, Rodbard HW, Winters SJ, Sherins RJ. Gonadotropin therapy in men with isolated hypogonadotropic hypogonadism: the response to human chorionic gonadotropin is predicted by initial testicular size. J Clin Endocrinol Metab 1988;66:1144.
64. Sokol RZ, McClure RD, Peterson M, et al. Gonadotropin therapy failure secondary to human chorionic gonadotropin-induced antibodies. J Clin Endocrinol Metab 1981;52:929–933.
65. Kirk JM, Savage MO, Grant DB, et al. Gonadal function and response to human chorionic and menopausal gonadotrophin therapy in male patients with idiopathic hypogonadotrophic hypogonadism. Clin Endocrinol 1994;41:57–63.
66. Nachtigall LB, Boepple PA, Prolong FP, et al. Adult-onset idiopathic hypogonadotrophic hypogonadism a treatable form of male infertility. N Engl J Med 1997;336:410.
67. Burris AS, Clark RV, Vantman DJ, Sherins RJ. A los sperm concentration does not preclude fertility in men with isolated hypogonadotropic hypogonadism after donadotropin therapy. Fertil Steril 1988;50:343.
68. Whitcomb RW, Crowley WF Jr. Clinical review 4: Diagnosis and treatment of isolated gonadotropin-releasing hormone defieciency in men. J Clin Endocrinol Metab 1990;70:3.

3 Sperm Preparation for Insemination

Grace M. Centola, PhD, HCLD(ABB)

Contents

INTRODUCTION

After the evaluation of both female and male partners and consequent diagnosis, a couple may be directed toward assisted reproductive technologies (ARTs), ranging from the more intensive and invasive in vitro fertilization (IVF) to minimally invasive intrauterine insemination (IUI). The direction to proceed depends on the individual couple, considering maternal age, sperm concentration and motility, treatable hormonal disturbances, and unexplained infertility *(1,2)*. Clearly, a woman with blocked fallopian tubes may proceed directly to IVF unless she is a candidate for tubal repair. Men with severe oligozoospermia, perhaps with less than 1 million motile sperm, may also proceed directly to IVF. Similarly, men with obstructive or nonobstructive azospermia would undergo testicular sperm retrieval and use in IVF with sperm injection.

Fertility potential can be reduced by several factors, including reduced number of motile sperm in the ejaculate, poor progressive motility, cervical mucus that is "hostile" to sperm, insufficient quality or quantity of cervical mucus, or structural irregularities of the cervical canal. These conditions may be circumvented by mechanical delivery of motile sperm onto and into the cervical canal (cervical insemination [AIH]) and/or into the uterine cavity (IUI).

IUI affords an easy technique with a reasonable chance of pregnancy that can be performed in an office setting. Patients may elect to use IUI, especially con-

From: *Contemporary Endocrinology: Office Andrology*
Edited by: P. E. Patton and D. E. Battaglia © Humana Press Inc., Totowa, NJ

sidering a potential chance of pregnancy, as well as financial considerations. The cost for IUI has been reported as approx $500 per cycle *(3)*.

Prior to proceeding with IUI, it is important to document tubal patency and ovulation, along with reasonable sperm parameters. Generally, 4 to 6 cycles of IUI would be recommended before IVF. Supplementation of the IUI with ovulation induction would be dependent on the ovulatory status of the female partner.

Cervical insemination is another form of artificial insemination often referred to as "AIH" and was primarily used for ejaculatory disorders or in cases where the spermatozoa could not be deposited in the vagina or on the cervix. These include impotence or types of sexual dysfunction, such as vaginismus or dyspareunia *(4)*. Cervical insemination was also previously utilized exclusively for the insemination of fresh or frozen-thawed donor sperm. Currently, it appears to be used less frequently, being replaced by IUI, which results in reasonable success rates and is easily accomplished in the physician's office.

Success rates for IUI have ranged from 0% to 60%, with an average of 20 to 35% *(5,6)*. Schlaff and Awoniyi reported a composite IUI pregnancy rate of 19.9%, which is close to the pregnancy rate for "normal" intercourse *(6)*. Agarwal et al. reported success rates of 5% for women over 35, and Dodson and Haney reported that 14% of patients became pregnant with IUI *(7,8)*. A large-randomized controlled clinical trial of 932 couples assigned to receive invasive cervical insemination (ICI), IUI, IUI with superovulation, or ICI with superovulation demonstrated that the highest pregnancy rate of 33% was achieved in the IUI with the superovulation group *(1)*. In the IUI (alone) group, the pregnancy rate was 18%, 19% with ICI and superovulation, and 10% in ICI alone. These authors concluded that treatment of infertile couples with superovulation and IUI was three times as likely to result in pregnancy as was ICI and twice as likely as IUI alone or ICI with superovulation *(1)*. Previous studies reported a chance of pregnancy with IUI and superovulation to be 5.6 times higher than no treatment *(9)*, 4% for IUI alone, 8% for superovulation alone, and 18% for IUI with superovulation *(9,10)*.

IUI is a viable means of treating the infertile couple and should be utilized prior to attempting the more invasive treatment options. Guzick et al. concluded that for couples in which the woman has no identifiable infertility factor, and the male has motile sperm, the combination of IUI and superovulation is an effective means of achieving pregnancy *(1)*. However, physicians should consider the risks of superovulation (i.e., hyperstimulation and multiple birth rate), female age, and costs. The capability of the practitioner to administer ovulatory medications, as well as monitor ovulation induction with hormone analyses and ultrasound should also be taken into account. The physician and the couple must cooperate in the decision-making process.

RATIONALE FOR SPERM PROCESSING

The ejaculate contains a mixed population of cells, debris, hormones, and pathogens suspended in seminal fluid. Intercourse normally deposits seminal fluid within the vagina and on the cervix where motile sperm migrate from the external os through the cervical canal and into the uterine lumen. Migration leaves behind all seminal fluid and nonmotile cells. The selection process continues in the uterus where the sperm with the most aggressive motility and most "normal" morphology pass through the cervical canal, then actively and passively transport to the ampulla of the fallopian tube—the site of fertilization.

Introduction of the raw ejaculate into the uterine cavity is inappropriate because seminal fluid contains smooth-muscle stimulants, such as prostaglandins capable of causing severe discomfort from uterine cramping. Additionally, the ejaculate contains many nonmotile sperm, nonsperm cells, and other particulate matter, e.g., microbes, which represent a nonphysiological and immunological challenge in the uterine cavity. Because these latter cell types are not usually introduced into the uterus, the procedure of sperm washing attempts to mimic the function of the cervical mucus. The motile sperm, suspended in sterile culture media known to be supportive to human sperm motility, longevity, and fertilization can then be released into the uterine cavity by use of a small catheter placed through the cervical os.

Sperm separation techniques do not guarantee the removal of all cells (e.g., white blood cells [WBCs]), and pathogens, particularly hepatitis and HIV viruses, but the process does minimize the concentration. It is essential that the status of sexually transmitted disease risk be ascertained to provide appropriate counseling to the couple regarding the effects of these agents on treatment.

METHODOLOGY

Many techniques of sperm preparation for IUI have been employed over the years, some complex and expensive. Among the techniques are filtration of semen through a sephadex column, glass wool column, and albumin gradient, which are replaced by three major techniques used in most andrology and ART laboratories. Currently, the primary techniques include the simple centrifugation wash, swim-up, and density gradient centrifugation with advantages and disadvantages to each. The selection of the best method is dependent on the semen specimen, laboratory capability, and proficiency of the technical staff.

Laboratory Safety

All semen specimens are considered potentially infectious and are handled as if capable of transmitting HIV or hepatitis or other sexually transmitted diseases, (e.g., gonorrhea, *Chlamydia, Mycoplasma,* or *Streptococcus*) *(11)*. All laboratories that contain human specimens must institute a safety policy to protect the technical staff from potential risks of transmission of these pathogens. An exposure control plan must be developed according to the federal OSHA guidelines, which outlines safety measures, as well as actions to take in the event of accidental exposure. Personal protective equipment (PPE) consisting of gloves, fluid resistant lab coat, and face and eye protection (surgical mask and safety goggles) should be worn while performing these procedures. Ideally, a small laminar flow hood can be used to protect the technician from exposure to biohazardous specimens, as well as to protect the specimen and maintain sterility. All procedures must be performed in such a way as to minimize the creation of droplets and aerosols *(11)*. Eating, drinking, applying cosmetics, and smoking is strictly prohibited in the laboratory area. The work area should be cleaned before and after each procedure with disinfectant such as a 10% bleach solution. Hands should be washed after removal of disposable gloves. The lab coat should not be worn outside of the laboratory. All waste, particularly any materials that have come into contact with any human cells or fluid specimens must be disposed of according to safety practices in red biohazard containers.

General Equipment and Supplies

The following materials are used for IUI sperm preparation:

- Compound microscope
- Incubator set at 37°C
- Sperm counting chamber
- Centrifuge
- Refrigerator
- Gloves
- Pasteur pipet
- Sterile sperm wash media—HEPES-buffered
- Sterile 15-mL polystyrene centrifuge tubes
- Sterile plastic pipets
- Sterile specimen containers
- Biohazard waste containers
- Test-tube racks

The laboratory must have a standard refrigerator to store the media and supplies before use. The temperature should be checked and recorded daily as part of the laboratory's quality control protocol. All media must be prewarmed to body temperature prior to use (37°C), which can be done by incubating the media in a water bath, a block placed on a slide warmer, or in a dry incubator. Small and dry incubators that fit easily on the laboratory bench are the most advantageous vs other warming methods. The internal temperature of the incubator should similarly be checked on a daily basis. This incubator can also be used to hold the semen specimen during liquefaction time prior to initiation of processing and to hold the final prepared specimen before insemination.

A small clinical centrifuge is needed to process the specimens and must be able to spin the tubes at approx 300*g*. Various types and models of centrifuges are available—some with fixed speeds and others with adjustable speeds. A timer is also essential because the centrifugation procedure is timed at each step of the processing protocol. Specimens are centrifuged at room temperature.

Lastly, a light microscope is needed to assess the sperm specimens before and after the processing procedure. Generally, the specimens are examined at ×20 or ×40 magnification. Depending on the methodology employed (*see* Chapter 9), an appropriate counting chamber (Makler Chamber, disposable counting slide, hemocytometer) is used to perform the sperm count and motility *(11)*.

General laboratory supplies are also required to prepare semen for insemination. Sterile-graduated pipets, able to measure 1, 5, and 10 mL can be used or sterile 1- to 2-mL transfer pipets. Transfer pipets are equipped with a suction bulb, whereas the sterile-graduated pipets require a mechanical bulb or electric pipet-aid to aspirate the specimen into the pipet. Sterile polystyrene 15-mL centrifuge tubes are used to process the specimen, and sterile specimen containers (e.g., urinalysis containers) are necessary for specimen collection. Additional supplies include indelible markers to label each tube or a preprinted labeling system and racks to hold the centrifuge tubes. Additionally, worksheets, report forms, and a laboratory accession log is needed to maintain records of each specimen processed in the laboratory.

Media and Reagents

Sperm processing is accomplished by replacing the seminal fluid with a nutrient solution, which can support sperm cells until they are placed into the uterine environment. There are many different types of nutrient solutions commercially available *(11)*. However, the most commonly used for sperm processing is that which mimics the uterotubal fluids and is termed, "human tubal fluid" (HTF) medium (12.)The medium is supplemented with a protein source, usually human serum albumin, which is essential for sperm survival and function. The most typical type of buffering agent used for the culture medium is HEPES, which maintains the medium pH at approx 7.3 to 7.5. HEPES-buffered medium is best for an office laboratory because this type of buffer does not require a CO_2 incubator to maintain pH. When using this type, it is important to keep the tube caps tightly closed during any incubation or holding period. A second form of buffer for medium is bicarbonate buffer and relies on carbonic acid/bicarbonate equilibrium to maintain pH *(13)*. When using bicarbonate-buffered medium, it is necessary to loosen the tube caps and maintain the tubes for processing in a CO_2 incubator. Media commercially available are also supplemented with antibiotics, such as penicillin-streptocycin or gentamycin. The antibiotic, gentamycin, is currently the preferred antibiotic because a patient's sensitivity to penicillin is frequently unknown. The HTF type of media, supplemented with protein (human serum albumin) and antibiotic, are available in several volumes (50- or 100-mL bottles and 10- or 5-mL vials) from numerous commercial sources of ART supplies. Larger volumes need to be separated into smaller volumes in sterile tubes; the smaller volumes can be used directly from the supplied vial for an individual patient's specimen processing.

Semen Analysis

A sperm count and motility are performed on the raw semen specimen as well as the final specimen for insemination to determine the efficacy of the sperm preparation technique, along with pregnancy rates *(11)*. (*See* Chapter 9 for methodology.)

*Simple Wash Procedure (*Fig. 1*)*

The simple wash or pelleting procedure employs concentration of all sperm, both motile and nonmotile, as well as all other cells and debris into a pellet at the bottom of the centrifuge tube. The semen is usually diluted with 2 to 3× volume of sterile culture medium. The semen-medium mixture is then centrifuged at room temperature for 10 min at approx 280 to 300*g*. The supernatant fraction is carefully removed down to the pellet with a sterile pipet. The pellet is then resuspended in 2 mL of fresh culture medium and mixed well without formation of bubbles or frothing. The specimen is centrifuged a second time for 10 min and the supernatant removed. The final pellett is resuspended in culture medium for insemination (*see* pg. 49).

The disadvantage of the simple wash procedure is that all of the sperm are centrifuged together with dead sperm, contaminating cells, debris, and microbes. Mixing these elements with normal motile sperm may damage motile functional sperm. Dead cells and WBCs are known to produce reactive oxygen species (ROS; oxygen radicals), which can induce irreversible damage to sperm and impair fertilizing capability *(11)*. Therefore, the use of pelleting in unselected populations of sperm should be avoided. The simple wash procedure is suitable only in specimens with high-motile count and little or no debris or cells. A simple wash can also be attempted with specimens presenting with very low-sperm count, whereas a high-loss of motile sperm numbers would be incurred using the other procedures.

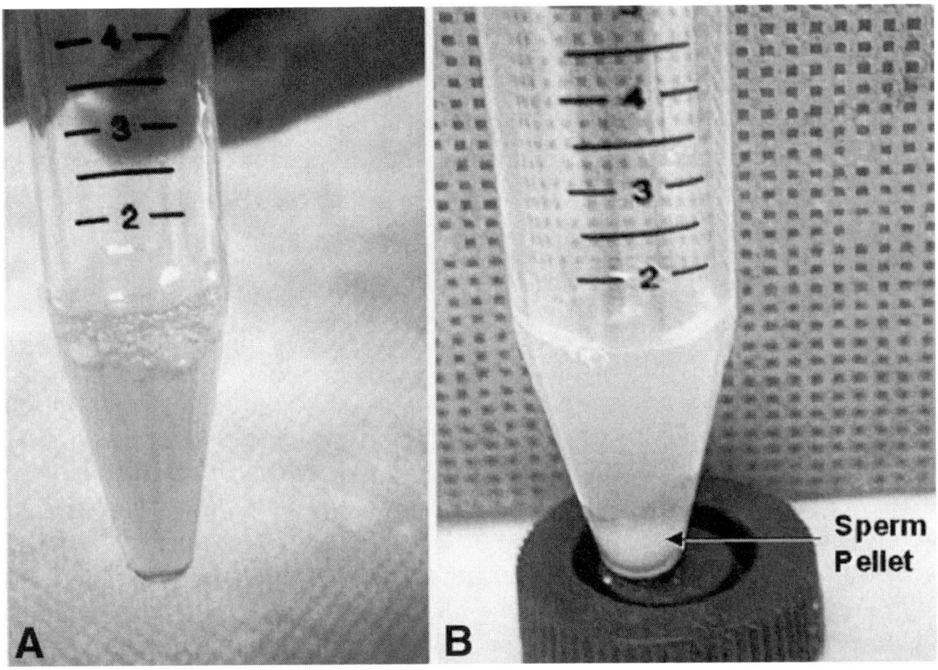

Fig. 1. Simple sperm wash technique. **(A)** Semen suspended in nutrient media prior to initial centrifugation. **(B)** After centrifugation, cells are concentrated in the pellet (*see* text). Photos courtesy of Michael Vernon, PhD, HCLD, Professor and IVF Lab Director, West Virginia University.

Migration Method

The migration procedure relies on the ability of motile sperm to migrate into a layer of nutrient medium *(13)*. This technique involves the swim-up of motile sperm from liquefied semen or a pellet *(11)*. For the swim-up procedure, approx 1 mL of semen is placed into a centrifuge tube and overlayered with nutrient medium. Alternately, the semen can be placed *under* 1 mL of nutrient medium in a centrifuge tube *(11)*. Multiple tubes are generally set up with no more than 2 mL of total volume to allow for sufficient interface between medium and sperm. The tubes are then placed at 37°C for 1 to 2 h to allow the motile sperm to swim into the medium. After incubation, the supernatant medium is removed and placed into a clean centrifuge tube. An equal volume of fresh medium is added, and the specimen is centrifuged at room temperature for 10 min at 280 to 300*g*. The supernatant is removed and the final pellet resuspended for insemination.

The swim-up method is preferred for specimens relatively free of contaminating cells and debris and with a high-sperm concentration because the recovery of motile sperm is low, particularly in the swim-up from pellet procedure *(11)*. However, after the swim-up procedure, the resulting inseminate is generally very clean, free of contaminating debris and cells, and contains more than 90% motile sperm. It is important to note that when the swim-up from a washed pellet is used, similar problems and damage from ROS must be considered.

*Density Gradient (*Fig. 2)

The density gradient procedure is the most popular method used to prepare sperm for insemination. Historically, Percoll, a product of polyvinylpyrrolidone-coated silica particles, was the most widely used density gradient solution in the early 1990s until it was removed from the market for human use. Subsequently, silane-coated colloidal silica particles have been used as a gradient solution. This gradient procedure uses centrifugal force to propel sperm and seminal debris into contact with the gradient material *(13)*. The motile sperm pass into the gradient, leaving dead sperm and contaminating material trapped at the interface. When more than one concentration of gradient layers is used, the sperm are progressively "cleaned" free of seminal contaminants, and the motile sperm are pulled into a pellet by the centrifugal force. The density gradient method is particularly advantageous for specimens with debris, high concentration of dead or nonmotile sperm, or increased concentration of WBCs or round cells.

A single gradient or multiple gradient layers may be used. A single gradient with a concentration of 80 or 90% is used for the majority of routine semen specimens. Multiple layers (e.g., 45% upper; 90% lower) are appropriate for routine specimens, but are also advantageous for specimens with low concentration of motile sperm. A poor specimen (low count, low motility, or poor progression) may not penetrate through the 80 or 90% density gradient separation solution; in these situations, 45% upper and 60% lower gradient may be used. If a double-layer gradient is used, care must be taken to layer the upper gradient (45%) over the lower gradient (90%) without significant mixing of both concentrations at the interface. Very poor samples may be subjected to 45% only or 60% density gradient separation solution only.

In practical terms, a single 80 or 90% gradient layer is the easiest and most cost-effective method for a physician's office laboratory, and is currently the most common method for preparation of sperm for IUI.

The gradient solution (80 or 90%) and culture medium should be warmed to 37°C. Generally, 1 mL of the gradient is placed into a centrifuge tube for each 1 mL of semen. For specimens with lower sperm concentration, 0.5 mL of the gradient can be used. The liquefied semen is then gently layered onto the gradient, being cautious not to mix the semen into the gradient. The tubes are then

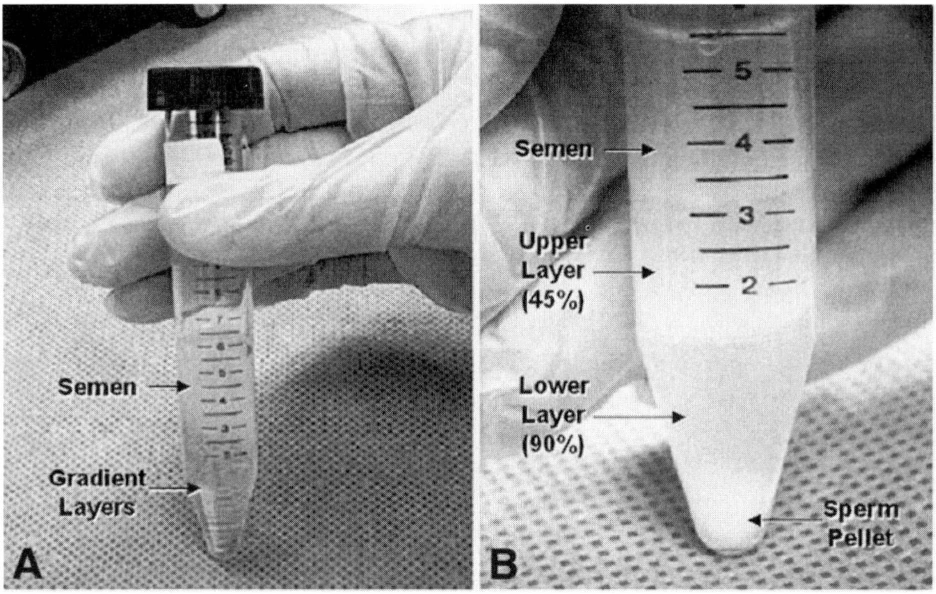

Fig. 2. Density gradient centrifugation technique. **(A)** Prior to centrifugation, semen is layered onto the double gradient (upper and lower layers). **(B)** After centrifugation, pellet is visible below the gradient layers. Note the remaining seminal fluid over the upper gradient layer. Photos courtesy of: Michael Vernon, PHD, HCLD, Professor and IVF Lab Director, West Virginia University.

centrifuged at 300*g* at room temperature for 20 min. Following centrifugation, the supernatant is removed, and the pellet resuspended in 2 mL of medium. The tube is centrifuged a second time, supernatant removed, and the pellet resuspended in fresh medium for the insemination. Alternatively, following the first gradient centrifugation, a sterile glass Pasteur pipet can be placed through the supernatant and the pellet aspirated. The pellet is then placed into a clean centrifuge tube and resuspended in culture medium. After a second centrifugation, the supernatant is removed, and the pellet is resuspended for the insemination.

Preparation of Thawed Semen for Intrauterine Insemination

Insemination of frozen-thawed donor sperm or a male partner's sperm can be done as either an ICI or IUI. The IUI method is by far preferred, and most commercial sperm banks "wash" the donor semen prior to freezing, thus making IUI-ready vials available to physician offices. IUI-ready specimens only need to be thawed, a slide made to insure the motile-sperm guarantee, and the thawed specimen inseminated. Some practices prefer to "wash" the IUI-ready vials upon thawing to remove the cryopreservative, but this is not necessary, and the commercial sperm banks will not guarantee survival of motile sperm if the IUI-ready specimens are further processed after thawing. Thawed sperm can be irreparably damaged from the freeze-thaw process and thus are labile to further manipulations. Therefore, care must be taken if thawed sperm are to be further processed in any way.

Thawed semen should be subjected to only one cycle of simple centrifugation wash to remove the seminal fluid and cryopreservative. After the vial is thawed, the semen should be placed into a sterile centrifuge tube, and a drop taken for a sperm count and motility analysis *(11)* (*see* Chapter 9). A volume of warmed culture medium equal to twice the volume of the thawed semen should then be added slowly, dropwise, to minimize any osmotic shock to the sperm. After addition of the culture medium, the specimen should then be centrifuged at 280 to 300*g* for 5 min, supernatant removed, and the pellet resuspended for the insemination.

Preparation of Retrograde Ejaculates for Insemination

Retrograde ejaculation occurs when the semen is forced into the bladder, instead of outward through the urethra. When the semen enters the bladder, the acidic urine renders the sperm nonmotile or dead. It is important in cases of retrograde ejaculation to neutralize the urine pH to lessen the damage to sperm and increase recovery of motile sperm from the urine. Alkalinization or neutralization of the urine requires cooperation with the patient's general practitioner or a urologist who can provide a regimen of oral bicarbonate and/or instill buffer into the bladder with a sterile catheter to neutralize the urine acidity. The patient is asked to masturbate and collect any antegrade ejaculate. A urine specimen would be collected into a separate container, and the laboratory would examine the urine for sperm. The urine is diluted further with culture medium and placed equally into sterile centrifuge tubes. Following centrifugation of the tubes for 10 min at 280 to 300*g* at room temperature, the supernatant is removed, and the pellets are combined and resuspended in culture medium for insemination.

Recovery

Recovery of motile sperm from the original ejaculate varies from 10 to 90%. It is not uncommon to demonstrate a 90% or more motility in the final inseminate, particularly after swim-up or density gradient centrifugation. The recovery percentage is dependent on the volume of the gradient layer(s), concentrations (%) of density gradient separation solution use, centrifugal force applied, total time of centrifugation, and motility characteristics of the sperm. Although changing the column and centrifugation parameters may increase the percent recovery of motile forms, the less motile sperm and debris of the ejaculate may also appear in the pellet.

INSEMINATION

An important factor in success of insemination is the timing of the insemination relative to ovulation. Timing of the insemination based on cycle length, i.e., inseminate on d 14 of a 28-d cycle, is not an accurate method, except in the most ideal cycles. The current, most acceptable methods of timing insemination utilize the at-home leuteinizing hormone (LH) predictor kits, serum LH analysis, or use of ultrasound, with or without administration of human chorionic gonadotropin (hCG). Generally, one insemination per cycle is done and performed the day after the LH surge, as detected by a positive LH-predictor test (using an afternoon urine specimen), or significant increase in serum LH. When using the ultrasound, an insemination is timed based on hCG administration (34–36 h post-hCG administration) when ultrasound findings indicate a mature follicle (18 mm).

The suggested number of cycles to try IUI before proceeding to either IUI with superovulation or other forms of assisted reproduction, such as IVF, is variable. In a report of 258 patients, those with a motile count of less than 1 million/IUI took 3.8 cycles to pregnancy, whereas patients with a motile count of between 1 and 10 million/IUI had 2.7 cycles to pregnancy *(14)*. Furthermore, the monthly chance of pregnancy was 5.3 and 17.8% in the two groups, respectively. It is generally accepted that no more than six cycles of IUI be undertaken before adopting other options. The physician must weigh the infertility factors, cost–benefit ratio, and risks with the couple when the treatment algorithm is developed. This should be done individually on a couple-by-couple basis. Ovulation medications (clomiphene; follicle-stimulating hormone [FSH], and so forth) with IUI can be initially considered when female factors include an ovulation disorder or luteal phase insufficiency. Ovulation induction is also attempted with male factor infertility, such as reduced sperm count *(1)*. Generally, four to six cycles of IUI are done prior to IVF, with the exception of obvious cases of severe oligozoospermia or tubal disease. In instances of sperm retrieval from testicular biopsy specimens or epididymal aspiration, IVF with sperm injection is used as IUI is not feasible.

The volume of the inseminate is usually approx 0.3 to 0.5 cc, which is easily accommodated by the uterine cavity. Some physicians have utilized tubal perfusion, where a larger final inseminate volume of 2 to 5 cc is *slowly* injected with light pressure into the uterus. With tubal perfusion, the inseminate would flow gradually into the fallopian tubes.

Catheter

The choice of catheter is based on the physician's comfort level with a particular type of catheter. Catheters are purchased sterile and are disposable. Many catheters are available for use with IUI from surgical suppliers, as well as from manufacturers of ART and andrology supplies.

CONCLUSION

In an office setting, it is relatively easy to set up sperm preparation for IUI with minimum routine laboratory equipment and readily obtainable supplies. The methodology as indicated previously is also easy to learn and perform by laboratory technologists or by the physician. However, it is clear that with *unusual* or *uncommon* specimens, referral to a specialized andrology laboratory or ART program is warranted. Such instances include severe oligozoospermia, use of epididymal or testicular sperm, sperm obtained by electroejaculation, and possibly even retrograde-ejaculated specimens. Semen specimens that present with increased viscosity may need more intense laboratory manipulation to recover sufficient numbers of motile sperm. Andrology suppliers market viscosity treatment systems that contain chymotrypsin, an enzyme that is used to treat elevated viscosity. Long-term experience in the andrology laboratory with sperm preparations will assist with decisions on how to manipulate difficult semen specimens.

Office laboratory quality control is an important aspect of andrology procedures. Furthermore, quality assurance analysis must be undertaken to analyze the efficacy of the procedures utilized (i.e., is motile sperm recovery sufficient?), and the pregnancy rates for IUI.

Although it might therefore appear to be relatively simple to set up sperm preparation for insemination procedures, technical expertise is essentially needed not only for laboratory manipulations, but also specifically for decision making based on the quality of the individual semen specimens. Should a gradient procedure, swim-up, or simple wash procedure be used? Should procedures be attempted to treat viscosity? How many cycles are appropriate for a particular couple? The physician in consultation with the laboratory staff and, of course, the couple, should develop an appropriate treatment algorithm.

REFERENCES

1. Guzick DS, Carson SA, Coutifaris C, et al. Efficacy of superovulation and intrauterine insemination in the treatment of infertility. N Engl J Med 1999;340:177–183.
2. Conaghan J. Basics of male and female infertility. In: Andrology and Embryology Review Course. American Association of Bioanalysts, St. Louis, MO, 2003.
3. Van Voorhis BJ, Sparks AE, Allen BD, et al. Cost effectiveness of infertility treatments: a cohort study. Fertil Steril 1997;67:830–836.
4. Byrd W. Processing human semen for insemination: comparison of methods. In: Centola GM, Ginsburg KA, eds. Evaluation and Treatment of the Infertile Male. Cambridge University Press, New York, NY, 1996, pp. 89–107.

5. Allen NC, Herbert CM III, Maxson WS, et al. Intrauterine insemination: a critical review. Fertil Steril 1985;44:569–580.
6. Schlaff WD, Awoniyi CA. Intrauterine insemination for male factor. In: Centola GM, Ginsburg KA, eds. Evaluation and Treatment of the Infertile Male. Cambridge University Press, New York, NY, 1996, pp. 72–88.
7. Agarwal SK, Buyalos RP. Clomiphene citrate with intra-uterine insemination: is it effective therapy in women above the age of 35 years? Fertil Steril 1996;65:759–763.
8. Dodson WC, Haney AF. Controlled ovarian hyperstimulation and intrauterine insemination for treatment of infertility. Fertil Steril 1991;55:457–467.
9. Tummon IS, Asher LJ, Martin JS, Tulandi T. Randomized controlled trial of superovulation and insemination for infertility associated with minimal or mild endometriosis. Fertil Steril 1997;68:8–12.
10. Guzick DS, Sullivan MW, Adamson GD, et al. Efficacy of treatment for unexplained infertility. Fertil Steril 1998;70:207–213.
11. Mortimer D. Practical Laboratory Andrology. Oxford University Press, New York, NY, 1994.
12. Quinn PJ, Kerin JF, Warnes GM. Improved pregnancy rate in human in vitro fertilization with the use of a medium based on the composition of human tubal fluid. Fertil Steril 1985;44:493–498.
13. Gliedt D, Ree ML. Preparation of gametes for assisted reproductive technologies. In: Andrology and Embryology Review Course, American Association of Bioanalysts, St. Louis, MO, 2003.
14. Centola GM. Successful treatment of severe oligozoospermia with sperm washing and intrauterine insemination. J Androl 1997;18:448–453.

4 Specialized Sperm Testing

Pros and Cons

Kirk C. Lo, MD, *Aron Johnson*,
Larry I. Lipshultz, MD,
and Dolores J. Lamb, PhD, HCLD

CONTENTS

INTRODUCTION

Infertility is traditionally defined as the inability of a couple to conceive following 1 yr of unprotected intercourse. It is not an uncommon problem, with nearly 15% of couples failing to establish a pregnancy without medical intervention. In those couples who seek evaluation from a reproductive specialist, 30 to 40% of males have an abnormality that significantly contributes to their infertility. In another 40% the female requires treatment, and in the remaining 20% the infertility is classified as "unexplained."

Routine Semen Analysis

Evaluation of the male partner begins with a complete history and physical examination and rapidly proceeds to a laboratory assessment. A problem that confronts physicians who treat infertile couples is the frequent inability to diagnose a defined cause of male infertility, when the male has normal circulating levels of sex steroids and pituitary hormones. An initial evaluation, which

From: *Contemporary Endocrinology: Office Andrology*
Edited by: P. E. Patton and D. E. Battaglia © Humana Press Inc., Totowa, NJ

includes at least two semen analyses (sperm concentration, motility, forward progression, and morphology), is the first test used to assess the male. This analysis cannot predict fertility; rather, it provides important information concerning sperm production by the testis, quality of genital tract secretions, and adequacy of ejaculation. The classic semen parameters considered to be "normal" as defined by the World Health Organization (WHO) *(1)* are: volume more than 2.0 mL; sperm concentration over 20×10^6/mL; motility greater than 50%; forward progression equal to or more than 2.0 (0–4), and WHO morphology over 30% also establish limits of "adequacy."

Volume (>2 mL)

Low-seminal volume can be caused by a variety of conditions, including blockage of the ejaculatory ducts, congenital absence of the *vas deferens*, hypogonadism, and retrograde ejaculation. It can also be a simple consequence of collection errors by the patient or a short-abstinence interval. Therefore, repeat testing is warranted before recommending an extensive evaluation. High-seminal volume can be caused by prolonged abstinence, which can result in an artificially lowered sperm concentration and morphology assessment. As a general rule, most laboratories request that the semen analysis be performed after only 2 to 3 d of abstinence to avoid these problems.

Sperm Count (>20×10^6/mL)

Sperm count or "sperm density" reflects the concentration of sperm in a given ejaculate. Counts lower than 20 million per milliliter represent oligozoospermia. Low-sperm counts can be caused by suboptimal testicular physiology. However, acute illnesses, or as yet poorly defined prescription drug interactions, can also lead to abnormal sperm counts. Because the recovery of sperm production and ultimately a normal sperm count may take up to 3 mo, a repeat semen analysis is recommended 3 mo after the last suspected compromise. Persistently low-sperm counts require the investigation of possible anatomic, genetic, or endocrinologic conditions (*see* Chapter 9).

Sperm Motility (>50%)

Normally, more than half of the sperm in an ejaculate are motile. Low motility can be caused by defects in the seminal fluid, antisperm antibodies, altered sperm production, and other causes. When samples are collected outside of the laboratory, exposure of the sample to excessive heat or cold can artificially reduce sperm motility. Additionally, a delay in analyzing the specimen can impact motility measures, thus a reputable laboratory will perform a motility assessment within 1 h of collection to provide accurate results.

Sperm Morphology (>30%)

Human semen contains a wide variety of morphologically variant cells. A "normal" sperm head is considered to have a distinct size and oval shape along with characteristic midpiece and tail dimensions. The percentage of normal-appearing sperm cells is believed by some to be an important predictor of fertility potential, but there is still considerable disagreement among practitioners. Abnormal sperm may be associated with numerous features, which are not particularly good indicators of fertility (e.g., amorphous shaped heads or tail abnormalities). Some laboratories perform an analysis called "strict morphology." Under this type of analysis, it is thought that (4 or >14%) of normal morphology is representative of the fertile population.

pH (>7.2)

A normal semen sample is slightly alkaline. Low pH is often an indicator of an obstruction of the seminal vesicles and is often seen with low-seminal volume as well. Instead of pH measurment, some laboratories test for the presence of fructose, which is low when there is seminal vesicle obstruction.

Leukocytes ($<1 \times 10^6$/mL)

The presence of highleukocyte levels in the semen is indicative of an inflammatory response or infection within the reproductive tract. The analysis of leukocytospermia is complex and covered in detail elsewhere in this book (*see* Chapter 13).

Clearly, situations exist in which two males have identical semen analyses and their partners have no female factors; yet, one couple is fertile, and the other is not. Men with normal count, motility, and morphology may have sperm with abnormal function, leading to infertility. Conversely, men with poor count or morphology may be fertile. A semen analysis is not a test of fertility potential unless a man has no sperm in the ejaculate. The greater the degree of abnormality of each semen parameter (or combination), the greater the chance the patient will be included in the infertile population. However, it is inappropriate to draw a *clinical* conclusion regarding male fertility status entirely on the basis of diminished semen parameters. In addition, fertility is a couple-related process that involves many steps to achieve pregnancy and eventual childbirth (Fig. 1).

Tests of Sperm Function

Most sperm function tests are bioassays that compare the performance of live-patient sperm to known fertile-donor sperm. A limitation of bioassays is the lack of acceptable universal industry standards (samples of live sperm from one source) to assess proficiency between different laboratories or maintain quality

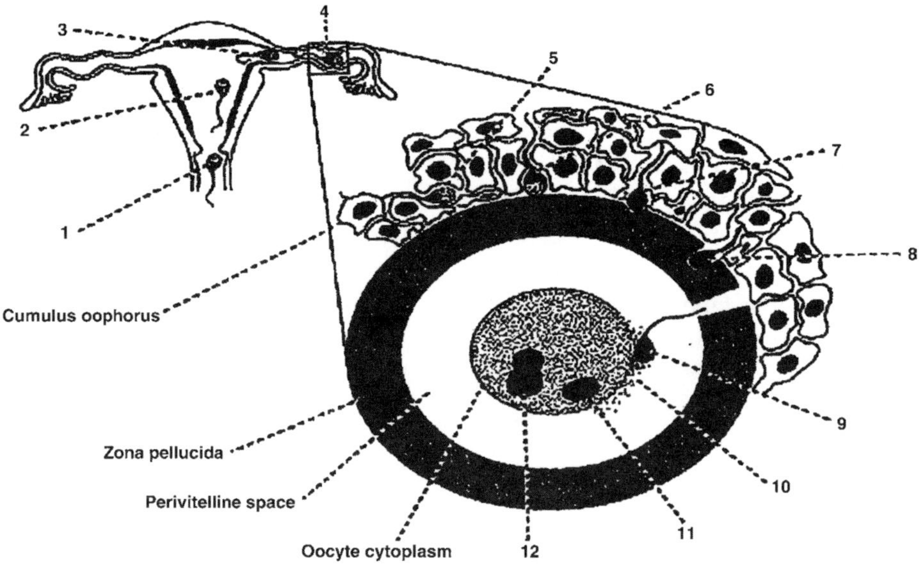

Fig. 1. Sperm requirements following ejaculation to fertilization. (1) Swim through cervical mucus. (2) Move through the uterus and fallopian tube to the ampulla of the oviduct. (3) Undergo capacitation. (4) spermatozoa–oocyte interaction. (5) Traverse the cumulus matrix. (6) Bind to the zona pellucida. (7) Undergo acrosome reaction. (8) Penetrate the zona and pass through the perivitelline space. (9) Bind and fuse with oocyte plasma membrane. (10) Activate the oocyte, and induce cortical granule exocytosis to block polyspermy. (11) Nucleus decondenses to form a pronucleus. (12) Fusion with the female pronucleus. (13) Embryo cleavage (not illustrated here). No single test can measure all the complex functional requirements that sperm need to complete their journey through the reproductive tract to achieve fertilization. Each test described determines functional competence of sperm to complete specific portions of the journey: postcoitus test, 1; hypo-osmotic swelling test, 2 to 8; hemi-zona assay, 4 to 6; sperm penetration assay, 7 to 10; sperm chromatin structure assay.

control using accepted principals of clinical chemistry. Laboratories use donors to provide fresh or frozen positive and negative controls. Although the use of fresh donors provides an acceptable means for quality control, it also reflects the normal biological variations of donor sperm. It does not permit assay standardization over time; accordingly, frozen standards have been developed to be used in every assay. In addition, as conditions for bioassays may vary between laboratories, universal definitions of normal ranges must be established in each laboratory.

Despite interlaboratory variability with bioassays, these tests do provide relevant diagnostic information and may lead to treatment to improve the sperm quality for potential spontaneous pregnancy or artificial insemination. Also, the results of some tests may be used as prognostic indicators for in vitro fertilization

(IVF) or intracytoplasmic sperm injection (ICSI) that can assist physicians and patients in their treatment decision making. This chapter discusses the pros and cons of some commonly prescribed sperm function tests and their application in reproductive medicine.

SPECIALIZED TESTING FOR SPERM INTEGRITY

Strict Morphology

The routine semen analysis usually includes the percentage of spermatozoa with "normal morphology." A percentage below the normal threshold is termed *teratozoospermia*. However, the normal value varies and depends on the andrology laboratory. In 1986, Kruger and colleagues proposed "strict" criteria for the determination of normal sperm *(2)*. These are based on measurements taken from spermatozoa that successfully migrated to the cervix. The clinical correlation between patterns of sperm morphology, judged with strict criteria, and successful fertilization rate for IVF, demonstrated that patients with under 4% normal forms had a fertilization rate of 7.6% in comparison to 63.9% when the normal forms ranged between 4 and 14%. ($p < 0.0001$) *(3)*. A subsequent structured literature review of the association with IVF by Coetzee et al. showed the majority of studies obtained a positive predictive value for the success of fertilization and pregnancy using the established strict morphology criteria *(4)*.

The prognostic value of the strict morphology assay in IVF has a major implication in the selection of the assisted reproductive techniques, namely IVF vs ICSI. Because ICSI consistently produces fertilization rates between 50 and 70% in cases with severe male factor causes, it is considered more efficacious and of cost-benefit for couples with a strict morphology of less than 4% normal forms to undergo this procedure *(3)*. However, it should be noted that because this test does not measure a function of the sperm, it is unclear why the subtle differences indicated in this analysis should impact sperm function.

Laboratory variations and false-positive results are significant pitfalls of strict morphology, that make this a potentially unreliable test. Therefore, it is of utmost importance to maintain good quality control in a laboratory. Automated sperm morphology analysis systems have been developed to circumvent the subjective variability by technicians in the evaluation of sperm morphology *(5)*. The computer's ability to classify normal morphology is promising, but more studies are necessary to establish accuracy and reproducibility.

Modified versions of strict criteria have been described, including the WHO that empirically set the minimum of normal sperm to be 30% *(1)*. However, criteria using this classification has been criticized for its high degree of subjectivity and lack of consensus regarding the clinical value and corresponding fertility thresholds *(4)*.

Sperm DNA Damage Test

The presence of DNA damage in the male genome has been shown in animal experiments in which there is transgenerational expression, resulting in various effects that range from miscarriages to carcinogenesis. The application of DNA-damage methodology to sperm provides a direct assessment of the gametes and may provide insight into the potential effects on human reproduction.

Three techniques have been used to examine DNA damage in spermatozoa. First, using a terminal deoxynucleotidyl transferase-mediated dUTP nick-end labeling (TUNEL) technique, Sakkas et al. found that DNA damage may arise from inefficient apoptosis of germ cells during spermatogenesis *(6)*. Oxidative stress, toxic insults, and potentially shearing forces to sperm during ejaculation could damage sperm DNA, especially if not properly condensed. Other mechanisms, such as failure to efficiently repair the chromatin breaks during spermatogenesis (when chromatin is being restructured for compaction in the sperm head), has also been proposed *(7)*. From a clinical perspective, Sun et al. reported that a significant negative association exists between the percentage of sperm DNA fragmentation and fertilization rate ($p = 0.008$) and embryo cleavage rate ($p = 0.01$) in 143 IVF samples *(8)*.

The Comet assay, another test commonly used for diagnosis, uses the property of DNA migration away from the nucleus during electrophoresis as a consequence of the release of broken ends of the DNA and relaxation of supercoils by DNA breakage. The resulting fluorescent imaging of the sperm DNA resembles a comet (Fig. 2). This technique allows the detection of double-stranded DNA breakage in a neutral buffer or the addition of single-stranded breakage in an alkaline buffer. DNA damage is higher in sperm samples from men with a low sperm count *(9)*. Morris et al. also reported a multivariant analysis showing a significant correlation between DNA damage with male age, sperm motility, and concentration, and the failure of fertilized oocyte to cleave in patients undergoing ICSI *(10)*.

The third technique is the sperm chromatin structure assay (SCSA) that stains sperm DNA with an intercalating dye—acridine orange. The resulting DNA fluorecses green in the normal double-stranded form, but shifts to red if DNA is denatured or is single-stranded. The level of DNA damage is estimated as a ratio of red-to-green fluorescence using a fluorescent-activated cell sorter (FACS). Reports suggested that DNA damage was elevated in the semen of men attending an infertility clinic and may be associated with miscarriage and impaired fetal development *(11,12)*, but these studies need further clinical validation.

Regardless of technique, sperm DNA damage assays provide a diagnostic tool for couples with recurrent miscarriages and an independent prognostic factor for IVF/ICSI. In addition, with the frequent use of ICSI, the genetic consequences of transgenerational expression in the event of sperm DNA damage should be

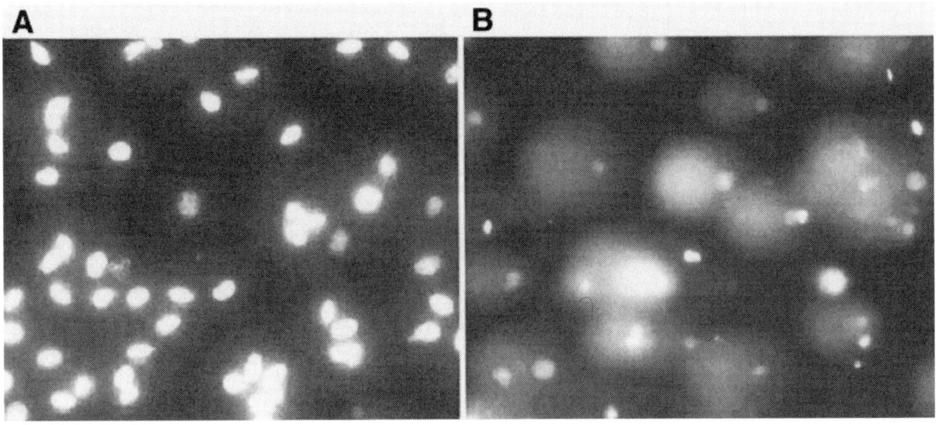

Fig. 2. Comet assay to detect sperm DNA damage. Ejaculated sperm from a fertile donor (**A**) and a patient with a high degree of sperm DNA damage (**B**) are shown here. (**A**) Bright oval-shaped sperm heads represent the normal compacted sperm nucleus when examined under florescent microscopy. (**B**) Fragmented DNA "migrates" away from the sperm head and forms a "tail" that resembles a comet.

addressed and incorporated into the counseling for couples planning to undergo IVF/ICSI.

A lack of consensus and standardization for the methods used to evaluate sperm DNA damage limits the widespread use of the test. Some techniques, such as SCSA, are difficult to reproduce in different laboratories. Although the results may have prognostic value for IVF/ICSI, the etiology of the damage is still unclear. Hence, there is no standard treatment for patients with a high percentage of sperm DNA damage. Some have tried antioxidant administration and/or anti-inflammatory treatments. However, in general, a high incidence of DNA damage in sperm would be expected to be an abnormal finding and unlikely to be positive for reproductive efficiency.

Fluorescent In Situ *Hybridization*

Since the early 1990s fluorescent *in situ* hybridization (FISH) in decondensed sperm nuclei has been used to study the chromosome constitution of human spermatozoa. The technique involves the initial fixation and decondensation of the sperm. After proper incubation, multicolor FISH is performed: triple-color FISH for chromosome 18, X and Y, and dual-color FISH for chromosomes 13 and 21. The slides are analyzed under an epifluorescence microscope, and the spermatozoa are scored according to defined criteria (*see* Fig. 3). Prevalence of numerical chromosomal abnormalities in spermatozoa has been reported in a wide range of individuals, including carriers of chromosome anomalies—fertile

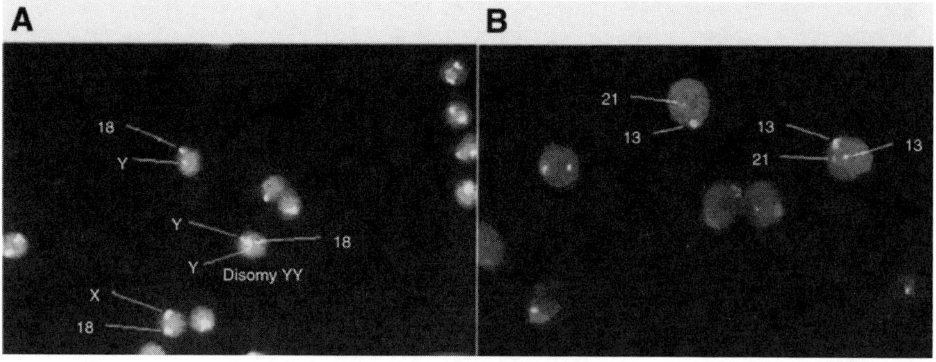

Fig. 3. Fluorescent *in situ* hybridization (FISH) technique to detect sperm chromosomal aneuploidy. **(A)** Three-color FISH detecting chromosome 18, X and Y. Normal sperm should have only one complement of each sex chromosome (e.g., X or Y), however, disomy can occur as shown in this case (YY). **(B)** Nondisjuction of autosomes can also be detected using FISH as shown here (two chromosome 13s).

and infertile males. In fertile controls, the percentage of aneuploid (abnormal chromosome number) sperm is estimated to be at least 6% *(15)*. The mean frequencies of disomy for the autosomes and sex chromosomes in this population are 0.13 and 0.37%, respectively. The presence of diploid sperm can also be detected in 0.06 to 0.24% of subjects *(16)*.

In infertile men with normal karyotype, significantly higher aneuploidy rates in sex chromosomes and diploid nuclei in spermatozoa have been reported *(17,18)*. Using FISH, Vegetti et al. reported that the risk of chromosomal aneuploidy in spermatozoa is inversely correlated to sperm concentration and total progressive motility *(18)*. Studies on testicular tissue samples from infertile men confirmed to have impaired spermatogenesis of unknown cause also showed increased incidence of aneuploidy among diploid nuclei *(19)*. This suggests that chromosome instability results from deficient genetic control during cell division and proliferation during spermatogenesis. Because these patients are the most frequent candidates for IVF/ICSI, information on meiotic studies and sperm chromosome analysis by FISH should be considered for reproductive counseling.

The use of FISH with specific DNA probes can determine chromosomal segregation pattern and aneuploidy levels in sperm from carriers of chromosomal structural reorganization or translocation *(20–22)*. In most patients with numeric sex chromosome anomalies (e.g., Klinefelter's syndrome), FISH studies show increased frequency of sex chromosome hyperhaploid and diploid sperm *(17)*. Owing to the fact that these patients are an important referral group for preimplantation genetic diagnosis (PGD), it is suggested that FISH should be performed to establish a prognosis prior to PGD *(23,24)*.

A study by Rubio et al. suggests a correlation between sperm chromosomal abnormalities and couples with first trimester miscarriages *(25)*. Thus, sperm analysis by FISH may have both diagnostic and prognostic value for couples with a history of recurrent miscarriages.

The major drawback for the wide use of FISH in infertility evaluation, in addition to cost, is the large variability in the reported frequencies of chromosomal abnormalities from different clinical and research groups. These results could reflect interindividual differences. However, technical differences in sperm-decondensing protocols, scoring criteria, number of sperm analyzed, and characteristics of the probes used may be the main factors that lead to the variability of the reported results. Standardization and rigorous controls from each laboratory are essential in the development of this technique. Nevertheless, FISH is a useful tool in the diagnosis and understanding of genetic causes of infertility.

Hypo-Osmotic Swelling Test/Viabiity Stain Assay

The hypo-osmotic swelling test (HOS) test and viability stain assay are designed to evaluate sperm viability. The HOS test is based on the principle that living spermatozoa can maintain an osmotic gradient under hypo-osmotic conditions (150 mOsm/L), whereas a dead cell cannot *(26)*. In a normal semen sample, more than 60% of spermatozoa react to a hypo-osmotic challenge.

The principle of a viability stain assay is that live sperm can exclude dye, and the damaged dead cells cannot. The most commonly used stains are eosin Y and trypan blue. The results of this assay correlate well with those of the HOS test because both evaluate the integrity of the plasma membrane.

The primary use of this test is to differentiate necrospermia (dead sperm) from nonmotile sperm from defects in the microtubles/dynen of the sperm tails (e.g., immotile ciliary syndrome). Another potential use of HOS is to evaluate the viability of testicular-extracted sperm for ICSI when there is little or no sperm motility. A retrospective analysis of 120 couples who underwent intrauterine insemination (IUI) showed a significantly lower pregnancy rate and a higher miscarriage rate in couples with a HOS below 50% ($p < 0.05$) *(27)*. Despite the trend of increased miscarriages in couples that underwent IVF when the HOS test was abnormal, results did not reach statistical significance *(28)*. Overall, the clinical application for HOS and vital staining is limited; the main use is for viability assessment of immotile sperm from testis biopsies obtained for ICSI.

SPECIALIZED TESTING FOR INTERACTION BETWEEN SPERM, FEMALE GENITAL TRACT, AND OOCYTE

Cervical Mucus/Sperm Interaction Assays

Although a semen analysis provides clues to some aspects of male infertility, the postcoital test (PCT) evaluates the interaction between the spermatozoa and cervical mucus. It is useful in evaluating a couple with male factor issues, such as hyperviscosity, abnormal penile anatomy, or unexplained infertility. Many methods are available, but the PCT is performed by examining the mid-cycle cervical mucus for the presence of sperm shortly after intercourse. The mucus is examined microscopically for presence of ferning and "channels" in the mucus and the sperm's forward motility. A normal PCT would show 20 or more spermatozoa per high power field. An abnormal test is most commonly caused by inappropriate timing of coitus. Other causes include antisperm antibodies, poor-semen quality, anovulation, abnormal hormonal milieu, genital tract infection, and male sexual dysfunction.

The PCT can also provide prognostic information in the treatment decision for infertility. In the Walcheren primary study, abnormal PCT outcome has been shown as the variable with the greatest influence on spontaneous live birth prognosis in 726 couples in a primary care situation *(29)*. Many other reports also showed a strong relationship between PCT and pregnancy rates *(30–32)*. In addition, the PCT is associated with human IVF results in couples with unexplained infertility *(33,34)*.

A major drawback of traditional PCT is the lack of specificity to distinguish between the male and female factor. To partially circumvent this problem, *Penetrak,* a commercially available test using bovine cervical mucus in place of the human mucus, can be used. In this assay, thin glass tubes filled with bovine cervical mucus are placed in a small pool of semen. After incubation, the distance traveled by the "vanguard" sperm (farthest swimming) is microscopically measured. This test specifically assesses the sperm's ability to penetrate cervical mucus.

The clinical usefulness of the PCT is also the subject of intense debate in the era of assisted reproductive technology *(35)*. Though a survey in 16 European countries showed that the PCT is still wildly applied (92% overall and routinely in 68% of the institutions), it is rated as one of the least useful of the standard fertility investigations *(36)*. Some criticize its prognostic value from the perspective of evidence-based medicine *(37)*, whereas others question the cost-effectiveness in light of the widespread use of IUI *(35)*. Although an abnormal PCT is a clear indication for IUI with or without ovulation stimulation, IUI is widely used in unexplained infertility regardless of the PCT results.

A counter argument for the benefit of PCT is the potential to avoid superovulation. Although IUI with ovarian stimulation generally has a higher efficacy than IUI alone, the possible hazard of superovulation in terms of multiple pregnancies should be considered *(38)*. In addition, a recent report suggests that IUI can be as effective without superovulation in cases of male subfertility and normal female partners *(39)*. Therefore, the PCT can contribute to the decision to perform IUI with or without hyperstimulation.

Tests to Assess Sperm-Zona Pellucida Binding

Analysis of human sperm–zona interaction is challenging because it is species-specific and requires access to human zona pellucida (ZP). In 1976, Overstreet et al. first studied sperm–ZP binding and penetration using nonviable human oocytes from cancer patients *(40)*. They suggested that sperm–ZP interactions might predict subtle sperm defects that cause infertility, and cannot be diagnosed by standard semen analysis. In the late 1980s, the hemizona assay developed in the Jones Institute (Norfolk, VA) was used in a predictive manner to diagnose isolated defects in sperm–zona interaction *(41)*. This test requires technical expertise and costly equipment, as the zona must be isolated and cut in half by micromanipulation. Donor and patient sperm are incubated with the zona, and the number of bound sperm is counted and expressed as a ratio of patient-to-donor sperm bound per zona half. Subsequently, Liu and Baker developed a modification of this technique called a "competitive sperm zona-binding assay," in which patient and donor sperm are stained with two different vital dyes prior to sperm binding to the zona *(42)*. The zona in this test is not cut in half but is left intact. The sperm are examined under two different wavelengths to visualize the fluorescent vital dyes (red and green), and again a ratio of patient-to-donor sperm bound is evaluated. The advantage of this test is that it can be performed after IVF to determine whether a sperm defect or an egg (zona) defect caused the failure of sperm to bind to the ZP. Other sperm–ZP interaction tests have also been developed, including ZP-induced acrosomal reaction (AR), sperm–ZP penetration, and sperm–oolemma binding.

The relationship between sperm defects (i.e., strict morphology and zona–binding assay) and failure of fertilization in IVF has been extensively studied *(43)*. Statistical analysis showed that the proportion of ZP penetrated, number of sperm bound to the ZP, and percentage normal sperm morphology were the factors most strongly related to fertilization rates in vitro, whereas other sperm characteristics were less significant.

These tests are not widely performed because the advent of ICSI has brought a shortage of excess ova from failed IVF cases. Several methods currently under development will provide a standardized method to assess sperm–egg interactions. These tests are advantageous in that they do not require access to human ZP, but should provide insight into this sperm function similar to that provided by the hemizona and competitive sperm-binding assay previously described.

Sperm Penetration Assays

The sperm penetration assay (SPA) measures the ability of sperm to fuse with the egg membrane and disperse the tightly packed DNA that leads to the formation of the male pronucleus. Fresh-ejaculated sperm must undergo a series of complex time-dependent cell surface changes that normally occur as they proceed through the female reproductive tract. These membrane changes are collectively termed sperm "capacitation" or acquiring the "capacity" to fertilize *(44)*. Human sperm are able to bind and penetrate conditioned hamster oocytes only after undergoing capacitation. Therefore, in theory, measuring the degree to which sperm penetrate hamster oocytes, can better determine the functional competence of the sperm membrane. Because there is a significant crossover population of fertile males with poor-semen quality and infertile males exhibiting good semen parameters, the SPA evolved to better distinguish the infertile population on the basis of sperm-fertilizing potential rather than bulk semen parameters.

In 1976, Yanagimachi *(45)* attempted to produce hybrid zygotes in vitro. He noted that when the ZP of hamster oocytes was removed, human sperm (as well as the sperm of other species) would fuse and penetrate the plasma membrane. The zona-free hamster oocytes would also accommodate not just one, but multiple, sperm fusions. Yanagimachi postulated that this system had the potential to discern functional from dysfunctional sperm and could become the foundation of a diagnostic test of male fertility. In 1979, Barros *(46)* reported a significantly higher mean zona-free hamster oocyte penetration rate when comparing a group of fertile and infertile patients. Later that same year, Rogers (47) reported that a value of 10% of the oocytes penetrated as the most sensitive discriminator between fertile and infertile populations.

As IVF was becoming established as a high-tech therapeutic approach to overcome female-factor infertility in the early 1980s, many clinicians hoped that the SPA would predict IVF outcome more accurately than routine semen analyses. Investigators who performed the SPA realized IVF would be a perfect procedure to test the diagnostic relevance of SPA results.

Initial studies confirmed that when over 10% of the zona-free hamster oocytes were penetrated, there was a high likelihood of acceptable IVF, regardless of the quality of the original semen (SPA true-negatives). However, many SPA laboratories experienced a high degree of false-negatives (i.e., 10% or less of the hamster oocytes penetrated but incorrectly corresponding to good-quality human IVF). A problem with these earlier approaches was that not all sperm in an ejaculate undergo capacitation at the same time, and patients may produce predominately early or late capacitating sperm *(48)*. Because of varying capacitation patterns among patients, a single fixed period of capacitation time was certain to produce errors in a heterologous population of sperm. Poor predictive value of positive SPA results motivated researchers to refine the assay technique. The aim was to minimize the false-positives by increasing sperm penetration rates, without increasing false-negatives, thereby increasing assay sensitivity. These second-generation assays preincubated sperm either with biological compounds or using conditions to promote sperm capacitation, (i.e., progesterone, follicular fluid, platelet-activating factor, high salt, pentoxifylline, calcium ionophore A23187, and low-temperature long-term conditioning in a cryoprotectant). The changes increased sperm penetration rates, assay sensitivity, and prognostic value with varying degrees of success.

Our laboratory developed a second-generation assay, termed an "optimized SPA," establishing unique, controlled conditions for processing both the sperm and oocytes, in an effort to standardize the SPA and increase assay sensitivity *(49)*. The optimized SPA-maximized penetration rates and established a method of quality control that provided acceptable reproducibility for a bioassay of this complexity *(50)*. This method preconditions the sperm at 4°C for 42 h in the presence of a cryoprotectant (test yolk buffer [TYB]), producing a 10- to 50-fold increase in penetration rates. Cold-temperature storage of sperm effectively synchronizes the capacitation event for the early, middle, and late capacitating sperm in the specimen. All sperm able to undergo capacitation are simultaneously recruited to react with the oocyte membrane, resulting in very high sperm penetration rates. A common misconception is that calcium and egg yolk phospholipids in the cryoprotectant are influencing sperm penetration. The cryoprotectant does not confer any penetrating capabilities because simple water achieves the same penetration rates *(51)*. The acrosome reaction is somewhat elevated following this treatment, but not nearly enough to account for the dramatic difference in penetration rates *(51)*.

Most of the patients' sperm penetrate all the oocytes; thus, the score is determined by the average number of penetrations per oocyte (p/o), also termed the "sperm capacitation index" (SCI), rather than the percentage of oocytes penetrated. Other SPA systems typically have none, one, or two sperm penetrating each oocyte compared to the 10, 30, or 50 penetrations per oocyte achieved in the optimized SPA (Fig. 4). Positive scores are values of 5 or greater penetrations per oocyte (statistically consistent with the fertile population). Another important advantage of this SPA method is that it allows patient semen to be shipped overnight to a centralized laboratory without altering the testing process. The submitting clinic initiates the 42-h sperm conditioning by mixing the TYB cryoprotectant with the semen for overnight delivery using ice packs in a Styrofoam mailer. If the performing laboratory accepts specimens sent overnight, then its SPA clinical cutoff values must also be derived by the same method, i.e., the semen of all local patients must also be put through the same set of conditions as those mailed in.

It is critical for the laboratory performing the SPA to demonstrate acceptable assay reproducibility between runs. Because no commercial controls are available for the SPA, quality control is especially important when running this complex bioassay. The live sperm and oocytes are very sensitive to processing

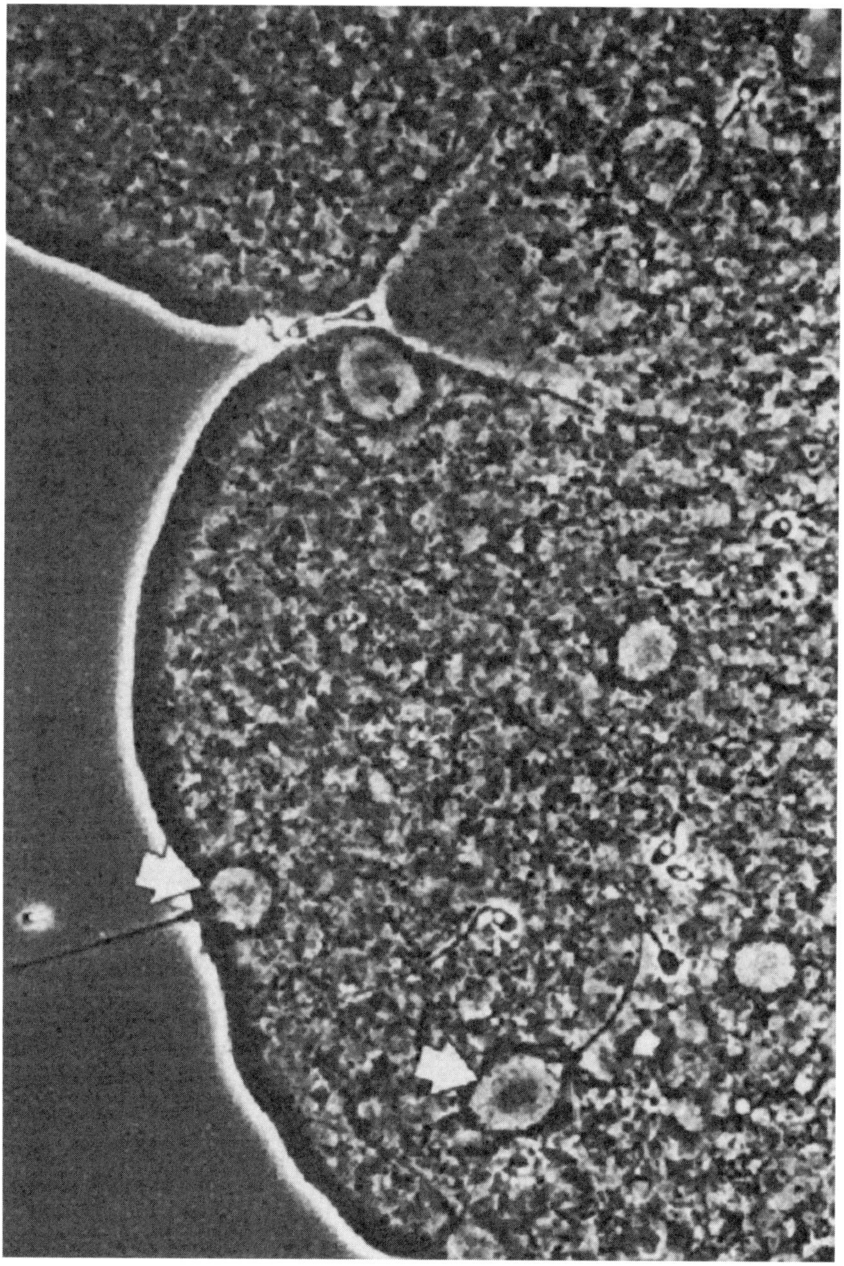

Fig. 4. Sperm decondensation within a zona-free hamster oocyte. The mean number decondensated sperm heads (arrows) within an oocyte is expressed as the sperm capacitation index.

variations that can easily influence the penetration score. Some laboratories mistakenly use freshly collected donor semen to confirm that a given SPA run achieves an acceptable penetration level. The use of fresh donor semen as a control is unreliable because donor sperm function varies over time *(50)*. A few laboratories have established more sensitive methods to determine if an assay run is in control by using aliquots from a frozen single ejaculate in every test run. Testing frozen controls in each run and comparing those results to all the previous frozen scores can confirm the SPA run to be in or out of control with classic rules of statistical acceptance *(52)*.

Although the SPA provides the physician with new prognostic information that cannot be gained by other means, it is only a test of sperm capacitation, and there are other conditions that might prevent fertilization. SPA results are most effectively interpreted in association with other testing, as no single test is able to predict male fertility with complete efficiency.

The SPA serves as a good model for IVF because of the obvious procedural similarities. However, three major biological differences are important to consider: the incubation concentration of sperm in the SPA is more than 30 times greater than that used in IVF; the sperm capacitation method is more rigorous; and sperm are not required to cross the ZP in the SPA. It is more proper to regard the zona-free hamster oocyte less as a model for a human oocyte and more as a membrane capable of fusing capacitated sperm.

Our laboratories have SPA/IVF comparisons both pre- and post-ICSI consistently using the optimized SPA. We derived a cutoff value of 5.0 SCI (or 5.0 p/o, the average sperm penetrations in each oocyte assayed) by subtracting 2 standard deviations (SD) from the SPA scores obtained from 30 pregnancy-proven donors (35 SCI ± 15 SD). SPA result 5.0 or less SCI were considered statistically excluded from the fertile population (positive test result), i.e., they were predicted to *have* a penetrating deficiency. Using this cutoff value, we analyzed a series of 138 IVF cycles performed in 1986 through 1987 *(49)*. A positive SPA correlation was considered to be any IVF cycle that experienced a fertilizing deficiency, defined as 30% or less of the human ova fertilized (Table 1). The high specificity and predictive value of negatives is fairly consistent with other SPA/IVF reports.

ICSI has become so successful that some clinicians contemplate the time when all IVF cases utilize ICSI. Clearly, as conventional IVF is replaced by ICSI, sperm function tests are bypassed. However, the complicated genetic and economic benefit–risk consequences of injecting sperm versus allowing sperm to be selected more "naturally" (by demonstrating the qualities needed to cross the last biological barriers of the egg) are still being questioned (*see* Chapter 16). If there is a hidden detriment to injecting sperm into eggs, then there will be a return to

Table 1
Optimized Sperm Penetration Assay Relevance to Predicting In Vitro Fertilization

138 IVF cases	*+ Positive fertilization deficiency IVF ≤ 30%*	*– Negative fertilization deficiency IVF > 30%*
+ Positive penetration deficiency SPA ≤ 5.0 SCI	18 True-positives	8 False-positives
– Negative penetration deficiency SPA > 5.0 SCI	5 False-negatives	107 True-negatives
Sensitivity 78%	Predictive value of positives	69%
Specificity 93%	Predictive value of negatives	96%

IVF, in vitro fertilization; SCI, sperm capacitation index.

using conventional IVF whenever possible. If so, the SPA may again have a valuable diagnostic influence.

CONCLUSION

Bioassays exhibit inherently more variability than to more common clinical diagnostic tests, such as a basic metabolic blood panel. For this reason, it is important to interpret test scores using the normal ranges defined by each laboratory. Test results obtained in different laboratories are not directly comparable beyond being in the normal or abnormal range.

"Double" bioassays, such as the PCT, hemi-zona assay, and SPA, use cells or biological materials from males and females for analysis. Substrates for these assays are not commercially available. Consequently, protocol differences between laboratories produce fluctuations in measurements. The lack of commercially available reagents and standardized laboratory methodology, combined with a high level of technical expertise required to process biological material, has resulted in considerable controversy in the literature regarding both laboratory values and interpretation of results.

Nevertheless, specialized sperm testing still has a role in determining the etiology of the couple's infertility and in optimizing the treatment available for patients.

REFERENCES

1. World Health Organization. WHO Laboratory Manual for the Examination of Human Semen and Sperm-Cervical Mucus Interaction, 4th ed. Cambridge, UK; New York, NY, 1999, Published on behalf of the World Health Organization [by] Cambridge University Press, pp. x, 128.

2. Kruger TF, Menkveld R, Stander FS, et al. Sperm morphologic features as a prognostic factor in in vitro fertilization. Fertil Steril 1986;46:1118.
3. Kruger TF, Acosta AA, Simmons KF, et al. Predictive value of abnormal sperm morphology in in vitro fertilization. Fertil Steril 1988;49:112.
4. Coetzee K, Kruge TF, Lombard CJ. Predictive value of normal sperm morphology: a structured literature review. Hum Reprod Update 1998;4:73.
5. Kruger TF, du Toit TC, Franken DR, et al. Sperm morphology: assessing the agreement between the manual method (strict criteria) and the sperm morphology analyzer IVOS. Fertil Steril 1995;63:134.
6. Sakka D., Mariethoz E, Manicardi G, et al. Origin of DNA damage in ejaculated human spermatozoa. Rev Reprod 1999;4:31.
7. Kierszenbaum AL. Transition nuclear proteins during spermiogenesis: unrepaired DNA breaks not allowed. Mol Reprod Dev 2001;58:357.
8. Sun JG, Jurisicova A, Casper RF. Detection of deoxyribonucleic acid fragmentation in human sperm: correlation with fertilization in vitro. Biol Reprod 1997;56:602.
9. Irvine DS, Twigg JP, Gordon EL, et al. DNA integrity in human spermatozoa: relationships with semen quality. J Androl 2000;21:33.
10. Morris ID, Ilott S, Dixon L, et al. The spectrum of DNA damage in human sperm assessed by single cell gel electrophoresis (Comet assay) and its relationship to fertilization and embryo development. Hum Reprod 2002;17:990.
11. Evenson DP, Jost LK, Marshall D, et al. Utility of the sperm chromatin structure assay as a diagnostic and prognostic tool in the human fertility clinic. Hum Reprod 1999;14:1039.
12. Larson KL, DeJonge CJ, Barnes AM, et al. Sperm chromatin structure assay parameters as predictors of failed pregnancy following assisted reproductive techniques. Hum Reprod 2000;15:1717.
13. Evenson DP, Larson KL, Jost LK. Sperm chromatin structure assay: its clinical use for detecting sperm DNA fragmentation in male infertility and comparisons with other techniques. J Androl 2002;23:25.
14. Alvarez JG, Sharma RK, Ollero M, et al. Increased DNA damage in sperm from leukocytospermic semen samples as determined by the sperm chromatin structure assay. Fertil Steril 2002;78:319.
15. Egozcue J, Blanco J, Vidal F. Chromosome studies in human sperm nuclei using fluorescence in-situ hybridization (FISH). Hum Reprod Update 1997;3:441.
16. Downie SE, Flaherty SP, Matthews CD. Detection of chromosomes and estimation of aneuploidy in human spermatozoa using fluorescence in-situ hybridization. Mol Hum Reprod 1997;3:585.
17. Egozcue S, Blanco J, Vendrell JM, et al. Human male infertility: chromosome anomalies, meiotic disorders, abnormal spermatozoa and recurrent abortion. Hum Reprod Update 2000;6:93.
18. Vegetti W, Van Assche E, Frias A, et al. Correlation between semen parameters and sperm aneuploidy rates investigated by fluorescence in-situ hybridization in infertile men. Hum Reprod 2000;15:351.
19. Huang WJ, Lamb DJ, Kim ED, et al. Germ-cell nondisjunction in testes biopsies of men with idiopathic infertility. Am J Hum Genet 1999;64:1638.
20. Blanco J, Egozcue J, Clusellas N, et al. FISH on sperm heads allows the analysis of chromosome segregation and interchromosomal effects in carriers of structural rearrangements: results in a translocation carrier, t(5;8)(q33;q13). Cytogenet Cell Genet 1998;83:275.
21. Martini E, von Bergh AR, Coonen E, et al. Detection of structural abnormalities in spermatozoa of a translocation carrier t(3;11)(q27.3;q24.3) by triple FISH. Hum Genet 1998;102:157.

22. Van Hummelen P, Manchester D, Lowe X, et al. Meiotic segregation, recombination, and gamete aneuploidy assessed in a t(1;10)(p22.1;q22.3) reciprocal translocation carrier by three- and four-probe multicolor FISH in sperm. Am J Hum Genet 1997;61:651.
23. Van Assche E, Staessen C, Vegetti W, et al. Preimplantation genetic diagnosis and sperm analysis by fluorescence in-situ hybridization for the most common reciprocal translocation t(11;22). Mol Hum Reprod 1999;5:682.
24. Escudero T, Lee M, Carrel D, et al. Analysis of chromosome abnormalities in sperm and embryos from two 45,XY,t(13;14)(q10;q10) carriers. Prenat Diagn 2000;20:599.
25. Rubio C, Simon C, Blanco J, et al. Implications of sperm chromosome abnormalities in recurrent miscarriage. J Assist Reprod Genet 11999;16:253.
26. Jeyendran RS, Van der Ven HH, Perez-Pelaez M, et al. Development of an assay to assess the functional integrity of the human sperm membrane and its relationship to other semen characteristics. J Reprod Fertil 1984;70:219.
27. Tartagni M, Schonauer MM, Cicinelli E, et al. Usefulness of the hypo-osmotic swelling test in predicting pregnancy rate and outcome in couples undergoing intrauterine insemination. J Androl 2002;23:498.
28. Biljan MM, Buckett WM, Taylor CT, et al.: Effect of abnormal hypo-osmotic swelling test on fertilization rate and pregnancy outcome in in vitro fertilization cycles. Fertil Steril 1996;66:412.
29. Snick HK, Snick TS, Evers JL, et al. The spontaneous pregnancy prognosis in untreated subfertile couples: the Walcheren primary care study. Hum Reprod 1997;12:1582.
30. Cohlen BJ, te Velde ER, Habbema JD. Postcoital testing. Postcoital test should be performed as routine infertility test. BMJ 1999;318:1008.
31. Eimers JM, te Velde ER, Gerritse R, et al. The validity of the postcoital test for estimating the probability of conceiving. Am J Obstet Gynecol 1994;171:65.
32. Hull MG, Savage PE, Bromham DR. Prognostic value of the postcoital test: prospective study based on time-specific conception rates. Br J Obstet Gynaecol 1982;89:299.
33. Balasch J, Jove I, Ballesca JL, et al. Human in vitro fertilization in couples with unexplained infertility and a poor postcoital test. Gynecol Endocrinol 1989;3:289.
34. Hull MG, Joyce DN, McLeod FN, et al. Human in-vitro fertilisation, in-vivo sperm penetration of cervical mucus, and unexplained infertility. Lancet 1984;2:245.
35. Balasch J. Investigation of the infertile couple: investigation of the infertile couple in the era of assisted reproductive technology: a time for reappraisal. Hum Reprod 2000;15:2251.
36. Oei SG, Keirse MJ, Bloemenkamp KW, et al. European postcoital tests: opinions and practice. Br J Obstet Gynaecol 1995;102:621.
37. Oei SG, Helmerhorst FM, Bloemenkamp KW, et al. Effectiveness of the postcoital test: randomised controlled trial. BMJ 1998;317:502.
38. Guzick DS, Carson SA, Coutifaris C, et al. Efficacy of superovulation and intrauterine insemination in the treatment of infertility. National Cooperative Reproductive Medicine Network. N Engl J Med 1999;340:177.
39. Goverde AJ, McDonnell J, Vermeiden JP, et al. Intrauterine insemination or in-vitro fertilisation in idiopathic subfertility and male subfertility: a randomised trial and cost-effectiveness analysis. Lancet 2000;355:13.
40. Overstreet JW, Hembree WC. Penetration of the zona pellucida of nonliving human oocytes by human spermatozoa in vitro. Fertil Steril 1976;27:815.
41. Burkman LJ. Coddington CC, Franken DR, et al. The hemizona assay (HZA): development of a diagnostic test for the binding of human spermatozoa to the human hemizona pellucida to predict fertilization potential. Fertil Steril 1988;49:688.

42. Liu DY, Clarke GN, Lopata A, et al. A sperm-zona pellucida binding test and in vitro fertilization. Fertil Steril 1989;52:281.
43. Liu DY, Baker HW. Evaluation and assessment of semen for IVF/ICSI. Asian J Androl 2002;4:281.
44. Bedford JM. Significance of the need for sperm capacitation before fertilization in eutherian mammals. Biol Reprod 1983;28:108.
45. Yanagimachi R, Yanagimachi H, Rogers BJ. The use of zona-free animal ova as a test-system for the assessment of the fertilizing capacity of human spermatozoa. Biol Reprod 1976;15:471.
46. Barros C, Gonzalez J, Herrera E, et al. Human sperm penetration into zona-free hamster oocytes as a test to evaluate the sperm fertilizing ability. Andrologia 1979;11:197.
47. Rogers BJ, Van Campen H, Ueno M, et al. Analysis of human spermatozoal fertilizing ability using zona-free ova. Fertil Steril 1979;32:664,.
48. Perreault SD, Rogers BJ. Capacitation pattern of human spermatozoa. Fertil Steril 1982;38:258.
49. Smith RG, Johnson A, Lamb D, et al. Functional tests of spermatozoa. Sperm penetration assay. Urol Clin North Am 1987;14:451.
50. Johnson A, Bassham B, Lipshultz LI, et al. A quality control system for the optimized sperm penetration assay. Fertil Steril 1995;64:832.
51. Jacobs BR, Caulfield J, Boldt J. Analysis of TEST (TES and Tris) yolk buffer effects on human sperm. Fertil Steril 1995;63:1064.
52. Westgard JO, Barry PL, Hunt MR, et al. A multi-rule Shewhart chart for quality control in clinical chemistry. Clin Chem 1981;27:493.

5 Genetic Testing for Male Infertility

Robert D. Oates, MD

CONTENTS

INTRODUCTION

The end result of mitosis, meiosis, and spermiogenesis is the production of a functionally competent and genetically normal spermatozoon. These processes are under strict genetic regulation and a variety of genetic mishaps may therefore eventuate in disruption of the spermatogenic process. In addition, the reproductive ductal structures must form properly for the released spermatozoa to be transported successfully to the ejaculate. Permutations and mutations in the genes underlying this complex sequence and series of events can lead to reproductive failure. Darwinian evolution is commonly thought to reflect changes in the genome that confer upon the organism an adaptive advantage. These alterations are maintained in subsequent offspring, leading to "improvement" in a species or the eventual formation of a new species altogether. However, the maintenance of reproduction is also of great importance, as these new genetic and phenotypically beneficial changes must not come at the expense of the reproductive axis. The fidelity of this axis must be preserved (or even improved) and is an underlying, but equally significant, theme of the evolutionary process.

A genomic variation will be ephemeral if it is adaptive in terms of survival but maladaptive to procreation. A genomic variation can only persist if it does not impair any one of a number of steps crucial to reproduction. In other words,

From: *Contemporary Endocrinology: Office Andrology*
Edited by: P. E. Patton and D. E. Battaglia © Humana Press Inc., Totowa, NJ

for evolution to proceed and a lineage to flourish, the reproductive axis, and all the genes that control it, must be stable or only change in ways that are advantageous. It is distinctly unusual, and certainly not salutary, therefore, that an individual is born with suboptimal or absent reproductive function (1).

This chapter reviews some known genetic etiologies of male reproductive failure, a promiscuous phenomenon that spares no race, ethnic group, or individual population. These constitute only a small fraction of what will eventually be discovered as underlying reasons. Common sense relates that the most severe forms of reproductive failure are genetically based, even though the genetic reasons are not yet identified at this point. The ability to treat severe male reproductive failure, thereby allowing continuation of a man's genetic lineage that nature otherwise would not have, has far exceeded knowledge of the etiologic basis. For some conditions, discoveries have been made and couples can be thus informed, gathering information to help decide about continuing to try to procreate. For other conditions, it is not known yet, and couples are in a nebulous world of uncertainty. Conception using advanced technologies is, in a sense, a big experiment, with the subject of that experiment acting as the "child." What will the child's future hold? What genetic anomaly may have been passed along, not just in terms of reproduction, but also relating to somatic health? Research is moving forward; hopefully, in the near future, couples can be given the knowledge they need to make the best and most informed decision possible. Reproduction using one's own gametes is not a mandate but rather a choice.

This chapter focuses on those known genetically based disorders of male reproduction either diagnosed by physical examination in the office, readily available genetic testing, or semen analysis alone.

GENETIC EVALUATION OF MEN WITH NONOBSTRUCTIVE AZOOSPERMIA

A 36-yr-old male presents with a 2-yr history of infertility. His 32-yr-old wife has a normal d 3 follicle-stimulating hormone (FSH), a normal hysterosalpingogram, and no evident cycle irregularities. His semen analysis shows a volume of 3 cc but with no sperm, even upon centrifugation. His testes are small in size and slightly soft in consistency; his vasa are easily palpable; and his epididymides do not feel congested or full. He is adequately virilized. His serum FSH is 9. After explaining the known genetic basis of azoospermia, a karyotype and Y chromosomal microdeletion assay were drawn. The karyotype was normal 46, XY, whereas the Y chromosomal assay revealed a microdeletion of the b2/b4 (AZFc) region. After genetic counseling and much reflection, the couple proceeded along to testicular sperm extraction (TESE) where sperm were identified and used as the source of sperm for an intracytoplamic sperm injection (ICSI) cycle. A healthy baby girl was delivered at term.

Nonobstructive azoospermia (NOA) can be easily diagnosed in males when the ejaculate volume is normal, testes are small and soft, and reproductive ductal structures are present. Most often, the serum FSH is elevated as well. However, there is no upper limit that the FSH must be for nonobstructive azoospermia to occur. As spermatogenesis declines owing to testicular factors, there is compensatory output of FSH from the pituitary. Therefore, if the FSH value is above the lower aspect of a reference range, it is usually indicative of spermatogenic compromise. These clinical clues lead to the diagnosis of spermatogenic failure, either in the azoospermia setting or in cases of severe oligospermia. It is always necessary to centrifuge the semen specimen to definitively confirm azoospermia. In approximately one-third of cases, a few sperm may be found in the centrifuged pellet. If motile, they may be used as the source of sperm for ICSI. Because spermatogenesis must reach a certain level for spermatozoa to spill out into the ejaculate, approx 50% of men with nonobstructive azoospermia may be found to have individual spermatozoa within the testicular parenchyma *(2,3)*.

TESE is the technique used to harvest these spermatozoa for use in conjunction with ICSI. It is critically important to understand the genetic basis for severe male oligospermia or nonobstructive azoospermia because there may be a treatment that allows a pregnancy to be achieved. For such men, a karyotype and Y chromosomal microdeletion assay should be obtained prior to continuing with therapy to elucidate the genetic basis and allow either a prediction of genetic issues in the offspring or of the success of TESE *(4–6)*. When certain aberrations are discovered, TESE may not be a worthwhile venture or may not be chosen by the couple as a desirable avenue.

Y Chromosomal Microdeletions

The Y chromosome contains approx 60 million base pairs. It is divided into a short arm (Yp) and long arm (Yq), separated by the centromere (Fig. 1). The euchromatic region consists of all of Yp and approximately half of Yq. The heterochromatic region appears to be transcriptionally devoid. Distal Yp and Yq contain pseudoautosomal regions that pair with the X chromosome during mitosis and meiosis. Most of the euchromatic Y chromosome is the male-specific region (MSY), which contains numerous genes involved in the spermatogenic process *(7)*. It is within this region that illegitimate homologous recombination may take place leading to the elimination of segments of the Y chromosome that may be the proximate cause of spermatogenic deficiency.

In 1976, Tiepolo and Zuffardi recognized that there was a region on the Y chromosome that must be involved in the spermatogenic process *(8,9)*. They

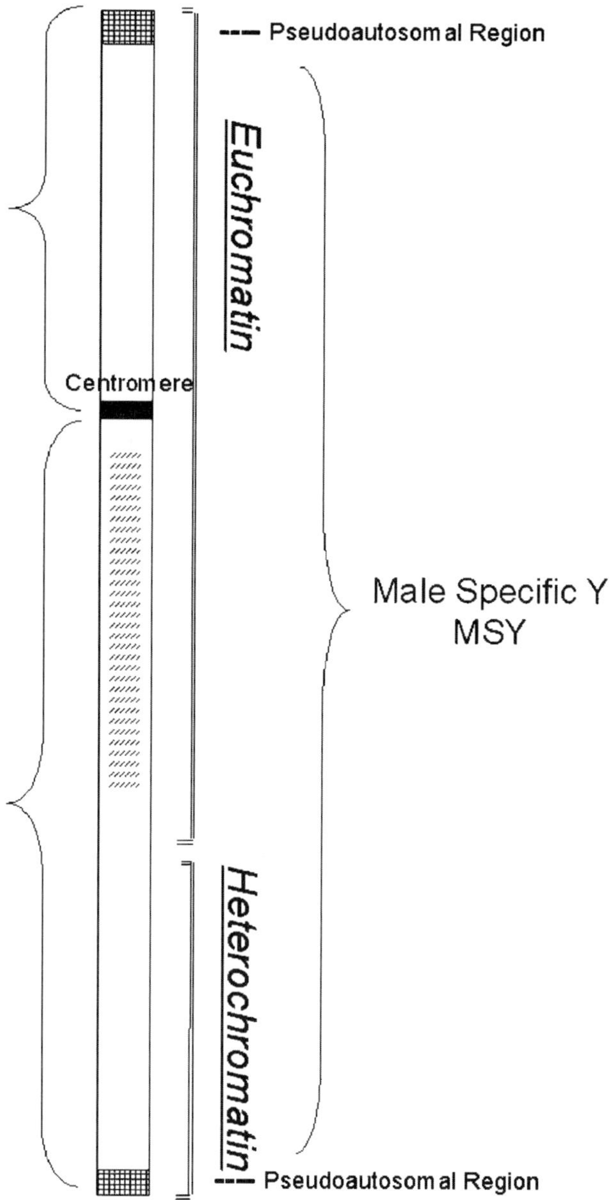

Fig. 1. The Y chromosome with a short arm (Yp) and a long arm (Yq) separated by the centromere. The male-specific region (MSY) occupies most of the total length. The shaded area is the region where *AZFa*, *AZFb*, and *AZFc* are located.

termed this region the "azoospermia factor" (AZF). It is now known that there are essentially two subregions of the MSY prone to deletion and fulfill the con-

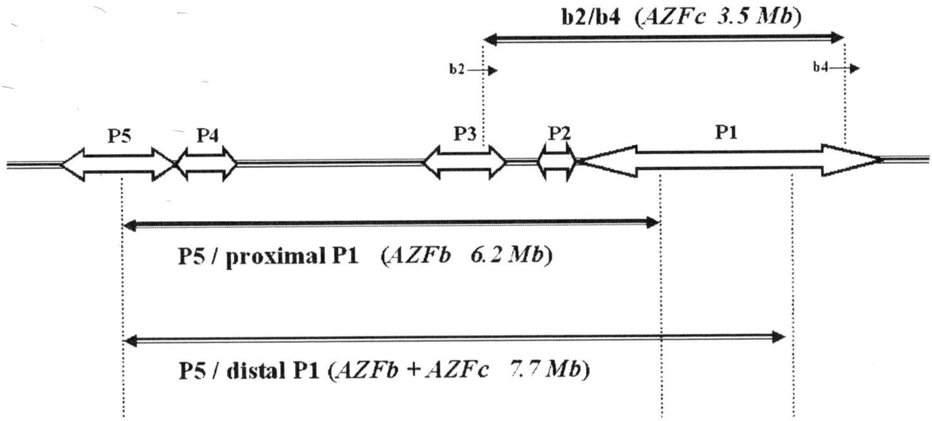

Fig. 2. A schematic of the portion of the Y chromosome that contains the *AZFb* and *AZFc* regions. When homologous recombination occurs between two direct sequences (b2 and b4), all of the intervening chromosome (a small amount of the palindrome P3, all of the palindrome P2, and nearly all of the palindrome P1) is lost. This defines the *AZFc* region and the *AZFc* microdeletion. Longer stretches of deletion may occur (P5/proximal P1 or P5/distal P1). Patients with a P5/proximal P1 or P5/distal P1 microdeletion will not have sperm in their ejaculate or in their testis tissue, whereas those with a b2/b4 microdeletion may have a severe oligospermia or spermatozoa in their testis tissue.

cept of AZF *(10)*. The first region is still commonly referred to as *AZFa*, and the second consists of what was formerly referred to as *AZFb* and *AZFc* (Fig. 2). This is actually one continuous stretch of DNA with variable segments that may be found to be microdeleted. In this area, the Y chromosomal structure is intriguing because there are multiple palindromic sequences (variable length stretches of exactly similar base pairs that radiate from a central point—they read in one direction as in the other direction). For example: CTGAGCCTA•ATCCGAGTC. There are also direct repeats (variable length sequences of base pairs separated by some distance that read exactly the same in the same direction). For example, AATCGTACTG … …AATCGTACTG. On occasion, these direct sequences may undergo illegitimate homologous recombination with the "excision" of the intervening material. In Fig. 2, b2 and b4 are 229-kb direct repeats, b2 located in the P3 palindrome and b4 in the P1 palindrome. When b2 and b4 undergo illegitimate homologous recombination, the intervening segment, which consists of all of P2 and nearly all of P1 (3.5 Mb) is eliminated in the resultant chromosome. Within this region are three genes that probably have a role in the spermatogenic process: *DAZ*, *BPY2*, and *CDY1*. Of course, these genes are lost when a b2/b4 microdeletion occurs. This region, and the microdeletion, is referred to as "*AZFc*" or the "*AZFc* microdeletion." An *AZFc* microdeletion is found in approx 1:4000 men and constitutes the most common molecular etiology for NOA. The clinical characteristics of *AZFc*-microdeleted men were summarized by Oates et al. when reviewing 42 men with an *AZFc* microdeletion as the proximate cause of their NOA or severe oligospermia *(11)*:

- The patients were phenotypically normal with no increased incidence of cryptorchidism, hypospadias, or testis cancer.
- Nearly all microdeletions were *de novo* events, occurring first in the individual spermatozoa of the patient's father, which was the source of the patient's Y chromosome. In other words, the father of the patient was not microdeleted himself, just the sperm that eventually fertilized the egg that became the affected patient.
- There was no paternal age effect as the fathers of the patients were neither older nor younger than average.
- Whether the patient was severely oligospermic or azoospermic with sperm in the testis tissue baseline sperm production appeared stable over time. There was no indication that an immediate pursuit of fertility was necessary lest sperm production decline to sterile levels, as had been previously suggested *(12)*.
- Of those requiring TESE, 70% will have sperm found in their tissue.
- Not all men with this diagnosis will choose to pursue ICSI with either ejaculated or testis-derived sperm.
- If spermatozoa are found in the ejaculate or testis tissue, they are fully capable of fertilization, embryo development, and pregnancy. Children conceived were all somatically healthy *(13)*.
- Male offspring will inherit the b2/b4 (*AZFc*) microdeletion and are predicted to be infertile or sterile upon reaching reproductive maturity. The deletion length did not increase to more proximal regions of the Y chromosome (Fig. 3) *(14)*.

The *AZFb* region was once thought to be distinct and separate from *AZFc*, but as shown in Fig. 2, they are really just overlapping regions *(15,16)*. When homologous recombination takes place between a short sequence located in P5 and an exactly similar sequence in proximal P1, a microdeletion can occur that eliminates the distal half of P5, all of P4, P3, and P2, and the proximal half of P1—a total length of approx 6.2 Mb. Within this region are a host of genes believed necessary for optimal spermatogenesis, including *CDY2*, *SMCY*, and *RBMY1*, among others. A longer deletion may also occur between a direct repeat in P5 and one in distal P1. Other deletions have been predicted, found, and reported that remove variable stretches—both long and short—with variable spermatogenic consequences *(17)*. However, if the microdeletion encompasses the P5/proximal P1 or P5/distal P1 intervals, it is doubtful that sperm will be found in either the ejaculate or testis tissue, perhaps because of impaired meiotic X-Y pairing *(18)*. When compared to an *AZFc* microdeletion, a longer and more expansive length deletion offers little hope, and the Y chromosomal microdeletion assay is unfortunately prognostic; no TESE needs to be performed *(19)*.

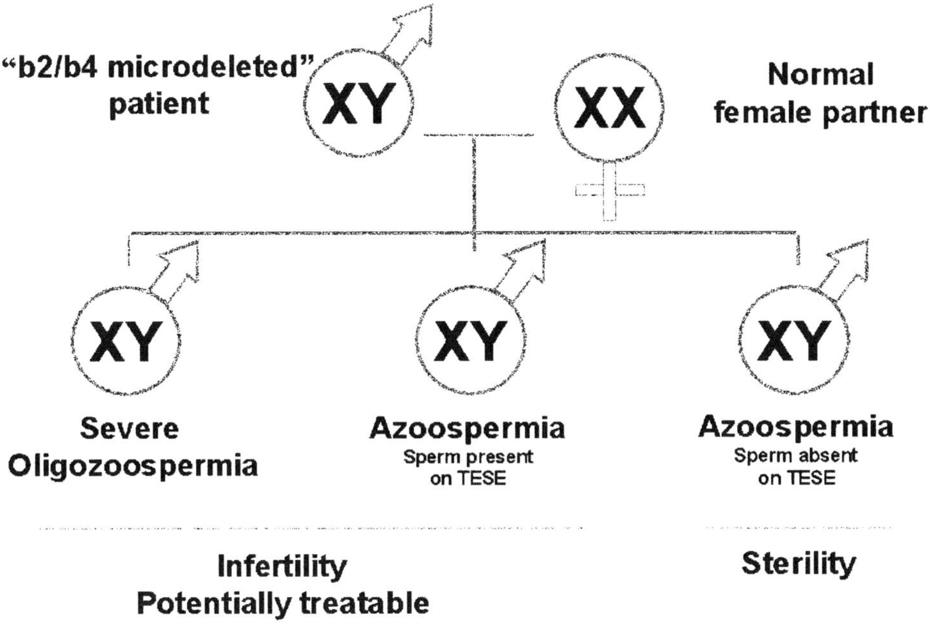

Fig. 3. Predicted outcome for male offspring of a patient with a b2/b4 (*AZFc*) microdeletion in whom sperm are available, either from the ejaculate or from testis tissue. The reproductive spectrum of any male conceived will most likely be similar to that observed in *AZFc*-microdeleted men, some of whom have no sperm available.

The *AZFa* region is found to be microdeleted in approx 1% of men with NOA. Deletion results from homologous recombination between two proviral sequences that flank the *AZFa* region. Within *AZFa* are two genes of importance: *USP9Y* and *DBY*. As with P5/P1 deletions, the prognosis is grave for sperm production, and TESE will not be beneficial *(19)*.

Testing for Y chromosomal microdeletions is critically important to accomplish before any therapy is offered. Basically, using sophisticated polymerase chain reaction (PCR)-based molecular biology, very short stretches of known sequence sprinkled strategically about the MSY are searched for *(20,21)*. Failure to identify (amplify) them implies their absence and a microdeletion. Depending on the combination of results, an isolated b2/b4 (*AZFc*) microdeletion, an isolated *AZFa* microdeletion or one that is more extensive, i.e., a P5/P1 microdeletion, can be discovered. Few reference and/or genetics laboratories have the capability to perform a proper Y chromosomal microdeletion assay, but it is necessary to seek them out. This assay should be ordered on any male with either NOA or a sperm density less than 5 million per cc. If the patient is NOA, and the microdeletion is b2/b4 (*AZFc*), the patient can be counseled about its significance and TESE outcome using the previous information. If the patient is NOA, and the deletion is more extensive (P5/P1) or involves the *AZFa* region, he can be informed that the chance for sperm recovery from the testis is extremely poor, if not nonexistent. This may sway him away from TESE and save unnecessary surgery and cost. If the patient is severely oligospermic, an *AZFc* microdeletion will be found in 6% of such cases, and he can be informed of the genetic basis of his condition prior to undergoing therapy. This allows him and his partner to make an informed decision for themselves, including the consideration of more severe consequences for the children that we do not yet recognize *(22)*. The Y chromosomal microdeletion assay may therefore be informative and prognostic and should be, for those two reasons alone, ordered prior to therapy in any male with a sperm density below 5 million per cc *(23)*.

Karyotypic Anomalies

A peripheral karyotype demonstrates the structure and number of chromosomes present in the somatic compartment of an individual. Although a host of unusual abnormalities may be found, there are three findings that are not uncommonly seen in the severely oligospermic or azoospermic male (Fig. 4).

46, XX male syndrome may be present in an NOA male who has no phenotypic findings to suggest the diagnosis. Although extremely rare, XX males will not have sperm production and, in this instance, the karyotype is prognostic if obtained before surgical testicular intervention. A small portion of the distalmost aspect of Yp is usually present in the genome, most often attached to one of the two X chromosomes. This Y segment contains the *SRY* gene, one of the components of the cascade of genes determining gonadal, and as a consequence, external genital sex. The male has two testes and a normal male external phenotype but will have absent spermatogenesis. He is missing the complete MSY, therefore including all of the *AZFa*, *AZFb*, and *AZFc* regions.

Translocations of large chromosomal segments may occur and disrupt the spermatogenesis process, either by directly interfering with a specific gene function or impairing the pairing of homologous chromosomes/chromatids during mitotic and meiotic stages of spermatogenesis. A karyotype demonstrates translocations in approx 1 to 3% of the male population with significant spermatogenic deficiency. Preconception counseling will then be mandatory to educate the couple as to their therapeutic success, genetic possibilities for their offspring, and option of preimplantation genetic diagnosis/screening of embryos.

Klinefelter (47, XXY) syndrome occurs in 1:500 male births, the extra X chromosome arising from failure of X:Y separation during meiosis in either the maternal or paternal gamete. Consequently, it is one of the most common genetic anomalies found in the azoospermic male. Most patients have a pure 47, XXY karyotype. Typically, men have small, firm testes and are azoospermic;

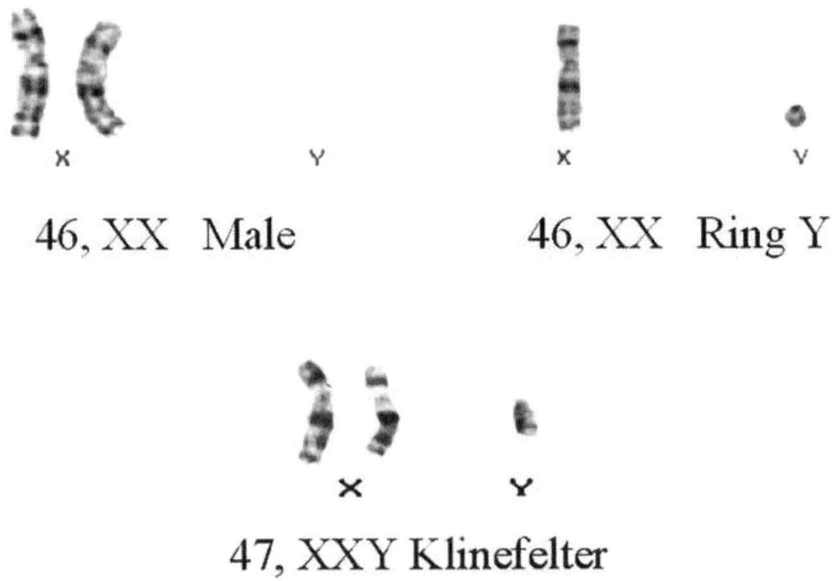

Fig. 4. Sex chromosomes in three different conditions: 46, XX male syndrome in which no formal Y chromosome is present; ring Y in which the Y chromosome has circularized after a break occureed at some point along its length; 47, XXY Klinefelter syndrome in which there is an extra X chromosome.

they may or may not have gynecomastia. There is a wide spectrum of Klinefelter males, which depends on the androgenic axis. If the androgenic axis is severely affected and testosterone output is minimal, the patient may present as a teenager with failure to virilize. This is the classic presentation, the case most often noted in textbooks. A boy may be taller than expected with little facial hair and very small testes. Typically, he presents to his pediatrician or pediatric endocrinologist. Testosterone therapy may be important to stimulate pubertal development. It is unclear whether this type of Klinefelter male will have any possibility of ongoing spermatogenesis. It is debatable whether TESE (with cryopreservation of any sperm) should be carried out in an attempt to preserve future fertility *(24)*. An alternative presentation is that of the less severely affected Klinefelter male who initially comes to diagnosis at the time of infertility evaluation. Typically, this patient is adequately virilized and has escaped detection, as there was no particular reason to present to the medical establishment because puberty went as expected; virilization was not an issue; libido was excellent; and his intellectual capacity did not show obvious impairment *(25)*. When TESE is carried out, sperm can be found in approx 50% of cases. When used, fertilization and pregnancy may occur, where all babies born to date display a normal karyotype. Although it is theoretically possible that an extra X chromosome will be found in an offspring, it has not been clinically seen thus far *(26–30)*. These men may still have androgenic axis compromise, and it is crucial to diagnose them prior to TESE *(31)*. If spermatozoa are found, they are in such tiny numbers that a frozen thawed approach is not reasonable. A combined approach, in which testis tissue extraction is performed on the same date as oocyte retrieval, is most prudent. The patient must be aware that androgenic axis compromise, to the point of testosterone replacement necessity, may be a postoperative untoward outcome.

Other Y chromosome macroaberrations may be found on karyotype. In a small percentage of cases, truncated Y chromosomes, ring Y chromosomes, and isodicentric Y chromosomes may be found *(32,33)*. Ring and isodicentric Y chromosomes usually do not predict spermatogenic potential. However, depending on the point at which the isodicentric fusion has occurred, spermatogenesis may be possible. If sperm are available, the outcomes (in regards to a male offspring) are unknown but may include more severe infertility/sterility and/or external genital abnormalities. This is based on whether the isodicentric Y is lost in a variable percentage of embryonic somatic and germ cells. All men with isodicentric Y chromosomes should also have a Y chromosomal microdeletion assay, which may reveal how far along the Y chromosome the point of fusion is. If the loss of the distal aspect of the Y chromosome begins anywhere proximal to the *AZFc* region, the likelihood of sperm present during TESE would be very small indeed.

Therefore, a karyotype should be obtained in all severely oligospermic or azoospermic men before the institution of any invasive diagnostic or therapeutic intervention. A karyotype can be obtained in many reference or genetic laboratories. Genetic counseling is mandatory when an abnormality is discovered. As mentioned previously, preimplantation genetic screening may be applicable for those couples in whom a translocation has been detected. Some also believe that preimplantation genetic diagnosis (PGD) has a role when the male has Klinefelter syndrome *(34,35)*.

GENETIC EVALUATION OF MEN WITH OBSTRUCTIVE AZOOSPERMIA

A 28-yr-old male presents with a 12-yr history of infertility. His 27-yr-old wife has a normal d-3 FSH, no evident cycle irregularities, and a normal uterine/ pelvic ultrasound. His azoospermic semen analysis shows a volume of 0.6 cc and a pH of 6.5. His testes are normal in size and consistency. There are no palpable varicoceles, hydroceles, or cord lipomas. The vasa are not palpable, and his epididymides consist of only a distended caput. He is adequately virilized. His transrectal ultrasound, performed to document the status of his abnormal seminal vesicles, shows complete absence of the seminal vesicle and vasal ampulla on the left side, an absent vasal ampulla on the right side, and a 4 × 3-cm cystic, hypoechoic seminal vesicle remnant on the right. Renal ultrasonography demonstrated kidneys in normal anatomic position bilaterally. Cystic fibrosis (CF) mutation analysis revealed ΔF508 and 5T, whereas his partner's CF mutation screen was negative. The couple went on to pursue microsurgical epididymal sperm aspiration (the harvested sperm were cryopreserved in several vials) coupled with a later ICSI cycle. They conceived a healthy male child with palpable vasa.

Congenital bilateral absence of the vas deferens (CBAVD) is found in approx 1% of the infertile male population and is one of the leading causes of non-vasectomy obstructive azoospermia. The principle findings are normal-sized testes (spermatogenesis is unaffected), absent vasa deferentia bilaterally, and deficient length to the epididymal remnant (the caput is always present and distended). Attentive palpation on physical examination in the office is the key to an easy diagnosis. The seminal vesicles are typically atrophic or dysplastic but occasionally may be large and cystic. It is important to document this abnormal anatomy in an asymptomatic young man so that if ever visualized again, thoughts of something more ominous will not be entertained. Transrectal ultrasonography serves this purpose quite well. Because the seminal vesicles contribute 70% of the fluid to the ejaculate, the ejaculate volume is typically quite low (< 1 cc) in CBAVD cases. Because the alkalinity of the seminal fluid derives from the seminal vesicle output, the semen is acidic (pH < 7.0) with CBAVD. The ejaculate is only comprised of prostatic secretions. Therefore, in the setting of a low-volume, acidic, azoospermic semen specimen, CBAVD is high on the differential diagnosis list, competing just with complete bilateral ejaculatory duct obstruction. Careful palpation of the cords, noting the presence or absence of the vasa, easily distinguishes these two potentials. As the caput derives from an embryologic precursor different from the distal two-thirds of the epididymis, entire vas deferens, and the seminal vesicle, the caput is always present in vasal aplasia syndromes—either owing to mutations in the CF genes or defects in mesonephric duct development (vide infra). Renal anatomy is normal in those with CF mutation-based CBAVD but may show unilateral renal agenesis in non-CF mutation-based etiologies.

Since 1992, it has been known that approx 65 to 80% of CBAVD cases result from mutations in the CF genes *(36)*. The CF gene is located on chromosome 7 and codes for a protein termed "cystic fibrosis transmembrane conductance regulator" (CFTR). CFTR is responsible for maintaining an optimal fluid milieu in epithelial-lined tubes, such as those that occur in the respiratory tree and pancreatic exocrine system through its selective Na+/Cl– ion pump function. When the total CFTR pool (the contribution from both the maternally inherited gene [allele] and paternally inherited gene [allele]) is normal, the individual has completely perfect CFTR levels and function and will not express any degree of CF-related disease. If one of the alleles is mutated and the total functional pool of CFTR drops to 50%, the person will still not demonstrate disease and is said to be a carrier (one affected allele, one unaffected allele, and no phenotypic consequences). However, when both alleles carry deleterious mutations, the person will exhibit disease—the severity of which depends on the combination of mutations which, in turn, determines the degree of dysfunction/function of the CFTR pool. Specifically, the more severely the two mutations impair the level or function of CFTR, the more severe the phenotypic consequences will be (Fig. 5). If the mutations in combination are "mild," only vasal aplasia may result with normal function of both the respiratory and pancreatic systems. If the mutations in combination are "severe," then pulmonary and pancreatic disease, along with vasal aplasia, will be manifest. Therefore, it appears that the condition of CBAVD represents the mildest expression of CFTR dysfunction clinically recognizable.

It is mandatory to have both partners tested for CF mutations. A specific mutation termed "5T" is found frequently in men with CBAVD and in 5% of the general population of Northern European descent *(37)*. Most assays performed for mutations found in clinical CF will not assay for 5T. It must be clearly stated that the clinical condition of the patient is CBAVD, and milder mutations must be searched for (those that would not ordinarily be found in patients with severe disease but may be found in those with milder disease, e.g., CBAVD *[38]*). The male partner is tested and, when mutations are detected, he should be offered genetic counseling to allow for the proper screening of appropriate family members, such as brothers and sisters who may be of reproductive age. In this circumstance, the patient may be the first person in the family to have CF mutations discovered, and it is appropriate to have his siblings informed and screened as well. The female partner requires a CF mutation assay prior to the couple moving to therapy to define and refine the couple's risk of passing along either CF or CBAVD (Fig. 6). If she is a carrier, genetic counseling is mandatory before therapy (microsurgical sperm aspiration coupled with ICSI) as they may choose one of four options: avoid therapy altogether; move ahead with therapy with no testing until a child is born; amniocentesis of any pregnancy with termination of a fetus who will be predicted to have clinical CF; PGD of each embryo with transfer of only those embryos without two CF mutations.

Because it appears that the vasal deficiency from CF mutations and aberrant function of CFTR develops in the latter stages of fetal life and early in infancy, the development of the mesonephric duct in the initial stages of embryo growth is probably normal. The mesonephric duct "divides" around wk 7 of gestation and leads to two separate subdivisions: (1) the ureteral bud that drives formation of the kidney and ureter and (2) the reproductive ductal structures including the

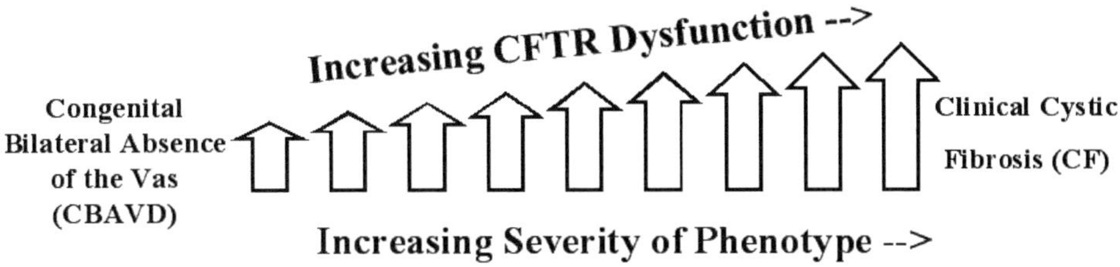

Fig. 5. The clinical spectrum consequent to mutations in the cystic fibrosis (CF) genes depends on the exact nature of those mutations. If both are "severe," cystic fibrosis transmembrane conductance regulator (CFTR) function will be so poor that clinical CF results, but if the combination of mutations is "milder," CFTR function will be less compromised and perhaps only vasal aplasia (congenital bilateral absence of the vas deferens) will result.

Male CF Mutation Status

Female CF Mutation Status	ΔF508	5T allele
ΔF508	ΔF508 / ΔF508 Cystic Fibrosis	ΔF508 / 5T CBAVD
+	ΔF508 / + Carrier of ΔF508	5T / + Carrier of 5T

Fig. 6. Punnett square showing the possible outcomes for offspring if the female partner of a man with congenital bilateral absence of the vas deferens (CBAVD) is a carrier for ΔF508, the most common cystic fibrosis (CF) mutation. The offspring may have clinical CF if he/she inherits both the maternal and paternal ΔF508 mutations, will be a carrier if only one paternal mutation is inherited and the maternal ΔF508 mutation is not, and may present with CBAVD if a male.

seminal vesicle, entire vas deferens, and the distal two-thirds of the epididymis. Therefore, in CF mutation-based CBAVD, the kidneys would be predicted to be normal, and they routinely are. However, there is a second likely etiology for CBAVD, which involves dysfunctional mesonephric duct development prior to wk 7 of gestation. This defect may be responsible for some cases of bilateral renal agenesis, but in the CBAVD population, this presumed genetic flaw may lead to a combination of CBAVD and unilateral renal agenesis. The phenotypic manifestation is slightly less than that which occurs in bilateral renal agenesis and, because at least one renal unit is present, the individual can grow normally and present later in life with infertility. Nature would not allow passage of this genetic aberration, regardless of what it might be, but our newfound technologies will. McCallum et al. presented a series of such patients and noted one male conceptus with bilateral renal agenesis (pregnancy terminated) and 10 healthy offspring with two renal units each *(39)*. Therefore, the genetic basis of this second etiology for CBAVD is unknown, and the risk of transmission is unclear, but the couples require counseling regarding the possibility. Renal ultrasound is necessary in all cases of CBAVD upon diagnosis.

Finally, there are cases of unilateral absence of the vas (one is palpable; one is not) that occur in low-volume, acidic, azoospermic semen specimens. Similar to CBAVD, these patients most likely have bilateral vasal deficiency and require CF mutation analysis. Most likely the vas that is palpable probably ends blindly in the inguinal or pelvic area, and the seminal vesicles are atrophic/dysplastic. CF mutations are often found *(40)*.

DISORDERS READILY IDENTIFIABLE ON SEMEN ANALYSIS

Round-headed sperm, or globozoospermia, is an easily recognizable condition in that the spermatozoa have absolutely round, circular heads (Fig. 7). This results from an absence of the acrosome, perhaps owing to a genetic defect involving the golgi apparatus from which the acrosomal membrane originates, rendering the sperm functionally impotent and unable to penetrate the outer investments of the oocyte proper. Genetic testing is not presently available. Although this disorder has no known genetic basis, it must be stressed to the couple that the few babies born to date appear to be phenotypically normal *(41,42)*. Of equal importance in terms of solidifying the diagnosis is that the embryology laboratory processing the sperm for ICSI has knowledge of the condition beforehand. There is some evidence that the early fertilization events that occur immediately following injection of the sperm into the egg may be impaired and that "activation" of the oocyte with calcium ionophore may be required to maximize the chances of proper fertilization in cases of globozoospermia *(43)*.

Immotile cilia syndrome is the end result of a mishap in the function of the spermatozoan motor apparatus (the axoneme), most likely caused by a defect in any one of the many components comprising the axonemal substructure *(44)*. Sperm density is normal, but there is a complete absence of motility. The exact genetic basis has not yet been elucidated *(45)*. ICSI can be used with some success, but couples must be warned that very few offspring have been reported thus far, and the consequences of using these sperm are therefore unknown *(46)*.

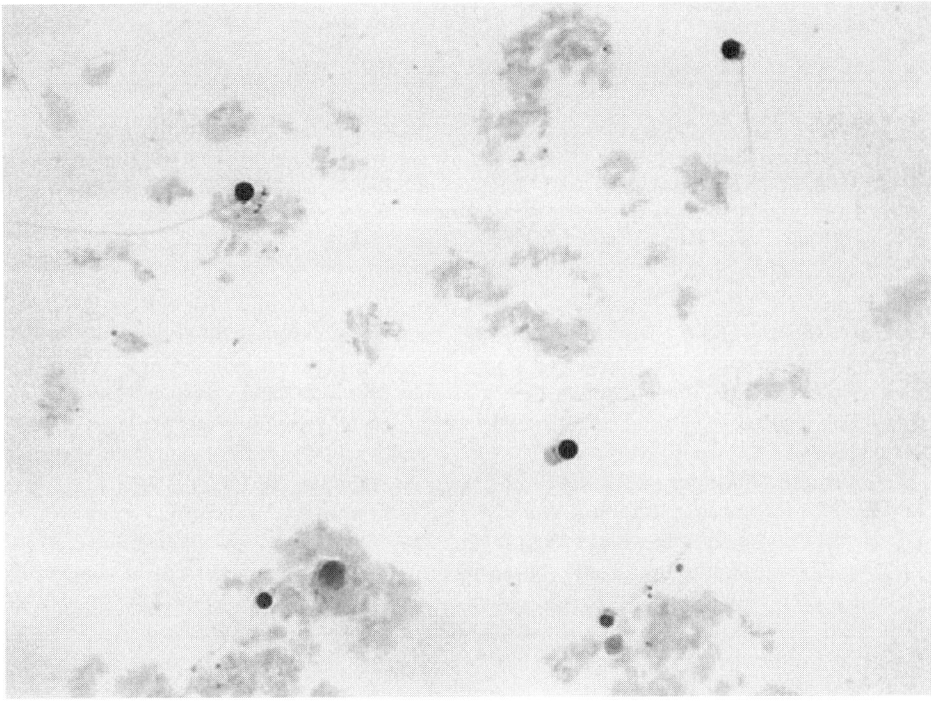

Fig. 7. Microscopic view of globozoospermia. Notice how the sperm heads are all perfectly round and not tapered as would be normal. The condition arises because of the lack of an acrosomal membrane.

CONCLUSION

There are many unusual etiologies of male reproductive failure, most of them with a genetic basis. Some have been defined, whereas the majority has not. However, what can be determined for a patient seen in a physician's office is growing as research defines these genetic bases and ways to test for them. Discussed are just a few disorders whose genetic considerations are significant to couples. A karyotype and Y chromosomal microdeletion assay should be ordered on all men with either severe oligospermia or NOA. Any man with one of the syndromes of vasal aplasia should be screened for mutations in the CF gene, and his partner should be as well. Finally, conditions, such as immotile cilia syndrome or globozoospermia, are rare but treatable. Couples should be informed of their presumed genetic etiology and that there have been only a few babies currently born from men with these maladies. Caution should be exercised on behalf of the not-yet-conceived.

REFERENCES

1. Oates R. Genetic considerations in the treatment of male infertility. In: Thornton K, ed. Infert Reprod Med Clin N Am. vol. 13. Elsevier Science, 2002, pp. 551–585.
2. Schlegel PN, Li PS. Microdissection TESE: sperm retrieval in non-obstructive azoospermia. Hum Reprod Update 1998;4:439.
3. Silber SJ. Microsurgical TESE and the distribution of spermatogenesis in non-obstructive azoospermia. Hum Reprod 2000;15:2278–2284.
4. Chiang HS, Wei HJ, Chen YT. Genetic screening for patients with azoospermia and severe oligoasthenospermia. Int J Androl 2000;23:20–25.
5. Kleiman SE, Maymon BB, Yogev L, et al. Prognostic value of Y deletion analysis: The prognostic role of the extent of Y microdeletion on spermatogenesis and maturity of Sertoli cells. Hum Reprod 2001;16:399–402.
6. Krausz C, Quintana-Murci L, McElreavey K. Prognostic value of Y deletion analysis: What is the clinical prognostic value of Y chromosome microdeletion analysis? Hum Reprod 2000;15:1431–1434.
7. Skaletsky H, Kuroda-Kawaguchi T, Minx PJ, et al. The male-specific region of the human Y chromosome is a mosaic of discrete sequence classes. Nature 2003;423:825–837.
8. Vogt PH, Edelmann A, Kirsch S, et al. Human Y chromosome azoospermia factors (AZF) mapped to different subregions in Yq11. Hum Mol Genet 1996;5:933–943.
9. Tiepolo L, Zuffardi O. Localization of factors controlling spermatogenesis in the nonfluorescent portion of the human Y chromosome long arm. Hum Genet 1976;38:119–124.
10. Kuroda-Kawaguchi T, Skaletsky H, Brown LG, et al. The human Y chromosome's AZFc region features massive palindromes, uniform recurrent deletions, and testis gene families. Nature Genet 2001;29:279–286.
11. Oates RD, Silber S, Brown LG, Page DC. Clinical characterization of 42 oligospermic or azoospermic men with microdeletion of the AZFc region of the Y chromosome, and of 18 children conceived via ICSI. Hum Reprod 2002;17:2813–2824.
12. Calogero AE, Garofalo MR, Barone N, et al. Spontaneous regression over time of the germinal epithelium in a Y chromosome microdeleted patient. Hum Reprod 2001;16:1845–1848.
13. Mulhall J, Reijo R, Alagappan R, et al. Azoospermic men with deletion of the DAZ gene cluster are capable of completing spermatogenesis: Fertilization, normal embryonic development and pregnancy occur when retrieved testicular spermatozoa are used for intracytoplasmic sperm injection. Hum Reprod 1997;12:503–508.
14. Page DC, Silber S, Brown LG. Men with infertility caused by AZFc deletion can produce sons by intracytoplasmic sperm injection, but are likely to transmit the deletion and infertility. Hum Reprod 1999;14:1722–1726.
15. Repping S, Skaletsky H, Lange J, et al. Recombination between palindromes P5 and P1 on the human Y chromosome causes massive deletions and spermatogenic failure. Am J Hum Genet 2002;71:906–922.
16. Ferlin A, Moro E, Rossi A, et al. The human Y chromosome's azoospermia factor b (AZFb) region: sequence, structure, and deletion analysis in infertile men. J Med Genet 2003;40:18–24.
17. Repping S, Skaletsky H, Brown L, et al. Polymorphism for a 1.6-Mb deletion of the human Y chromosome persists through balance between recurrent mutation and haploid selection. Nat Genet 2003;35:247–251.
18. Yogev L, Segal S, Zeharia E, et al. Sex chromosome alignment at meiosis of azoospermic men with azoospermia factor microdeletion. J Androl 2004;25:110–116.
19. Hopps CV, Mielnik A, Goldstein M, et al. Detection of sperm in men with Y chromosome microdeletions of the AZFa, AZFb and AZFc regions. Hum Reprod 2003;18:1660–1665.

20. Nakashima M, Koh E, Namiki M, Yoshida A. Multiplex sequence-tagged site PCR for efficient screening of microdeletions in Y chromosome in infertile males with azoospermia or severe oligozoospermia. Arch Androl 2002;48:351–358.
21. Simoni M. Molecular diagnosis of Y chromosome microdeletions in Europe: state-of-the-art and quality control. Hum Reprod 2001;16:402–409.
22. Patsalis PC, Sismani C, Quintana-Murci L, et al. Effects of transmission of Y chromosome AZFc deletions. Lancet 2002;360:1222–1224.
23. Dada R, Gupta NP, Kucheria K. Molecular screening for Yq microdeletion in men with idiopathic oligozoospermia and azoospermia. J Biosci 2003;28:163–168.
24. Damani MN, Mittal R, Oates RD. Testicular tissue extraction in a young male with 47,XXY Klinefelter's syndrome: potential strategy for preservation of fertility. Fertil Steril 2001;76:1054–1056.
25. Temple CM, Sanfilippo PM. Executive skills in Klinefelter's syndrome. Neuropsychologia 2003;41:1547–1559.
26. Staessen C, Tournaye H, Van Assche E, et al. PGD in 47,XXY Klinefelter's syndrome patients. Hum Reprod Update 2003;9:319–330.
27. Rosenlund B, Hreinsson JG, Hovatta O. Birth of a healthy male after frozen thawed blastocyst transfer following intracytoplasmic injection of frozen thawed testicular spermatozoa from a man with nonmosaic Klinefelter's syndrome. J Assist Reprod Genet 2002;19:149–151.
28. Poulakis V, Witzsch U, Diehl W, et al. Birth of two infants with normal karyotype after intracytoplasmic injection of sperm obtained by testicular extraction from two men with nonmosaic Klinefelter's syndrome. Fertil Steril 2001;76:1060–1062.
29. Greco E, Rienzi L, Ubaldi F, Tesarik J. Klinefelter's syndrome and assisted reproduction. Fertil Steril 2001;76:1068–1069.
30. Friedler S, Raziel A, Strassburger D, et al. Outcome of ICSI using fresh and cryopreserved-thawed testicular spermatozoa in patients with non-mosaic Klinefelter's syndrome. Hum Reprod 2001;16:2616–2620.
31. Tomasi PA, Oates R, Brown L, et al. The pituitary-testicular axis in Klinefelter's syndrome and in oligo-azoospermic patients with and without deletions of the Y chromosome long arm. Clin Endocrinol (Oxf) 2003;59:214–222.
32. Takihara H, Tsukahara M, Baba Y, et al. Dicentric Y chromosome in azoospermic males. Br J Urol 1993;71:596–599.
33. Velissariou V, Antoniadi T, Patsalis P, et al. Prenatal diagnosis of two rare de novo structural aberrations of the Y chromosome: cytogenetic and molecular analysis. Prenat Diagn 2001;21: 484–487.
34. Morel F, Bernicot I, Herry A, et al. An increased incidence of autosomal aneuploidies in spermatozoa from a patient with Klinefelter's syndrome. Fertil Steril 2003;79 Suppl 3:1644–1646.
35. Kahraman S, Findikli N, Berkil H, et al. Results of preimplantation genetic diagnosis in patients with Klinefelter's syndrome. Reprod Biomed Online 2003;7:346–352.
36. Anguiano A, Oates RD, Amos JA, et al. Congenital bilateral absence of the vas deferens. A primarily genital form of cystic fibrosis. JAMA 1992;267:1794–1797.
37. Costes B, Girodon E, Ghanem N, et al. Frequent occurrence of the CFTR intron 8 (TG)n 5T allele in men with congenital bilateral absence of the vas deferens. Eur J Hum Genet 1995;3: 285–293.
38. Wang Z, Milunsky J, Yamin M, et al. Analysis by mass spectrometry of 100 cystic fibrosis gene mutations in 92 patients with congenital bilateral absence of the vas deferens. Hum Reprod 2002;17:2066–2072.

39. McCallum TJ, Milunsky JM, Munarriz R, et al. Unilateral renal agenesis associated with congenital bilateral absence of the vas deferens: phenotypic findings and genetic considerations. Hum Reprod 2001;16:282–288.
40. Mickle JE, Milunsky A, Amos JA, Oates RD. Congenital unilateral absence of the vas deferens (CUAVD): a heterogeneous disorder with two distinct subpopulations based upon etiology and mutational status of the cystic fibrosis gene. Hum Reprod 1995;10:1728–1735.
41. Kilani ZM, Shaban MA, Ghunaim SD, et al. Triplet pregnancy and delivery after intracytoplasmic injection of round headed spermatozoa. Hum Reprod 1998;13:2177–2179.
42. Kim ST, Cha YB, Park JM, Gye MC. Successful pregnancy and delivery from frozen-thawed embryos after intracytoplasmic sperm injection using round headed spermatozoa and assisted oocyte activation in a globozoospermic patient with mosaic down syndrome. Fertil Steril 2001;75:445–447.
43. Carrell DT, Emery BR, Liu L. Characterization of aneuploidy rates, protamine levels, ultrastructure, and functional ability of round heaed sperm from two siblings and implications for intracytoplasmic sperm injection. Fertil Steril 1999;71:511–516.
44. Guichard C, Harricane M-C, Lafitte J-J, et al. Axonemal dynein intermediate-chain gene 9DNAI1) mutations result in situs inversus and primary ciliary dyskinesia (Kartagener's syndrome). Am J Hum Genet 2001;68:1030–1035.
45. Blouin J-L, Meeks M, Radhakrishna U, et al. Primary ciliary dyskinesia: a geneome wide linkage analysis reveals extensive locus heterogeneity. Europ J Hum Genet 2000;8:109–118.
46. Kay VJ, Irvine DS. Successful in-vitro fertilization pregnancy with spermatozoa from a patient with Kartagener's syndrome. Hum Repro 2000;15:135–138.

6 Optimizing Success in a Donor Insemination Program

Phillip E. Patton, MD

Contents

INTRODUCTION

Therapeutic insemination with donor sperm (TDI) is an established and highly effective technique in the treatment of uncorrectable semen deficiencies, inherited genetic disorders, and with single or homosexual women who desire pregnancy. The first documented TDI case was performed as early as 1884 *(1)*, but

From: *Contemporary Endocrinology: Office Andrology*
Edited by: P. E. Patton and D. E. Battaglia © Humana Press Inc., Totowa, NJ

it is speculated that donor semen has been used worldwide for centuries *(2)*. In the United States and abroad, both fresh and cryopreserved unquarantined donor sperm was used up until the late 1980s. Donor screening focused primarily on the selection of candidates who were monogamous and free from any inheritable genetic or infectious diseases. Although long-recognized that infectious disease agents could be transmitted through exposure of semen, samples were not quarantined to confirm that the donor remained seronegative before samples were released for clinical use. The medical practice of using unquarantined semen samples changed forever in 1985 when Stewart and co-authors reported that four of eight recipients who underwent TDI from an asymptomatic carrier of HIV developed antibodies to the virus *(3)*.

With the awareness that TDI recipients could be infected by HIV and other genital pathogens harbored in semen from men thought to be at low risk for sexually transmitted diseases, professional and medical societies, as well as state and federal organizations, established new guidelines and legislative regulations for TDI. As a result, the exclusive use of frozen quarantined donor sperm in suitably screened donors became the standard of care in programs that offered TDI *(4)*. The initial guidelines for fresh donor semen were published in 1986 by the American Society for Reproductive Medicine (ASRM; formerly the American Fertility Society), and those subsequent to 1986 acknowledge infectious disease risk and reflect ASRM's effort to mandate a safe product for consumers. A summary of the published guidelines is illustrated in Table 1.

SAFETY OF DONOR SEMEN FROM ANONYMOUS DONOR SPERM BANKS

With current guidelines in place, sperm from a commercial or university-based anonymous donor sperm banks carries a low risk for transmission of sexually transmitted disease. Although TDI programs practice a policy of self-regulation, the current system does not routinely mandate reporting sexually transmitted infection (STI) by artificial insemination. How can a physician know at this point in time that the semen provided by a sperm bank is safe?

1. A sperm bank has adopted the ASRM guidelines and/or should specifically describe screening and testing procedures that mimic these guidelines. A 180-d quarantine must be observed.
2. Documentation accompanying samples should state that the donor was negative or nonreactive when tested for HIV-1 and HIV-2, hepatitis C, hepatitis B core antibody, hepatitis B surface antigen, human t-cell lymphotropic virus (HTLV)-1 and HTLV-2, cytomegolovirus (CMV) (IgM), gonorrhea, syphilis, and chlamydia.
3. A physician with an MD or PhD directs the sperm bank.

Table 1
Screening of Donors and Recipients of Sperm

	Summary of ASRM guidelines for anonymous semen donors					*Recommended recipient screening*
	Fresh vs frozen	*Quarantine*	*Tests for STIs*	*Max. donor age*	*Year*	*Max. donor blood type*
1986	Fresh or frozen	Not required; if elected, 60 d	Syphilis, HBsAg, CMV, HIV (then called HTLV-III); *Neisseria Gonorrhoeae* and *Chlamydia Trachomatis*	50	Donor should not have a ny nontrivial malformations, nontrivial mendelian disorder, or familial disease with a known major genetic component; he should not carry an autosomal recessive gene known to be prevalent in his ethnic background for which heterozygosity can be detected, namely Thalassemia in Mediterranean and certain Southeast Asian and Chinese populations, sickle cell anemia in African-Americans, and Tay-Sachs in Ashkenazi Jews.	Antibodies, if the blood type is Rh negative *Chlamydia Trachomatis* titer—blood test Rubella IgG HIV-1, 2 HBsAg HBcAb HCV RPR Normal Pap smear within a year Cystic fibrosis mutation screen

(continued)

Table 1 *(continued)*

	Summary of ASRM guidelines for anonymous semen donors					*Recommended recipient screening*
	Fresh vs frozen	*Quarantine*	*Tests for STIs*	*Max. donor age*	*Year*	*Max. donor blood type*
1988	Frozen	180 d	Same	50		
1990	Frozen	180 d	Same, plus HBcAB, Mycoplasma (optional), Trichomonas (optional)	49		
1998	Frozen	180 d	Same, plus			
HCV						
CMV-IgM (Mycoplasma and Trichomonas not listed)				39		
2002	Frozen	180 d	Same, plus HTLV-I and -II, and HIV-2	39	Same as above, plus DNA analysis of specified panel of 25 CFTR mutations for cystic fibrosis. Because the chance is small among healthy young adults of having a chromosomal rearrangement that could be transmitted in unbalanced form to offspring, routine karyotyping of donors is optional.	

ASRM, American Society for Reproductive Medicine; STI, sexually transmitted infection; HBsAg, hepatitis B surface antigen; HBcAb, hepatitis B core antibody; HCV, hepatits C antibody; CFTR, cystic fibrosis tansmembrane regulator; CMV, cytomegolovirus; HTLV, human t-cell lymphotrophic virus; RPR, rapid plasma reagin.

4. Evidence of accreditation by the American Association of Tissue Banks (six are listed on their website in August 2003).

In the final analysis, human semen can never be claimed as 100% safe. Microorganisms other than those considered to be STIs may be present in semen, including *Enterobacter, Klebsiella, Haemophilus, Proteus,* or *Staphylococcus.* Samples may contain "sleeping viruses," that is, viruses not yet known to be present in semen, such as what occurred with HIV.

MAXIMIZING SUCCESS RATES: CLINICAL MANAGEMENT STRATEGIES

Despite obvious benefits, cryopreservation results in variable degrees of irreversible sperm damage, including structural damage to the cellular organelles (plasma membrane, acrosome, and chromatin) and functional changes at the cellular and molecular levels *(5)*. When compared to fresh sperm samples, there is a reduction in normal sperm morphology and up to a 25 to 50% decrease in sperm motility. Moreover, pregnancy rates are significantly lower when cryopreserved semen samples are used *(6–8)*. Investigators have identified multiple factors that influence success rates (*see* Table 2), but the analysis of the critical elements that predict success or failure are exceedingly complex because of the large number of prognostic issues, interdependence of variables, as well as the inherent heterogeneity in the female population undergoing TDI. Despite these limitations, a review of the substantive factors associated with success and failure is informative.

When TDI is unsuccessful after multiple attempts, either recipient- or sperm-related factors could exist. Given the range of influences that can impact pregnancy outcome, distinguishing between the two possibilities is not always a simple process, and an inevitable degree of uncertainty exists regarding the most effective approach in diagnosis and management. The following chapter presents the key fundamental issues pertaining to TDI and our strategic approach in the management of women who choose this reproductive option.

ASSESSING THE SPERM DONOR

Sperm banks are challenged to recruit suitable donors with consistently extraordinary sperm counts. In our program, the screening process (Table 3) requires a minimum of 8 wk. Following an initial questionnaire, rejection from the program occurs most frequently because the number of motile sperm present in the final product is not high enough secondary to the freeze-thaw process, dilution with cryoprotectants, or from the loss of cells during processing for intrauterine insemination (IUI). Consequently, the amount of motile sperm present in fresh samples must be extraordinarily high.

Table 2
Prognostic Variables for Therapeutic Insemination With Donor Sperm

Degree of recipient screening
Coexisting infertility disorders
Timing and route of insemination
Number and technique of inseminations
Sample quality
Differences in donor fecundity
Recipient age
Maternal infertility factors
Indication for insemination

Table 3
Recruitment of Semen Donors: Dropout Rates During Screening Process

	Time frame	*Approximate percent remaining after each step*
Initial interview	wk 1	95%
Semen analyses (2–3)	wk 1–2	25%
Medical geneticist review of family medical history	wk 3	20%
Cystic fibrosis mutation study and carrier status tests as indicated by ethnicity	wk 4–5	18%
Physical examination and health history	wk 6	17%
Screening for STIs	wk 7	16%
Accepted donors	wk 8	15%

STI, sexually transmitted infection.

In the ideal sperm bank, recipients could select a donor sample from a pool of donors, where individual donor fecundity rates are available for review. Indeed, convincing clinical evidence exists that donor fecundity rates are highly variable among donors *(9,10)*. In a retrospective survey conducted by Thyer and colleagues, individual donor fecundability rates were calculated in 20 sperm donors in more than 800 inseminations and ranged from 0.01 to 0.26. Fecundity rates could not be predicted on the basis of routine semen parameters, but could be ascertained after the completion of 15 insemination cycles. Realistically, few laboratories can provide information about donor fecundity. The calculation of individual donor fecundity rates requires that sperm banks receive accurate and timely notification concerning the use of a specific donor and outcome of the recipient following insemination. Very few sperm banks have access to this data. Furthermore, these analyses are invariably complicated by confounding factors, such as the use of specimens predominantly in women with advanced maternal age that would result in an artificially low fecundity rate in selected donors.

Whether specialized sperm testing assists in the selection of prospective semen donors is a subject of controversy. Although some have found the hamster egg penetration test useful in the prediction of reproductive potential of semen donors *(11)*, others have not *(9)*. In our program, specialized sperm testing is not used in the selection of prospective donors. We target donors with 90 million total motile sperm cells per unprocessed sample and assess donor fecundity rates after a suitable trial (15 cycles) of insemination. When outcome data are provided, samples from donors with very low fecundity rates are discontinued.

When multiple TDI cycles are unsuccessful, switching to an alternative donor is a common and reasonable practice, particularly when individual fecundity rates are available. In the absence of these data, we support the selection of an alternate donor in women who have completed careful screening for unrecognized ovulation, tubal or peritioneal factors after an unsuccessful trial of four to six inseminations.

ASSESSING THE DONOR SAMPLE

Pregnancy rates with cryopreserved sperm are lower when compared to sperm from a fresh ejaculate. In part, the decreased fecundity is attributed to a lower effective concentration of motile sperm cells compared to fresh ejaculates. Multiple investigators have demonstrated a positive correlation of total motile sperm concentration and outcome *(12–15)*. In a program that uses an IUI treatment protocol, Kang and Wu reported a 5% monthly fecundity rate with inseminations containing 5 million motile sperm or less, 11% with 5 to 10 million, 16% with 10 to 20 million, and 20% when samples contained greater than 20 million motile cells *(16)*. Presently, the threshold values (minimum and peak) necessary to achieve pregnancy are unknown. In our program, we guarantee a minimum of 12 million motile cells per inseminate, and pregnancy outcomes using this threshold compare favorably with the results from other institutions (Fig. 1).

Clinicians who purchase TDI products must adopt strategies to ensure that the products meet defined quality control standards. For example, Carrell and coauthors found roughly a 10-fold difference in the concentration of motile cells (range of 4.3–39 million) in cryopreserved samples analyzed from seven commercial sperm banks *(17)*. In addition, intradonor variation in sperm quality is a recognized and expected phenomenon that could impact clinical success rates

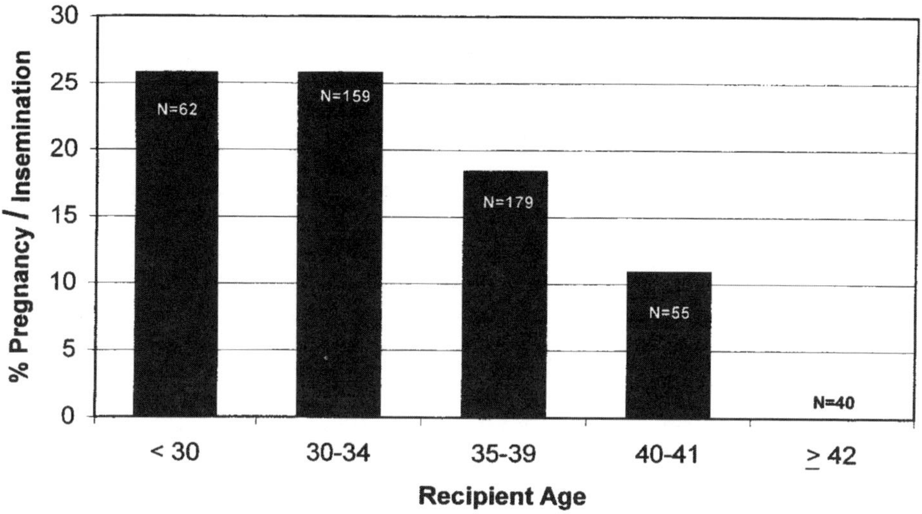

Fig. 1. Pregnancy outcome (fecundity rate) as a function of maternal age at the Andrology Laboratory at the Oregon Health and Science University.

(18). To address the issues of sperm quality, sperm banks guarantee a minimum number of motile sperm within a given sample, whether frozen samples are used for intracervical insemination (ICI) or IUI. At a minimum, we recommend that each sample be assessed for the percentage of motile cells before insemination. A more rigorous standard includes calculating the total number of motile sperm cells and the morphologic features present within each inseminate. When samples consistently fall below laboratory derived standards, then the pursuit of alternative sources of semen samples is encouraged.

WHAT PATIENTS NEED TO KNOW ABOUT SUCCESS RATES

Success rates can be defined as either a pregnancy rate per procedure (fecundity) or as a cumulative pregnancy rate derived from life-table analysis. In experienced programs, fecundity rates with cryopreserved samples range between 5 and 12% per cycle with ICI and a cumulative pregnancy rate that approaches 75% after 12 mo *(19,20)*. Fecundity rates for IUI are slightly higher and range between 9 and 24% per cycle with an 80% cumulative pregnancy rate at 12 mo *(21,22)*. An important insight derived from these studies is that average fecundity rates for the first six cycles are roughly twofold higher than those observed in the subsequent next six cycles. In a study by Kang and co-authors, 93% of the pregnancies occurred within the first seven cycles following IUI *(16)*. Other investigators confirm that the majority of pregnancies occur within a short interval (the first 6 mo) of treatment *(23–25)*. These findings provide a useful rationale for the initiation of screening tests to detect female-related infertility factors when TDI is unsuccessful.

RECIPIENT SCREENING AND ASSESSMENT

Table 1 summarizes the standard screening tests for men and women prior to TDI. Although there is little debate over the value of preconceptual testing for exposure and immunity to infectious diseases, there is considerable diversity within the medical community concerning the types of additional screening tests necessary before TDI. As a result, most clinicians use an individualized approach in the evaluation of TDI recipients.

The degree and extent of recipient screening is based on the findings taken from a directed history and physical examination. Most women pursuing TDI are fertile and conceive within four to six cycles of treatment; however, monthly fecundity rates are nearly 50% lower in women with coexisting infertility factors *(26)*. Therefore, a limited and focused survey prior to TDI that assists in the identification of infertility risk factors is recommended.

ASSESSING FOR ADNEXAL OR INTRAPERITONEAL DISEASE

Routine screening for tubal disease is of minimal value in most women at low risk. In a retrospective review, less than 5% of women undergoing TDI screened for tubal disease had an abnormal hysterosalpingogram (HSG) *(27)*. Tests designed to assess tubal disease are indicated when evidence exists of exposure to STIs, undiagnosed pelvic pain, or previous abdominal or pelvic surgery. We recommend a screening HSG prior to TDI in women with risk factors, women 35 years and older, or in women who fail to conceive after four to six insemination cycles. The predictive value of an HSG to diagnose distal tubal disease is high, and a test that demonstrates tubal patency is comforting. However, an HSG poorly predicts subtle tubal damage, proximal tubal disease, adhesions, or other intraperitoneal disease *(28)*. When historical findings or diagnostic studies are suspicious of undiagnosed tubal or intraperitoneal disease, laparoscopy is necessary to make a definitive diagnosis.

A history of progressive dysmenorrhea, painful intercourse, or undiagnosed bowel or bladder symptoms can suggest endometriosis or related intraperitoneal disease. In retrospective studies, the diagnosis of endometriosis correlates with decreased monthly fecundity rates in TDI programs *(29,30)*. However, the actual impact of endometriosis on TDI success is uncertain because the diagnosis is generally made following multiple unsuccessful inseminations. Therefore, fertile women with endometriosis who conceive quickly could escape detection and be filtered out from an analysis of TDI success. Presently, no large prospective studies confirm lower pregnancy rates in women with endometriosis diagnosed prior to TDI; thus, the impact of mild or minimal disease on success rates is unclear. Nevertheless, it is probable that advanced disease results in lower pregnancy rates, and surgical treatment improves reproductive outcome. As a screening tool, laparoscopy is unnecessary in most women before TDI, but it is advisable in selected cases with prevalent signs and symptoms of advanced intraperitoneal disease or after multiple cycles of unsuccessful TDI in carefully screened women.

SCREENING FOR OVULATORY FUNCTION

Various tools can be used to document ovulation, including basal body temperature (BBT) charting, cervical mucus changes, urinary leutinizing hormone (LH) predictor kits, luteal serum progesterone levels, and pelvic ultrasonography. BBT recording is an inexpensive and simple method to track ovulation. Oral temperatures are measured after 8 h of rest and recorded throughout the menstrual cycle. Ovulatory cycles are characterized by a biphasic temperature pattern, with the shift in temperature elevation ($\geq$0.3 degrees) beginning in the periovulatory period and maintained throughout the luteal phase. A monophasic BBT is consistent with anovulation, but it occasionally occurs with ovulatory cycles. The accurate interpretation of BBT records correlates with serum LH surge activity, subsequent ovulation, and progesterone production *(31)*. The BBT is sometimes used to detect subtle ovulatory disturbances. A temperature elevation of less than 11 d does correlate with the diagnosis of a luteal phase defect, but BBT charting is too insensitive for routine diagnostic use *(32,33)*.

A single mid-luteal serum progesterone value is a simple but slightly invasive tool to confirm ovulation. Following the LH surge, progesterone levels peak during the mid-luteal phase (7–8 d post-LH surge), and serum levels greater than 5 ng/mL indicate ovulation *(34)*. Urinary LH testing is another measure that can be used to evaluate ovulatory function. The appearance of urinary LH activity correlates not only with follicular collapse but also subsequent progesterone production during the luteal phase *(35)*. Estimates of luteal phase length (interval between LH surge and menses) can be compared to impressions from BBT records. In our practice, we use a combination of BBT records and urinary LH tests. Because no single technique is proven superior, individual clinicians may favor one method over another in the screening and treatment of ovulation disorders.

Ovulation disorders occur in many women undergoing TDI (10–60%) *(7,26,36)*, presenting as amenorrhea, irregular bleeding, or premenstrual spotting. Subtle changes in the menstrual cycle length may also indicate an underlying ovulatory disturbance. We aggressively treat ovulation disorders in women undergoing TDI. The oral agent, clomiphene citrate, is administered at a starting dose of 50 mg per day for 5 d beginning on d 3 or d 5 of the menstrual cycle. Higher doses may be necessary when the ovulatory defect is inadequately treated. There is good evidence that clomiphene treatment improves pregnancy outcome *(36)*, but monthly fecundity rates are still lower when compared to women with normal spontaneous menstrual cycles *(37,38)*. As a result, women taking clomiphene may require more treatment cycles to reach a given pregnancy rate in comparison to women with ovulatory cycles.

EMPIRIC USE OF OVARIAN STIMULANTS

The empiric use of ovarian stimulants during TDI cycles is a common, yet unproven, practice based on the premise that pregnancy rates are higher with the induction of multiple preovulatory follicles. Lashen and coworkers investigated fecundability rates in women undergoing TDI following a sequential step-up protocol using two types of ovarian stimulants *(39)*. TDI was initiated during spontaneous cycles, continued in cycles supplemented with clomiphene citrate, and completed in cycles where exogenous gonadotropins were used. A maximum of three cycles were fulfilled at each level before moving on to the next level. Cycles supplemented with gonadotropins had the highest fecundity rate (21%), whereas there was no difference between spontaneous cycles (13%) or clomiphene-supplemented cycles (10%). In a somewhat different study design, Mottoras and coauthors compared pregnancy outcome in women treated with either clomiphene citrate or gonadotropins in a randomized protocol where treatment was continued for up to six cycles in each arm *(40)*. The pregnancy rate per cycle using gonadotropins was significantly higher (14.4%) when compared to clomiphene cyles (6.1%) consistent with other retrospective studies *(41,42)*, but not all *(21)*.

The question of whether empiric use of ovarian stimulants enhances pregnancy outcome in TDI cycles remains unresolved because most supporting data are derived from retrospective reviews or small prospective studies. Nevertheless, the collective data indicates that pregnancy rates following gonadotropin treatment are about twofold higher when compared to spontaneous cycles. The major disadvantages with gonadotropin therapy are increased costs and treatment-related morbidity (cycle cancellation, multiple pregnancy, and ovarian hyperstimulation syndrome). The unexpectedly low fecundability rates observed in clomiphene-treated cycles could indicate potential adverse effects of the drug or, alternatively, the suboptimal results could be secondary to the design of treatment protocols where clomiphene is used following unsuccessful attempts of TDI during spontaneous cycles. In contrast to gonadotropin therapy, there is no clear advantage (and possibly a disadavantage) in using oral agents for empiric treatment.

THE INDICATION FOR TDI AS A RISK FACTOR FOR COEXISTING INFERTILITY DISORDERS

The primary indication for TDI is infertility secondary to a male factor where semen parameters demonstrate either azospermia or moderate to severe oligospermia. Cummulative pregnancy rates are 15 to 20% higher post-TDI in couples with azoopspermia when compared to oligospermia or other semen abnormalities *(1,26,38)*. In couples with azoospermia alone, cumulative pregnancy rates approach 80% after six cycles. In contrast, the corresponding pregnancy rate drops to approximately 30% in couples with subfertile male partners *(38)*. By inference, these data suggest that an aggressive screening strategy may be necessary to detect coexisting fertility factors in women with subfertile partners. However, in a large prospective study from the United Kingdom that included more then 50,000 cycles of TDI, the presence of a male factor did not adversely affect pregnancy outcome *(43)*, a finding supported by other studies *(42,44)*. Based on the inconsistencies in reported results, it is difficult to endorse a more aggressive screening policy in low risk women with subfertile partners prior to TDI. Therefore, we recommend a trial of TDI (3–6 cycles) before consideration of additional testing in women at low risk.

ASSESSING ROUTE OF INSEMINATION

Traditionally TDI was performed by the intracervical placement (ICI) of semen at the cervical os. Success rates with ICI were highly variable, ranging from 5 to 15% per insemination cycle *(45)*. In an effort to improve success rates, intrauterine placement of washed semen samples (IUI) was tested in small clinical trials, and higher pregnancy rates were achieved with IUI compared to ICI *(12,23)*. Although the benefits of IUI over ICI are continually debated, the findings of a recent Cochrane review are informative *(46)*. The study evaluated eight clinical studies comparing IUI and ICI in a population of women undergoing TDI. Overall, there was a significantly ($p < 0.001$) higher pregnancy rate per cycle for IUI (13.0%) in comparison to ICI (5.1%). The benefit of IUI was minimal in centers reporting high pregnancy rates with ICI. Using similar methodology, Goldberg and colleagues performed a metaanalysis of seven prospective studies of IUI vs ICI *(20)*. Consistent with the Cochrane review, a significantly higher monthly fecundity rate was seen with IUI compared to ICI with an odds ratio of 2.4 (confidence interval 1.5–3.8). Collectively, the published clinical experience endorses the use of IUI, particularly in programs where pregnancy rates are low after ICI. The recognized disadvantages of IUI include the need for additional equipment, personnel, and potential requirement to thaw additional samples to reach a minimum sperm concentration per insemination. Although a formal cost-effective analysis comparing IUI with ICI is unavailable at this time, we found that the advantages outweighed the disadvantages *(23)*.

In our TDI program, IUI is used in more than 95% of procedures. Inseminations are timed on the day following the appearance of the urinary LH surge or 36 to 40 h after human chorionic gonadotropin (hCG) administration. At the time of insemination, excess mucus is removed from the cervival os, and a flexible catheter is inserted in the external os and advanced into the uterine cavity. We stock a variety of catheters systems with variable stiffness because no single catheter system works in all patients. The washed sample (0.5 cc) is then slowly inserted over a 20- to 30-s period, and the patient remains recumbent for 15 min. Using this protocol, we and other authors have achieved results similar to those achieved with fresh sperm (Fig. 1).

MATERNAL AGE

Maternal age is a key variable in assessing future fertility potential. The results of population-based surveys and clinical experience indicate that fecundability rates in women decline with advancing age with a sharp drop noted in women more than 35 yr old *(47)*. Several studies confirm that pregnancy rates after TDI also decline with advancing age *(26,38,42,48)*. Cumulative pregnancy rates approach 90% in women less than 35 yr of age compared to 65% in women 35 to 40 and 41% in women over 40 yr of age after seven cycles of TDI. Monthly fecundity rates also demonstrate a corresponding age-related reduction with the lowest values occurring in women moe than 40 yr old (range of 4-8%) *(21,26,49)*.

Based on the decline in fertility potential in older women, we advocate a more aggressive screening strategy beginning in women more than age 35. In this population, it is reasonable to consider early hysterosalpingography or laparoscopy, particularly in women who fail to conceive after three TDI cycles or in females with risk factors for intraperitoneal disease. Testing ovarian reserve is useful in the prediction of pregnancy potential in older women. The testing paradigms are based on the observation that follicle-stimulating hormone (FSH) levels increase with increasing maternal age, and rising FSH levels are associated with decreasing reproductive potential. In women age 35 or older, we routinely perform a clomiphene citrate challenge test as described by Navot and coauthors *(50)*. Serum FSH levels are measured on cycle day (CD) 3 and CD 10 after the administration of 100 mg of clomiphene citrate from CD 5 to 9. An elevated FSH value on either day is associated with a decreased ovarian reserve and generally poor reproductive potential. Because of the variability in FSH assay methodology, it is necessary to establish laboratory specific threshold values of FSH to provide accurate counseling. In older women who have undergone appropriate screening, a greater number of inseminations may be indicated. Alternatively, gonadotropin therapy or the use of assisted reproductive technology may be a suitable option in this population.

ASSESSING THE TIMING OF INSEMINATION

In vivo studies demonstrate that cryopreserved and thawed sperm exhibit an immediate and significant decrease in postthaw motiltily when compared to fresh semen. More importantly, there is a rapid decline in the functional lifespan of thawed samples. On the basis of these observations, it is probable that accurate insemination timing is a critical component in the success of stored semen

The periovulatory period can be estimated by BBT charting, cervical mucus changes, serial ultrasonography, or urinary or serum LH assays. Choosing the best method for TDI timing is a debatable subject. BBT charting or cervical mucus changes are thought to be relatively imprecise methods in the prospective identification of ovulation *(51,52)*, as the BBT nadir or optimal cervical mucus coincides with LH surge activity in less than 50% of cycles. However, in a prospective randomized study comparing ICI timing with BBT charting and urinary LH kits, there was no significant difference in conception rate between the two groups *(53)*. Whereas one study found an overall cost savings by timing ICI with LH kits, others have not *(54, 55)*. A methodological weakness in these studies (and most studies of this kind) was that only a single insemination was used when timing was based on LH, and multiple inseminations were generally performed when BBT records were used. Whether different results would occur following a single ICI is unknown. The timing of ICI relative to LH detection may be important, particularly when ICI is performed on the day after LH surge detection (LH + 1). Previous work indicates that cervical mucous scores peak on the day of LH and in nearly 50% of cycles, cervical mucus scores are unfavorable on LH + 1 *(15,56)*.

Serial ultrasonography as a means to track preovulatory follicle growth is an appealing method to time insemination. However, the event of follicle rupture occurs at variable sizes. In a prospective randomized trial, timing by ultrasound findings was not significantly better than serum LH testing *(57)*. In our experience, the simplest and most practical method of insemination timing is through the use of urinary LH assays. Based on the previous cycle lengths or BBT charts, the kits are inititated once daily generally beginning 3 d before the expected time of ovulation. For IUI cycles, we time the insemination 24 h after the onset of the surge. Whether pregnancy rates are different when IUI is performed on LH + 0 or at other times is unknown. In contrast, ICI procedures are usually performed on LH + 0 and/or LH + 1 in an attempt to bracket favorable mucus production.

ONE OR TWO INSEMINATIONS

To overcome the reduced functional life span and decreased pregnancy rates associated with stored sperm, multiple ICI inseminations procedures may be recommended. Multiple inseminations may be beneficial, particularly in situations where the cervical mucus is receptive for only a short duration during the periovulatory period. Higher pregnancy rates are reported when more than one ICI insemination is performed *(58,59)*; however, in a retrospective analysis of 869 cycles, there were no detectable differences in pregnancy rate between single (8.2%) or multiple (5.7%) inseminations *(60)*.

In prospective studies of IUI vs ICI, two ICI inseminations offered no advantage over a single IUI *(46)*. Although multiple inseminations may be beneficial in programs where ICI is used, there is no documented advantage for multiple IUIs. When using ICI, the initial insemination should be timed on the basis of peak cervical mucus production or alternatively on LH + 0 using urinary asays. Generally, the second insemination is performed on the following day. In a program that predominately uses an IUI, a single insemination on LH + 1 results in acceptable pregnancy rates.

FUTURE OF ANONYMOUS DONOR SPERM

Carefully designed clinical trials should answer many of the unresolved issues concerning the optimal treatment regimens for TDI. Until then, treatment strategies will be representative of the best available data and clinical experience. Realistically, legislative actions will influence TDI more in the future than will scientific discovery. Sperm banks in the United States have voluntarily, conscientiously, and successfully self-regulated and provided a safe product at a reasonable cost. Federal regulation, projected to begin on January 1, 2004, will require the registration of "manufacturers" of human tissue, including reproductive tissues, e.g., gametes provided anonymously. Inspection and accreditation will follow registration. The Food and Drug Administration will require policies and procedures on donor screening, testing for STIs, maintenance of equipment, types of media used, personnel training, verification and routine quality control of computer systems, methods for storage in liquid nitrogen, labeling of vials, and so on, with detailed documentation. The process is designed to ensure a safer product, but the regulations will not likely improve sample quality or improve success rates. Because of the increased cost associated with the new regulations, the future of university or commercial sperm banks is uncertain. New federal standards may promote the closure of some sperm banks, thereby limiting access to semen samples. As a result, the cost of TDI may increase as an economic function of supply and demand in an open marketplace.

REFERENCES

1. Emperaire JC, Gauzere-Soumireu E, Audebert AJ. Female fertility and donor insemination. Fertil Steril 1982;37:90–93.
2. Sims JM. Clinical Notes on Uterine Surgery. Gryphon Editions, Birmingham, AL, 1990.

3. Stewart GJ, Tyler JP, Cunningham AL, et al. Transmission of human T-cell lymphotropic virus type III (HTLV-III) by artificial insemination by donor. Lancet 1985;2:581–585.
4. Centers for Disease Control. Semen banking, organ and tissue transplantation and HIV antibody testing. Morbidity Mortality Weekly Rep 1988;37:58,59.
5. Nijs M and Ombelet W. Cryopreservation of human sperm. Hum Fertil 2001;4:158–163.
6. Richter M, Haning R, Shapiro S. Artificial donor insemination fresh versus frozen semen: the patient as her own control. Fertil Steril 1984;41:277–280.
7. Smith KD, Rodriguez-Rigau LJ, Steinberger E. The influence of ovulatory dysfunction and timing of insemination on the success of artificial insemination donor (AID) with fresh or cryopreserved semen. Fertil Steril 1981;36:496–502.
8. Subak LL, Adamson GD, Boltz NL. Therapeutic donor insemination: a prospective randomized trial of fresh versus frozen sperm. Am J Obstet Gynecol 1992;166:1597–1604; discussion 1604–1606.
9. Marshburn PB, McIntire D, Carr BR, Byrd W. Spermatozoal characteristics from fresh and frozen donor semen and their correlation with fertlity outcome after intrauterine insemination. Fertil Steril 1992;58:179–186.
10. Thyer AC, Patton PE, Burry KA, et al. Fecundability trends among sperm donors as a measure of donor performance. Fertil Steril 1999;71:891–895.
11. Navarrete T, Johnson A, Mixon B, Wolf D. The relationship between fertility potential measurements on cryobanked semen and fecundity of sperm donors. Hum Reprod 2000;15:344–350.
12. Byrd W, Bradshaw K, Carr B, et al. A prospective, randomized study of pregnancy rates following intrauterine and intracervical insemination using frozen donor sperm. Fertil Steril 1990;53:521–527.
13. Gerris JM, Delbeke LO, Punjabi U, Buytaert P. The value of intrauterine insemination with washed husband's sperm in the treatment of infertility. Hum Reprod 1987;2:315–320.
14. David G, Czyglik F, Mayaux MJ, Schwartz D. The success of A.I.D. and semen characteristics: study on 1489 cycles and 192 ejaculates. Int J Androl 1980;3:613–619.
15. Nielson NC, Risum J, Bogaard Hansen K, Nissen U. Obtained pregnancies by AID using frozen semen in relation to specific qualities of the semen. Gynecol Obstet Invest 1984;18:147–151.
16. Kang BM, Wu TC. Effect of age on intrauterine insemination with frozen donor sperm. Obstet Gynecol 1996;88:93–98.
17. Carrell DT, Cartmill D, Jones KP, et al. Prospective, randomized, blinded evaluation of donor semen quality provided by seven commercial sperm banks. Fertil Steril 2002;78:16–21.
18. Wijchman JG, de Wolf BT, Graafe R, Arts EG. Variation in semen parameters derived from computer-aided semen analysis, within donors and between donors. J Androl 2001;22:773–780.
19. Le Lannou D, Lansac J. Artificial procreation with frozen donor semen: experience of the French Federation CEDOS. Hum Reprod 1989;4:757–761.
20. Goldberg JM, Mascha E, Falcone T, Attaran M. Comparison of intrauterine and intracervical insemination with frozen donor sperm: a meta-analysis. Fertil Steril 1999;72:792–795.
21. Botchan A, Hauser R, Gamzu R, et al. Results of 6139 artificial insemination cycles with donor spermatozoa. Hum Reprod 2001;16:2298–2304.
22. Williams RS, Adlerman J. Predictors of success with the use of donor sperm. Am J Obstet Gynecol 2001;185:332–337.
23. Patton PE, Burry KA, Thurmond A, et al. Intrauterine insemination outperforms intracervical insemination in a randomized, controlled study with frozen, donor semen. Fertil Steril 1992;57:559–564.
24. Hurd WW, Randolph JF Jr, Ansbacher R, et al. Comparison of intracervical, intrauterine, and intratubal techniques for donor insemination. Fertil Steril 1993;59:339–342; comment in Fertil Steril 1993;60:376,377.

25. Khalil MR, Rasmussen PE, Erb K, et al. Intrauterine insemination with donor semen. An evaluation of prognostic factors based on a review of 1131 cycles. Acta Obstet Gynecol Scand 2001;80:342–348.
26. Ebbiary NAA, Martin K, Gibbs A, et al. Spontaneous ovulatory cycle donor insemination programme: prognostic indicators of a successful pregnancy. Hum Reprod 1994;9:1852–1858.
27. Nach D, Haning R, Shapiro S. Value of hysterosalpingogram prior to donor artificial insemination. Fertil Steril 1979;31:378–380.
28. Opsahl MS, Miller B, Klein TA. The predictive value of hysterosalpingography for tubal and peritoneal infertility factors. Fertil Steril 1993;60:444–448.
29. Hammond MG, Jordan S, Sloan CS. Factors affecting pregnancy rates in a donor insemination program using frozen semen. Am J Obstet Gynecol 1986;155:480–485.
30. Bergquist CA, Rock JA, Miller J. Artificial insemination with fresh donor semen using the cervical cap technique: a review of 278 cases. Obstet Gynecol 1982;60:195–199.
31. Guermandi E, Vegetti W, Bianchi MM, et al. Reliability of ovulation tests in infertile women. Obstet Gynecol 2001;97:92–96.
32. Jordon J, Craig K, Clifton DK, Soules MR. Luteal phase defect: the sensitivity and specificity of diagnostic methods in common clinical use. Fertil Steril 1994;62:54–62.
33. Downs KA, Gibson M. Basal body temperature graph and the luteal phase defect. Fertil Steril 1983;40:466–468.
34. Ross GT, Cargille CM, Lipsett MB, et al. Pituitary and gonadal hormones in women during spontaneous and induced ovulatory cycles. Recent Prog Horm Res 1970;26:1–62.
35. Guida M, Tommaselli GA, Palomba S, et al. Efficacy of methods for determining ovulation in natural family planning program. Fertil Steril 1999;72:900–904.
36. Corson SL. Factors affecting donor artificial insemination success rates. Fertil Steril 1980;33:415–422.
37. Bradshaw KD, Guzick DS, Grun B, et al. Cumulative pregnancy rates for donor insemination according to ovulatory function and tubal status. Fertil Steril 1987;48:1051–1054.
38. Chauhan M, Barratt CLR, Cooke SMS, Cooke ID. Differences in the fertility of donor insemination recipients—a study to provide prognostic guidelines as to success and outcome. Fertil Steril 1989:51:815–819.
39. Lashen H, Afnan M, Kennefik A. Early resort to ovarian stimulation improves the cost-effectiveness of a donor insemination programme. Hum Reprod 1999;14:1983–1988.
40. Matorras R, Diaz T, Corcostegui B, et al. Ovarian stimulation in intrauterine insemination with donor sperm: a randomized study comparing clomiphene citrate in fixed protocol versus highly purified urinary FSH. Hum Reprod 2002;17:2107–2111.
41. Depypere HT, Gordts S, Campo R, Comhaire F. Methods to increase the success rate of artificial insemination with donor semen. Hum Reprod 1994;9:661–663.
42. Shenfield F, Doyle P, Valentine A, et al. Effects of age, gravidity and male infertility status on cumulative conception rates following artificial insemination with cryopreserved donor semen: analysis of 2998 cycles of treatment in one centre over 10 years. Hum Reprod 1993;8:60–64.
43. Human Fertilisation and Embryology Authority. The Publication of Centres' Success Rates for In Vitro Fertilization and Donor Insemination: Consultation document. Human Fertilisation and Embryology Authority, 1995.
44. Kovacs GT, Leeton JF, Matthews CD, et al. The outcome of artificial insemination compared to the husband's fertility status. Clin Reprod Fertil 1982;1:295–299.
45. Shapiro SS. Therapeutic donor insemination. In: Keye WR Jr, Chang RJ, Rebar RW, Soules MR, eds. Infertility Evaluation and Treatment. W.B. Saunders Company, Philadelphia, PA, 1995, pp. 712–728.

46. O'Brien P, Vandekerckhove P. Intra-uterine versus cervical insemination of donor sperm for subfertility. Cochrane Database Syst Rev 2003;1:CD000317.
47. Patton PE. Measurement of reproductive potential in the human female. In: Wolf DP, Zelinski-Woolen M, eds. Contemporary Endocrinology. Assisted Fertilization and Nuclear Transfer in Mammals. Humana Press, Totowa, NJ, 2001, pp. 81–93.
48. Schwartz D, Mayaux MJ. Female fecundity as a function of age: results of artificial insemination in 2193 nulliparous women with azoospermic husbands. Federation CECOS. N Engl J Med 1982;306:404–406.
49. Ferrara I, Balet R, Grudzinskas JG. Intrauterine insemination with frozen donor sperm. Pregnancy outcome in relation to age and ovarian stimulation regime. Hum Reprod 2002;17:2320–2324.
50. Navot D, Rosenwaks Z, Margalioth EJ. Prognostic assessment of female fecundity. Lancet 1987;2:645–647.
51. Lenton EA, Weston GA, Cooke ID. Problems in using basal body temperature recordings in infertility clinic. Br Med J 1977;1:803–805.
52. Templeton AA, Penney GC, Lees MM. Relation between the luteinizing hormone peak, the nadir of basal body temperature and the cervical mucus score. Br J Obstet Gynaecol 1982;89:985–988.
53. Barratt CLR, Cooke S, Chauhan M, Cooke ID. A prospective randomized controlled trial comparing urinary luteinizing hormone dipsticks and basal body temperature charts with time donor insemination. Fertil Steril 1989;52:394–397.
54. Federman CA, Dumesic DA, Boone WR, Shapiro SS. Relative efficiency of therapeutic donor insemination using a luteinizing hormone monitor. Fertil Steril 1990;54:489–492.
55. Odem RR, Durso NM, Long CA, et al. Therapeutic donor insemination: a prospective randomized study of scheduling methods. Fertil Steril 1991;55:976–982.
56. Pistorius LR, Kruger TF, de Villiers A, van der Merwe JP. A comparative study using prepared and unprepared frozen semen for donor insemination. Arch Androl 1996;36:81–86.
57. Vermesh M, Kletzky OA, Davajan V, Israel R. Monitoring techniques to predict and detect ovulation. Fertil Steril 1987;47:259–264.
58. Centola G, Mattox J, Raubertas R. Pregnancy rates after double versus single insemination with frozen semen. Fertil Steril 1990;54:1089–1092.
59. Le Lannou D, Gastard E, Guivarch A, et al. Strategies in frozen semen procreation. Hum Reprod 1995;10:1765–1774.
60. Lincoln SR, Long CA, Cowan BD. One artificial insemination per cycle with donor sperm is as efficacious as two inseminations. J Assist Reprod Genet 1995;12:67–69.

7 Ethical and Legal Considerations of Donor Insemination in the United States

Karen E. Adams MD, FACOG

Contents

INTRODUCTION

Donor insemination (DI) for humans was first reported in 1884, when not even the mother of the child conceived was informed that she had been inseminated with the sperm of another man *(1)*. In 1945, Mary Barton, a gynecologist, published an article in the *British Medical Journal* about her DI program that copied the already established veterinary practice in animal husbandry *(2)* and was met with outrage and widespread condemnation of the practice. In response to Barton's article, committees investigating DI generally recommended that it be considered a criminal offense *(3)*. Reasons for rejecting the procedure included religious concerns, fears of eugenic implications, and the association of DI with agriculture *(4)*. Sperm donors were viewed with suspicion, and the technique remained burdened in secrecy for four decades. It was not until the latter half of

From: *Contemporary Endocrinology: Office Andrology*
Edited by: P. E. Patton and D. E. Battaglia © Humana Press Inc., Totowa, NJ

the 20th century that a rapid growth occurred in the use of DI for family building *(5)*. By 1988, approx 80,000 women per year utilized DI, and more than 30,000 children were born each year in the United States *(6)*. Despite the widespread use of DI, the majority of adults and children conceived are unaware that the person they know as their father is not their genetic parent. Secrecy continues to surround the practice of DI.

SECRECY OR DISCLOSURE?

Despite increasing use by infertile couples, utilization of donor sperm is easy to hide. Because the child is usually the genetic product of the mother, it is possible to present the child to the world as the couple's biological child *(7)*. Using of donor sperm to achieve pregnancy can thus be easily disguised to preserve the appearance of a family created in the usual way *(8)*. For much of the 50 yr that DI has been a recognized medical procedure, physicians have supported and even encouraged secrecy. A 1992 bulletin from what was then called the American Fertility Society concluded: "Many physicians maintain that there is no reason for the child to know about the procedure" *(9)*. During these years, profound social forces influenced the couples' desire for secrecy, and the medical profession cooperated with this desire.

Most couples undergoing DI wanted to avoid stigma and appear as a "normal" family, stressing the social influences and minimizing the genetic reality *(10)*. Some men interpret infertility as a lack of virility or masculinity and are anxious to prevent friends and family members from gaining knowledge of their condition *(11)*. Keeping DI hidden therefore protected the feelings of the infertile husband. Also, couples often expressed concerns for the child. Fearing that the child would suffer taunts and isolation at school or grow up with a sense of uncertainty about his or her identity, parents commonly maintained secrecy to safeguard their child from the potential social ramifications of being conceived through DI. In addition, they feared the child's relationship with the social father would be undermined if the child knew that there was no genetic link with the husband *(12)*. Problems with legal paternity also contributed to the preference for privacy. For many years, DI was a practice that, although not unlawful, was carried out covertly. Both members of the couple were listed on the birth certificate, the husband of the woman receiving the treatment had no legal responsibility or duties toward the child. The husband was generally anxious to assume the parental role and create the image of a "normally" conceived family, but there were no statutes specifying him as the responsible party or relieving the donor of any responsibility in raising the child. In this context, donor anonymity could be seen as a necessary practice both to protect the donor from parental responsibility and allow the husband parental rights *(13)*. Faced with an inexpensive, simple, immediate, and successful "cure" for infertility, DI was seen by physicians as a straightforward and hopeful solution *(14)*. Multiple studies by physicians from 1956 to 1990 reported that DI reduced the stress of infertility, and couples were satisfied and well-adjusted after the birth of their child *(15–24)*. Yet, these studies were based on anecdotal reports, often from families requesting repeat insemination to attempt a second pregnancy. Most physicians treating infertility until the 1990s accepted that no sufficient data existed regarding how secrecy affected the families involved in DI. As Robert Nachtigall commented, "Until we have more specific and detailed information, we will have to trust the judgment of our patients about secrecy, just as we trust their ability to make other decisions about reproductive choice" *(25)*.

The debate regarding whether or not to disclose the genetic origin to a DI child has gained momentum in the past decade. Previously, there was little discussion about revealing the truth to family, friends, and most importantly, the child conceived; it was simply assumed that secrecy was best for all concerned. An increasing body of literature is now available to guide parents and DI programs in considering this issue. The debate regarding disclosure or nondisclosure originally derived from experience with adopted children, and it is useful to consider the similarities and differences between a situation in which a child is adopted into the family and a child conceived through DI. This chapter considers the similarities and differences between adoption and DI and also explores other issues related to the disclosure decision. Relevant issues in the debate include: the impact on family relationships and psychological adjustment of children both in disclosing and nondisclosing families; the potential for inadvertent disclosure by someone other than the parent with resulting psychological ramifications for the child; the availability of accurate genetic information for medical care of the conceived child and future offspring, and the issue of rights, including the right of all persons to know as much as possible about one's true origins. This chapter also presents the most current perspective of DI families: who is disclosing, who is not, and the reasons behind these decisions. Finally, the legal landscape regarding DI in the United States and other countries is considered, concluding with future directions for research and long-term recommendations for counseling couples who are considering DI as a means to build a family.

THE MODEL OF ADOPTIVE FAMILIES

Traditionally in adoption, parents had been counseled not to tell the child the truth of his or her genetic origin. Secrecy was believed to be in the best interests of the child. In writing of the nature of secrets, Karpel states that they involve information that is either withheld or differentially shared among persons *(26)*. Witholding a secret from someone represents power over that person and also a conflict of interest between two parties *(27,28)*. This conflict is managed by "information control"—the exchange of information. The challenges inherent in secrecy involve the control of information regarding the child's origins. Secrecy may be difficult to maintain: although it provides the appearance of avoiding any possible problems, it may actually become a difficult struggle for an impossible result *(29)*. For adoption, family therapists claim that openness and honesty are preferred, and basing family life on deception can cause stress and anxiety within the family *(30,31)*. When other individuals know the truth of the child's conception, there is great risk that the child will inadvertently discover the truth. Jennifer Spears states, "Social workers know very well that secrets are seldom kept, they arise for dubious reasons, and they store up trouble for the future. We know, because we get involved in helping sort out the resulting unhappiness, rage, and confusion" *(32)*. One physician/adoptee argues that after discovering such information, affected children may legitimately question what other secrets lie undiscovered and may regard their parents as adversaries instead of advocates. Their reality shaken, they may experience a sense of profound difference from peers whose biologic origins are clear *(29)*.

Nevertheless, for many years, privacy in adoptive families was the norm. It seemed unnecessary to complicate a child's life with such confusing and potentially unsettling information *(33)*. Secrecy was seen to be in the best interests of the child, to prevent the child from being stigmatized as unwanted or illegitimate and to ensure that the birth parent(s) would not interfere in the relationship between the child and adoptive family. The inadvertent result of such an approach was to convey attitudes of evasiveness, shame, and stigma about adoption *(34)*. Opinions toward secrecy have shifted, and most adoption agencies currently advise parents to disclose adoption, but some states still mandate sealed records *(35–39)*.

A similar shift is occurring for disclosure to children conceived using donor gametes. But, because the adopted child's search for identity is closely associated with feelings of abandonment *(40)*, the psychologic analogy between adoption and DI may be imprecise *(25)*. Donor offspring are seen to be more akin to a naturally conceived child than an adopted child, and correspondingly genetic unrelatedness has a different meaning for children conceived by gamete donation than for children in adoptive families *(41,42)*. For whatever reason, the adopted child was relinquished by his or her genetic parents and must psychologically confront this to understand the truth of his or her origins. The child born from the use of donor gametes would have to address different psychological issues, being created in the context of "donation" and a positive desire of the couple to raise the resulting offspring. Certainly, children by donor conception do not have to come to terms with their rejection by their birth parents *(43)*. The parents, too, particularly the mother of a child conceived by DI, may have much stronger feelings of a biological connection to a child she gestated and delivered than to a child carried by another. In his study of 86 women and 70 men who had conceived a child through DI, Robert Nachtigall found no evidence that DI parents identify with the adoption experience *(29)*. Because of the genetic relationship to one parent and control over the gestational environment, the recipient couple may feel that the donor gamete child is more "theirs" than an adopted child *(44)*. Nachtigall explains, "In contrast to the adoption model, which holds that children who are ignorant of their genetic heritage may have an incomplete sense of identity, the comments of donor insemination parents echo the tenets of 'attachment theory' *(29)*. This theory suggests that parental responsiveness, rather than biologic relatedness, is responsible for the quality of the child's attachment to the parent, which then fosters healthy social and emotional development" *(45)*.

PSYCHOLOGICAL ADJUSTMENT OF CHILDREN AND FAMILIES UTILIZING DONOR INSEMINATION

As late as 1993, reproductive endocrinologists and therapists lamented the paucity of information on the well-being of families created through DI, regardless of its widespread availability *(25)*. Although some social scientists speculated during 1980s and early 1990s about the long-term psychological consequences of DI on family functioning and child development, most attention was directed to the husband's infertility, which was seen as a potential source of serious distress in the family even after the birth of a child, instead of concern regarding the generally accepted practice of nondisclosure *(46–48)*. The generally accepted medical standard was to collaborate with the couple's desire to become a "normal" family, thereby allowing and even encouraging secrecy. But over time, criticism by psychologists, psychiatrists, social workers, and other therapists was directed at the practice of nondisclosure within families. They cautioned that secrecy about such essential items might negatively affect family relationships and undermine the relationship of trust between parents and children *(37,47,49–53)*.

A number of early studies addressed the characteristics of DI families through the use of anonymously written questionnaires *(19,54–57)*. In a large majority of cases, DI was believed to be a positive choice over adoption, and most fathers felt like "real fathers." Although the numbers of adults surveyed in this manner was quite large, the questionnaires were quite brief, and there were no control groups in any of the studies *(58)*. In a review of studies on parent–child relationships and child development in DI families, Brewaeys commented, "The rosy picture described above has been criticized by a number of researchers who reported the stress in DI couples after interviewing them. Stress was associated with coping, infertility, and the DI treatment itself. More particularly, patients cited the uncertainty and isolation resulting from the secrecy involved" *(58)*. However, most studies of this era demonstrated a consistent trend toward an average-to-high marital satisfaction and an average-to-low divorce rates in DI families *(15,19,54,57,59–61)*.

The earliest studies of child development and parent–child relationships in DI families were small and uncontrolled, but all demonstrated above-average intellectual, psychomotor, and language development in children conceived through DI *(15,20,55,56)*. One study did reveal that 14 of 53 DI children showed "hyperactive behavior" but gave no description of how that diagnosis was made *(20)*. In Brewaeys' review of six controlled studies of interpersonal relationships and child development in DI families, she found that DI parents showed a similar or higher quality of parent–child interaction when compared with control groups of naturally conceived families. DI mothers showed more emotional involvement toward their children than control mothers, and fathers did not differ in this respect from the controls *(58)*. One French study of 94 DI families with children between 3 mo and 3 yr old reported an "anxious overinvestment" in children by the parents and signs of increased emotional vulnerability, such as disturbed eating and sleeping patterns in the children *(62)*. However, this report was the exception to the norm that these parents and children appeared to be quite well-adjusted, at least by self-report—a possible source of bias in the studies. It is also important to recognize that these findings are preliminary owing to the young age of most of the children in the studies, with the oldest children being 8 yr old, too young for abstract thinking. It remains to be seen whether or not these children will have difficulties in adolescence and adulthood. In addition, response rates were low in most studies, raising the concern that families that were having problems did not participate *(58)*.

Two controlled studies evaluated family relationships and psychological adjustment of older children in DI families, including a follow-up report to Brewaeys' review, the European Study of Assisted Reproduction Families (The Netherlands, United Kingdom, Spain, and Italy) of children ages 11 to 12 *(63,64)*. In this study that compared a total of 94 DI families to 102 in vitro fertilization families, 102 adoptive families, and 102 natural conception families, there was no evidence of increased emotional or marital problems in the assisted reproduction (AR) couples as assessed by self-report measures of anxiety, depression, or marital state. The AR mothers did not differ from adoptive or natural conception mothers in expressed warmth, sensitivity toward the child, or affection, but the AR mothers did show greater emotional involvement with the child and a higher level of overprotective behavior. The AR fathers showed greater expressed warmth and emotional involvement than both the adoptive and natural conception fathers. There was also no difference in the frequency and severity of disputes between parents and children in any of the family types, and the children in AR families showed positive psychological adjustment with no signs of emotional or behavioral problems as assessed by mothers and teachers. Of interest, only 8 sets of parents (8.6%) told their child that he or she was conceived by DI. A total of 9 sets of parents (9.7%) planned to tell in the future, 11 (11.8%) were undecided, and 65 (69.9%) decided against telling the child. This study did not compare disclosure families to nondisclosure families in terms of the various outcome measures *(64)*.

The second controlled study on psychological adjustment and family functioning reported on 37 DI families, 49 adoptive families, and 91 families with a naturally conceived child (all from the United Kingdom) when the DI children were age 12. In this study, DI mothers showed higher levels of expressive warmth toward their children in comparison to the control groups. DI fathers were less likely to become involved in serious disputes with their children but showed the same level of expressive warmth as those in the adoptive families or naturally conceived families. The DI children did not show evidence of psychological difficulties. However, there was a lower-than-average separation rate for adoptive parents and a higher-than-average separation rate for DI parents. The adoption process differs from DI in that there is an intensive screening process for adoptive couples who are then expected to jointly commit to raising the child, compared with the role of the father in DI that is often marginalized, which the authors postulated may explain this finding. It is again striking that only 5% of the DI couples had revealed to the child the truth of his or her genetic origins *(65)*.

DISCLOSING VS NONDISCLOSING FAMILIES

The question of whether or not to tell children about their DI birth is one of the most important subjects in the DI literature. Most of what is known about disclosure within DI families is from recipients who used anonymous donors, and studies reveal considerable variation in the extent of actual or planned disclosure among families and across countries *(66)*. Brewaeys reviewed 23 studies between 1980 and 1995 and concluded that the vast majority of parents had not informed the child (range of 70–100%) and did not intend to do so in the future (range of 47–92%) *(67)*. Only 5% of couples told their 12-yr-old children about their true conception *(65)*, and only 8.6% had disclosed the child's origins in the four countries reported in the European Study of Assisted Reproduction Families, with an additional 9.7% planning to tell in the future *(64)*.

These high rates of nondisclosure in Europe may reflect the fact that relatively little information is available about the donor; thus, parents may wish to avoid disseminating incomplete knowledge to their children. In contrast, the United

States and New Zealand offer substantial information about the donor, particularly when open-identity donors are used. Counseling in DI programs is more oriented toward disclosure, with rates slightly higher in the United States than in Europe (20–30% with an additional 10–15% undecided) *(29,68,69)*. The results of a 1999 study from New Zealand were exceptional in that 30% of the parents had informed the child at a young age, and of the remaining parents, 77% intended to inform the child in the future. The authors explained: "The clinic offers counseling to all couples, and 94% of the study population took advantage of the opportunity to attend. At these sessions, counselors encouraged couples to disclose to children their conception circumstances and to do so at a young age." Of the 46 children in this study who had been told, 34 (74%) were age 3 or younger, 14 (30%) were less than 2, and 9 (20%) were talked to from birth *(70)*. Parents felt that they needed guidance, support, and an understanding of the possible consequences of disclosure, both to their children and to themselves. Nevertheless, the majority of parents in the study felt relieved that they had shared this information with their children.

Although only limited information about donors is available in Sweden, open-identity DI is legislated, and parents are counseled and expected to share conception information with children. In the first study that evaluated compliance with the law, Gottlieb and colleagues sent a questionnaire to all 194 couples who had conceived a child in Sweden via DI between 1985 and 1997. The response rate was 80%, and the mean age of the child was 3.5 yr. Of the couples who responded, 89% had not told their child, but about half of these indicated a plan to inform the child in the future *(71)*. This surprisingly low compliance is likely because open-identity is not voluntary and does not necessarily reflect the cultural acceptance of DI as a method of family creation *(66)*.

The focus of medical treatments and services for infertility has traditionally been on the infertile adult. The established approach in assisted reproduction technology is to favor anonymity of donors and to stress the confidentiality and privacy of the infertile adult patient *(72)*. However, more recently the focus has shifted to a consideration of the long-term outcome and consequences of these procedures on the children created and the adults they become, as well as future offspring. Although it has been argued that secrecy about the child's genetic origin would undermine family relationships, the evidence thus far points to the contrary. Studies in which family functioning is compared between DI and other families find that DI families generally have the same or more positive outcomes regarding children's psychological adjustment and familial relationships, despite the great majority of children who are uninformed about the circumstances of their conception *(64,65)*. To date, only one study has compared family characteristics between parents who had informed the child (30%) and those who had not (54%). In 94 families with adolescent children conceived through DI, no difference was found between the disclosers and nondisclosers regarding parental warmth, involvement, marital satisfaction, and marital intimacy. However, a negative relationship was found between the father's experienced stigma associated with infertility and his parental warmth and fostering of independence in his child, supporting the hypothesis that unresolved feelings about being infertile may affect the father–child relationship adversely *(29)*.

A subgroup of DI families worthy of noting is lesbian couples. When DI is the preferred method of conception, as it is among same-sex couples and single women, it is likely to result in higher disclosure rates. Among these types of families, disclosure or planned disclosure approaches 100% *(58,67,68,73)*. Because the couple will need to explain the absence of a father to the child, disclosure may come more naturally to lesbian couples, and they lack any concern of stigma that may be attached to male infertility *(66)*.

Several studies have examined disclosure and DI children's adjustment in lesbian families *(58,74,75)*. All have demonstrated excellent psychological health in the children and few behavioral problems up to age 17. In fact, lesbian mothers appear to show a higher quality of parent–child interaction when compared with two-parent heterosexual families, with no differences in the children's emotional or behavioral development *(58)*. One study showed that children in lesbian families experienced greater warmth and were more securely attached than heterosexual control group families. However, children from lesbian families were less self-confident than children from the control group, suggesting that the presence of a father might be important for the development of the child's self-esteem *(63)*. Regardless, children from lesbian families appear in all studies to be thriving, with nearly 100% knowledge of their genetic origins. When asked about the donor, about half of the children express interest and curiosity about "the man" or "unknown father" *(75)*. Because the majority of DIs come from anonymous donors, it is unlikely these children will gain significant information about the donor, and it remains to be seen whether this will impact their emotional and psychological well-being as they mature.

DIFFICULTIES WITH SECRECY: TRAUMATIC DISCLOSURE AND GENETIC INFORMATION

Evidence that secrecy does not seem to negatively impact family relationships suggests that the genetic tie between fathers and their children is less important for the development of a positive relationship than a strong desire for parenthood *(65)*. It is unclear, however, how the secrecy will affect the children in later adolescence and adulthood. In interviews with 23 couples regarding their perspective of infertility and the experience of undergoing DI, McWhinnie found that

> *"...secrecy is central to these families' functioning and their relationships with each other and with their wider family and friends...it emerged that the secrecy is maintained or 'managed' by denial of recourse to DI. DI is never talked of even between the parents in private conversations. Talking to the researcher was the first time it had been discussed since before the birth of the child"* (72).

McWhinnie poses the question: "But how easy or possible is it to maintain the secret in reality when the basic secret can be exposed by external events or comments, which to the parents can seem trivial?" She asserts that her study shows how daily events, such as questions the child brings home from school and the observations and comments from relatives (e.g., differences in eye color, height, aptitudes, and so on) can arise. Questions like "Whom does he/she look like?" or "Whom does he/she get that from?" are either evaded or answered obliquely. The dilemmas and evasions last a lifetime, into adulthood *(72)*.

Because of the extreme secrecy associated with DI, it is not possible to undertake a large study of adults conceived in this way. In a review of published material, three types of groups are apparent: (1) those who learned about their DI through a family disagreement, divorce, or from a step-parent; (2) those who were told by their parents because of some other event in the family, such as death or illness of the father; and (3) those who asked because something in the family relationships had puzzled them for years. Regardless of how the information was disclosed, the reported reaction was anger, resentment, and loss of a sense of self and identity *(72)*.

A study of 16 DI offspring recruited through DI support networks in the United Kingdom, United States, Canada, and Australia confirms the reaction of children who discover their DI origins as adults. Although this sample is biased toward those who sought out the services of support networks, the most significant factor was the withholding of information about their conception. All the participants reported feelings of mistrust within the family, poor self-perception, and feelings of frustration *(30)*.

Despite the fact that the majority of DI families maintain privacy, inadvertent disclosure is ever more likely given the growing role of genetics in medical diagnosis and treatment. More than 700 genetic tests are now available, and an increasing number of tests and an ever-more educated populace increase the risk that many children of DI will discover that they are not genetically related to their parents *(33)*. Thus, secrecy is difficult to maintain when 50% of the child's genetic and family history is unknown to the parents. Although parents have to lie or be evasive when confronted with questions from medical providers, they realize there could be circumstances in which they would need to disclose the truth of the child's genetic origins. Studies of adoptees and adult DI offspring show these revelations are traumatic and damaging to the self-image and identity

(30). It may not be possible for the DI child to obtain complete genetic information, but at the very least, knowledge of his or her origins is important *(33)*.

A recent event in The Netherlands underscores this concept. An apparently healthy sperm donor from 1982 to 1995 informed the hospital that he had recently been diagnosed with autosomal dominant cerebellar ataxia (ADCA), a severely debilitating neurological disease affecting 50% of offspring *(76)*. This disease remains latent for many years, and the donor had no family history of the disorder. His sperm had been used for the conception of 18 children in 13 women, all of who were eventually notified of the donor's diagnosis. In all donor gamete programs, a thorough family history is obtained, but it is possible in this case that the donor was not aware of the family history because of adoption or from the genetic mechanism known as "anticipation," whereby the age of symptom onset is earlier in successive generations, and, which is well-known in some ADCAs *(77)*. In Europe and the US programs, gamete donors are generally screened for common recessive conditions; yet, dominant conditions occurring in the absence of a family history are generally not. Therefore, it is of the utmost importance that careful records of donors and recipients be kept even if the donation is anonymous.

RIGHTS OF THE CHILD AND OTHER LEGAL AND POLICY ISSUES

Internationally, the vast majority of countries continue to endorse anonymous gamete donation *(41)*. However, in recent years there has been a trend toward open-identity DI *(78)*. This was legislated first in Sweden in 1985, with similar legislation following in Austria, Switzerland, the Australian state of Victoria, and most recently, The Netherlands *(66)*. In New Zealand, most programs have voluntarily switched to using exclusively open-identity donors despite the lack of legislation *(79)*. Central to this move toward nonanonymous donation is the right of the child to know his or her genetic origins *(41)*. Formal recognition of this right arises from the United Nations Convention on the Rights of the Child in 1989, which states in Article 7 "as far as possible the right to know. . .his or her parents" and in Article 8 "the rights of the child to preserve his or her identity" *(80)*. In the United States, open-identity DI increased with state statutes that protected the recipient's parental rights and clarified that the donor does not have any rights, obligations, or interest with respect to a conceived child, nor does the child have any rights, obligations, or interest with respect to the donor. Previous to the existence of such statutes, risks that the parental rights might be lost or shared with a donor were a significant barrier to the acceptance of open-identity inseminations. Lesbian couples were most likely to ask for open-identity DI, because they are most likely to disclose to the child his or her genetic origins, but only after the child reached age 18, when the child was no longer a legal dependent *(66)*.

The US standards put forth by the Ethical Considerations for Assisted Reproductive Technologies of the American Society for Reproductive Medicine are considered guidelines, and management of information regarding DI is not regulated by law. These guidelines require a genetic history as well as the provision for genetic tests to exclude potential donors with heritable diseases. In addition, the guidelines state that the genetic information collected without identifying information should be available on request to the infertile couple and the resulting child *(81)*. In states that do not provide DI children with a statutory right to genetic information, the child can sue to obtain that information. When such information is sought, most states permit disclosure under one of three conditions: if good cause is shown, the court determines the information is necessary, or the interested parties mutually consented to such disclosure *(82)*. However, from a practical standpoint, because state agencies are not involved in DI in the United States, it may be difficult to determine where the record is located. Because physicians attempt to protect the anonymity of donors, the record is unlikely to contain any identifying information that would allow the child, or even the physician providing the insemination, to recontact the donor for information *(82)*.

Issues like these have partly driven the US transition toward open-identity DI. The option was first created at The Sperm Bank of California (TSBC) in 1983 in response to recipients who wanted to be able to tell their children about their DI origins and donor identity when they reached age 18. This option was offspring-driven, with only the adult offspring being able to obtain identifying information. Although other programs in the United States offer such an option, the majority of programs are still completely anonymous. In 2003, TSBC undertook a survey of the offspring of lesbian, heterosexual, and single women who are now, on average, 14 yr old in preparation for the first planned release of donor identities from an American DI program when these children reach age 18 *(66)*. In this study, 93.3% had told the child the circumstances of his or her conception, with only three sets of parents who did not disclose. Two of the three planned disclosure at some point, and the third was undecided. Most disclosing parents (84.4%) felt that their child would try to contact the donor by letter, email, or phone. Parents knew or expected their child felt moderately positive toward the donor, but many (55.8%) reported that the child felt anxious about what the donor was like, whether he would be willing to meet, and whether he would like him or her. Parents usually thought the child's motivation was to learn more about the donor rather than looking for a parent, because they felt that it would help them learn more about themselves. Families in this study who used identity-release DI were positive overall regarding the decision and that their child had the option of identifying the donor at the age of legal majority.

In a 1997 survey of donors' attitudes with anonymity, Daniels and colleagues found that attitudes varied from country to country and even in clinics within the same country, and donors were almost evenly divided regarding sharing information with recipients *(83)*. Although donor characteristics and motivations have an impact on views regarding anonymity and tracing, results indicated that clinic policies and attitudes are likely to be highly influential. The authors suggested that official policies in countries where DI guidelines are legislated should reflect a less paternalistic approach, instead maximizing options for all the involved parties.

Some observers have advocated the establishment of a mandatory disclosure law, requiring that "by donation" be specified on birth certificates. Despite the fact that a policy of nonanonymous donation may help create a culture where more parents are able to tell their children the nature of their origins, it still does not guarantee that all children would receive such information *(7)*. Such a policy might decrease the pool of available donors or attract those who want to be abundantly involved in the child's life. A better choice would seem to be the existence of a "double-track" policy, which would allow participants to choose between an anonymous or open-identity program depending on their values and priorities *(78)*. Such a plan, though still leaving the disclosure decision to the parents, allows for the range of donor and recipient attitudes involved in DI. In the context of the humane practice of medicine, disclosure cannot be mandated. Such a mandate would represent an infringement on the intrinsic rights of the couple when no firm evidence of irreparable harm arising from nondisclosure exists *(43)*. However, educating recipient parents about the risks of nondisclosure, its consequences, and provision of sample "scripts" for disclosure should be mandatory. Disclosure does not end, but instead remains as an ongoing element within the parent–child relationship, and parents who choose this option need ongoing support. Upon entering a DI program, it is beneficial for potential parents to be aware of all relevant issues, which have been identified by earlier parents. Clinics should emphasize the importance of counseling and provide ongoing resources and support for parents following the birth of the child *(70)*.

CONCLUSIONS

Attitudes and practices regarding DI have changed dramatically in the past decade, despite the fact that the practice has been in existence for over a century. DI has traditionally been cloaked in secrecy, with parental rights of privacy, autonomy, and self-determination considered paramount. Additionally, secrecy was considered to be in the child's best interests, protecting him or her from the potential negative effects of such unsettling and confusing information. Only recently has emphasis shifted away from privacy concerns and toward the rights of the child. With the 1989 United Nations Convention on the Rights of the Child confirming each child's right to know their parents and understand their identity, some countries have begun to legislate open-identity donors. Data from DI families in these countries indicate poor compliance with the laws, largely because decision making regarding disclosure is viewed as a personal and individual decision of the parents. DI families who did not disclose are not suffering because of this decision, and function as well, if not better, than control families in terms of emotional and behavioral adjustment. Open-identity DI in the United States has grown as state statutes clarified the husband's role and limited the donor's rights and obligations. In centers in which open-identity DI is an option (but not required) recipients report great satisfaction with their choice and a generally positive response from the children. As DI households vary in their preference of disclosure or nondisclosure, donors similarly vary in their decision for anonymity or allowance to be traced.

As the debate surrounding secrecy and openness in DI expands, it seems clear that the best outcomes occur when donors and recipients are carefully counseled regarding anonymity and open-identity options and choosing what most closely seems to fit their needs. Genetic information regarding donors is critical and must be made available to parents and offspring, the child conceived will never know if the parents choose not to disclose, leaving parents in the ultimate position in having control of information. Nevertheless, it is the responsibility of DI programs to maintain those records in preparation for a potential request, and donors must be informed that such release may occur without identifying information attached. Release of further details about the donor should be left to the discretion of the parties involved, and mandatory disclosure should not be legislated. Those entering a DI program should be informed about the risks of nondisclosure and its consequences, provided with information and scripts regarding ways to inform their offspring of their genetic origins, and encouraged to make their own choice of anonymous or nonanonymous donation. DI programs should make such support available to all potential parents, and this support should continue after the child's birth.

This chapter has demonstrated the need for well-controlled studies to replace biases and supposition with data of outcomes of DI families. Research already established on DI families that continues as the children age will be an invaluable source of information about family functioning and the child's, then adult's and ultimately future generations' health and psychological adjustment.

REFERENCES

1. Achilles R. Donor Insemination: An Overview. Royal Commission on New Reproductive Technologies, Ontario, 1992, p. 8.

2. Barton M, Walker K, Wiesner B. Artificial insemination. Brit Med J 1945;13:40–43.
3. Frith L. Gamete donation and anonymity: the ethical and legal debate. Hum Reprod 2001;16: 818–824.
4. Pfeffer N. Artificial insemination, in-vitro fertilization and the stigma of infertility. In: Stanworth M, ed. Reproductive Technologies: Gender, Motherhood, and Medicine. Cambridge: Polity Press; 1987:81–97.
5. Johnston I. The donor. In: Wood C, Leeton J, Kovacs G, eds. Artificial Insemination by Donor. Brown Prior Anderson, Melbourne, 1980, pp. 10–17.
6. Office of Technology Assessment. Infertility: Medical and Social Choices. United States Congress, Washington, DC, 1988.
7. Cook R, Golombok S, Bish A, et al. Disclosure of donor insemination: parental attitudes. Am J Orthopsychiatr 1995;65:549–559.
8. Haimes E. Do clinicians benefit from gamete donor anonymity? Hum Reprod 1993:9:1518–1520.
9. The American Fertility Society. Therapeutic donor insemination: a guide for patients. The American Fertility Society, Birmingham, 1992; patient information series.
10. Snowden R, Mitchell GD, Snowden EM. Stigma and stress in AID. In: Artificial Reproduction: A Social Investigation. George Allen and Unwin, London, 1983, pp. 125–143.
11. Herz EK. Infertility and bioethical issues of the new reproductive technologies. Psychiatr Clin North Am 1989;12:117–131.
12. Schover LR, Collins RL, Richards S. Psychological aspects of donor insemination: evaluation and follow-up of recipient couples. Feril Steril 1992;57:583–590.
13. Dewar J. Fathers in law? The case of AID. In: Morgan D, Lee R, eds. Birthrights. Routledge: London, 1989;115–131.
14. Nijs P, Rouffa L. AID couples: psychological and psychopathological evaluation. Andrologia 1975;7:187–194.
15. Amuzu B, Laxova R, Shapiro SS. Pregnancy outcome, health of children, and family adjustment after donor insemination. Obstet Gynecol 1190;75:899–905.
16. Haman J. Therapeutic donor insemination: a review of 440 cases. Cal Med 1959;90:130–133.
17. Czyba JC, Chevert M. Psychological reactions of couples to artificial insemination with donor sperm. Int J Fertil 1979;24:240–245.
18. Portnoy L. Artificial insemination. Fertil Steril 1956;7:327–340.
19. Levie L. An inquiry into the psychological effects on parents of artificial insemination with donor sperm. Eugenics Rev 1967;24:240–245.
20. Clayton C, Kovacs G. AID offspring: initial follow-up study of 50 couples. Med J Aust 1982; 1:338,339.
21. Guttmacher AF. Role of artificial insemination in the treatment of sterility. Obstet Gynecol Surv 1960;15:767–785.
22. Kraus J, Quinn PE. Human artificial insemination—some social and legal issues. Med J Aust 1977;1:710–713.
23. Jackson MH. Artificial insemination (donor). Eugenics Rev 1957;48:205–209.
24. Warner MP. Artificial insemination review after thirty-two years experience. NY State J Med 1974;74:2358–2361.
25. Nachtigall RD. Secrecy: an unresolved issue in the practice of donor insemination. Am J Obstet Gynecol 1993;168:1846–1851.
26. Karpel MA. Family secrets: 1. Conceptual and ethical issues in the relational context. 2. Ethical and practical considerations in therapeutic management. Fam Process 1980;19:295–306.

27. Lauritzen P. DI's dirty little secret. Politics Life Sci 1993;12:188,189.
28. Tefft SK. Secrecy: a cross-cultural perspective. Human Science Press, New York, 1980, p. 69.
29. Nachtigall RD, Becker G, Quiroga SS et al. The disclosure decision: concerns and issues of parents of children conceived through donor insemination. Am J Obstet Gynecol 1998;178: 1165–1170.
30. Turner A, Coyle A. What does it mean to be a donor offspring? The identity experiences of adults conceived by donor insemination and the implications for counseling and therapy. Hum Reprod 2000;15:2041–2051.
31. Snowden R, Snowden E. The gift of a child: a guide to donor insemination. University of Exeter Press, Exeter, 1993, p. 141.
32. Spiers J. Children's rights to know their identity: social work perspective. In: Bruce N, Mitchel A, Priestley K, eds. Truth and the child: a contribution to the debate on the Warnock report. Family Care, Edinburgh, 1988, p. 37.
33. McGee G, Brakman S, Gurmankin A. Gamete disclosure and anonymity: disclosure to children conceived with donor gametes should not be optional. Hum Reprod 2001;16:2033–2038.
34. Sokoloff BZ. Alternative methods of reproduction: effects on the child. Clin Pediatr 1987; 26:11–17.
35. Brandon J, Warner J. AID and adoption: some comparisons. Brit J Soc Work 1977;7:338–340.
36. Pannor R, Baran A. Open adoption as a standard practice. Child Welfare League of America 1984;63:245–250.
37. Haimes E. Secrecy: what can artificial reproduction learn from adoption? Int J Law and the Family 1998;2:46–61.
38. Lamport A. The genetics of secrecy in adoption, artificial insemination, and in vitro fertilization. Am J Law Med 1988;14:109–124.
39. MacIntyre J. Resolved: children should be told of their adoption before they ask. J Am Acad Child Adolesc Psych 1990;29:828,829.
40. Berger D. Psychological aspects of donor insemination. Int J Psychiatry Med 1982;12:49–57.
41. Frith L. Beneath the rhetoric: the role of rights in the practice of non-anonymous gamete donation. Bioethics 2001;15:473–484.
42. Golombok S. New families, old values: considering the welfare of the child. Hum Reprod 1998;9:2342–2347.
43. Patrizio P, Mastroianni A, Mastroianni L. Gamete donation and anonymity: disclosure to children conceived with donor gametes should be optional. Hum Reprod 2001;16:2036–2038.
44. Klock SC. The controversy surrounding privacy or disclosure among donor gamete recipients. J Assist Reprod Genet 1997;14:378–380.
45. Main M, Kaplan N, Cassisy J. Security in infancy, childhood, and adulthood. Monogr Soc Res Child Dev 1985;50:233–256.
46. Berger D. Couples' reactions to male infertility and donor insemination. Am J Psychiat 1980;137:1047–1049.
47. Clamar AJ. Psychological implications of the anonymous pregnancy. In: Offerman-Zuckenberg J, ed. Families in Transition: A New Frontier. Plenum Press, New York, 1989, pp. 111–120.
48. Connolly K, Edelman R, Cooke I, et al. The impact of infertility on psychological functioning. J Psychosom Res 1992;36:459–468.
49. Baran A, Pannor B. Lethal Secrets: The Psychology of Donor Insemination, Problem and Solution. Amistead Press, New York, 1993, p. 158.
50. Daniels K, Taylor K. Secrecy and openness in donor insemination. Politics Life Sci 1993; 12:155–170.

51. Imber-Black E. Secrets in family and family therapy: an overview. In: Imber-Black E, ed. Secrets in Family and Family Therapy. W.W. Norton: New York, 1993, pp. 5–16.
52. Adair V, Purdie A. Donor insemination programs with personal donors: issues of secrecy. Hum Reprod 1996;11:2558–2563.
53. Bruce N. On the importance of genetic knowledge. Childr Soc 1990;4:183–186.
54. Rosenqvist H. Donor insemination: a prospective socio-psychiatric investigation of 48 couples. Dan Med Bull 1981;28:133–148.
55. Leeton J, Blackwell J. A preliminary psycho-social follow-up of parents and their children conceived by AID. Clin Reprod Fertil 1982;1:307–310.
56. Milson I, Bergman P. A study of parental attitudes after donor insemination. Acta Obstet Gynecol Scand 1982;61:125–128.
57. Kremer J, Frijling B, Nass J. Psychosocial aspects of parenthood by AI. Lancet 1984;i:628.
58. Brewaeys A. Review: parent-child relationships and child development in donor insemination families. Hum Reprod 2001;7:38–46.
59. Humphrey M, Humphrey H. Marital relationships in couples seeking donor insemination. J Biosoc Sci 1987;19:209–219.
60. Kloch S, Maier D. Psychological factors related to donor insemination. Fertil Steril 1991; 56:489–495.
61. Kloch S, Jacob M, Maier D. A prospective study of donor insemination recipients: secrecy, privacy, and disclosure. Fertil Steril 1994;62:477–484.
62. Manuel C, Facy F, Choquet M, et al. Les risques psychologiques de la conception par IAD pour l'enfant. Neuropsychiatrie de l'enfance 1990;38:642–658.
63. Golombok S, Brewaeys A, Cook R, et al. The European study of assisted reproduction families: family functioning and child development. Hum Reprod 1996;11:2324–2331.
64. Golombok S, Brewaeys A, Giavazzi MT, et al. The European study of assisted reproduction families: the transition to adolescence. Hum Reprod 2002:17;830–840.
65. Golombok S, MacCallum F, Goodman E, et al. Families with children conceived by donor insemination: a follow-up at age twelve. Child Dev 2002:73;952–968.
66. Scheib HE, Riordan M, Rubin S. Choosing identity-release sperm donors: the parents' perspective 13-18 years later. Hum Reprod 2003:18;1115–1127.
67. Brewaeys A. Review: donor insemination, the impact on child and family development. J Psychosom Obstet Gynecol 1996:17;1–17.
68. Klock S, Jacob M, Maier D. A comparison of single and married recipients of donor insemination. Hum Reprod 1996;11:2554–2557.
69. Leblum SR, Aviv AL. Disclosure issues and decisions of couples who conceived via donor insemination. J Psychosom Obstet Gynecol 1997;18:292–300.
70. Rumball A, Adair V. Telling the story: parents' scripts for donor offspring. Hum Reprod 1999; 14:1392–1399.
71. Gottlieb C, Lalos O, Lindblad F. Disclosure of donor insemination to the child: the impact of Swedish legislation on couples' attitudes. Hum Reprod 2000;15:52–56.
72. McWhinnie A. Gamete donation and anonymity: should offspring from donated gametes continue to be denied knowledge of their origins and antecedents? Hum Reprod 2001;16: 807–817.
73. Leiblum SR, Palmer MG, Spector IP. Non-traditional mothers: single heterosexual/lesbian women and lesbian couples electing motherhood via donor insemination. J Psychosom Obstet Gynecol 1995;16:11–20.
74. Chan R, Raboy B, Patterson C. Psychosocial adjustment among children conceived via donor insemination by lesbian and heterosexual mothers. Child Dev 1998;69:443–457.

75. Vanfraussen K, Ponjaert-Kristoffersen I, Brewaeys A. An attempt to reconstruct children's donor concept: a comparison between children's and lebian parents' attitudes towards donor anonymity. Hum Reprod 2001;16:2019–2025.
76. Gebhardt D. Sperm donor suffers years later from inherited disease. J Med Ethics 2002;28:213.
77. Delatycki M. Sperm donor suffers years later from inherited disease: commentary. J Med Ethics 2002;28:214.
78. Pennings G. The double track policy for donor anonymity. Hum Reprod 1997;12:2839–2844.
79. Daniels KR, Lewis GM. Openness of information in the use of donor gametes: developments in New Zealand. J Reprod Infant Psychol 1996;14:57–68.
80. United Nations Convention on the Rights of the Child. Geneva, 1989.
81. The American Society for Reproductive Medicine. Ethical Considerations for Assisted Reproductive Technology. Available at www.asrm.org. Accessed October 22, 2003.
82. Andrews L, Elster N. Adoption, reproductive technologies, and genetic information. J Law Med 1998;8:1–20.
83. Daniels KR, Lewis GM, Curson R. Information sharing in semen donation: the views of donors. Soc Sci Med 1997;44:673–680.

8 Laboratory Accreditation

William Byrd, PhD, HCLD

Contents

INTRODUCTION

Regarding health, each person should receive the highest quality of laboratory service and test results. Thoughts differ on how this is best accomplished. Over the years, laboratory professionals have argued that they understand quality and can best provide it by establishing their own laboratory standards. Indeed, the first group that approached the issue of quality in the laboratory was pathologists. Voluntary, nongovernmental clinical laboratory accreditation in the United States predates any federal government attempt at quality regulation. Proficiency testing (PT) was the first attempt at improving the quality of laboratory results. This is merely a quality control device that relies on an unknown analyte to be tested that is provided by an outside source. When a laboratory participates in a PT, unknown specimens are tested the same as patient samples are. These results would then be reviewed by the outside agency to determine the accuracy of the test results as compared to other laboratories. The first PT program began in 1946 as a regional program in Philadelphia *(1,2)*. After this initial event, the College of American Pathologists (CAP) offered PT surveys beginning in 1947. Accord-

From: *Contemporary Endocrinology: Office Andrology*
Edited by: P. E. Patton and D. E. Battaglia © Humana Press Inc., Totowa, NJ

ing to Sunderman *(2)*, the results were not released perhaps because of the variability in test results. Recognizing the inherent variability in laboratory testing, many wanted to improve their performance. It was recognized that the best mechanism to reach this goal was through the use of professional groups. Some of the earliest standards for laboratories were proposed by the CAP shortly after World War II *(3)*. In this early effort, CAP first proposed the concept of evaluating laboratories with the use of laboratory standards, PT, and the physical on-site accreditation of laboratories. This voluntary accreditation program was initiated in 1961; the first laboratory inspection/accreditation occurred in January 1964. This program has grown from an initial group of 200 laboratories to more than 6000 laboratories worldwide *(4)*. A key component of the CAP inspection is that professional peers—not paid inspectors—conduct the inspections.

Since this early attempt by the CAP, the Joint Commission Accreditation Health Care Organizations (JCAHO) has developed a program for accrediting laboratories. Although JCAHO usually inspects hospitals, it does have a laboratory component. In 1979, JCAHO officially recognized CAP accreditation and indicated that it would no longer inspect CAP accredited laboratories in JCAHO-accredited facilities. JACHO does not have its own PT program. Laboritories that are in JCAHO must subscribe to another PT program. Smaller andrology laboratories may choose to become accredited by the Commission on Laboratory Accreditation (COLA). This nonprofit organization is an accrediting organization for physician office laboratories. COLA was initially developed by the American Academy of Family Physicians, American Medical Association, American Society of Internal Medicine, and College of American Pathologists. The COLA program promotes education for the physician and office staff through its self-assessment process, written materials, and on-site surveys. The program was modified so that it could be by approved by Health Care Financing Administration (HCFA) for Clinical Laboratory Improvement Amendment (CLIA) certification.

Based on some rather outdated information on the quality of laboratory testing, the Congress decided in the 1960s that it was time to legislate laboratories, despite considerable opposition from laboratory professionals *(3)*. Through an act of Congress, the HCFA, which is now termed the Centers for Medicare and Medicaid Services (CMS), was the governmental agency that first regulated clinical laboratories through the CLIA of 1967 *(5)*. This act was limited in that it only applied only to laboratories engaged in interstate commerce, and many laboratories were not covered by this act. In the 1980s, following reports like those reported by the *Wall Street Journal (6–8)* about the quality of Pap smears and other tests, Congress passed the CLIA of 1988 (CLIA 88), which covered all laboratories providing clinical testing *(9)*. The CLIA 88 regulations (the final rules were implemented in 1992) regulated testing in all laboratory settings, including physician office laboratories. CLIA identified three different levels of testing based on the complexity of the test and its risk of harm to patients if not properly done. Laboratories performing only waived tests could receive a certificate of waiver and are not subject to routine testing or inspection. Laboratories using moderate-to-high complexity testing are subject to inspection to ensure they are meeting standards. All sites must pay a fee based on the level of testing. The influence of this latest amendment on the practice of medicine was significant. More than 64% of physicians surveyed in a 1995 study said that they either reduced or eliminated in-office testing in response to CLIA 88 *(10)*. Particularly influenced were pediatric and rural practices in which 70% of practices reduced or eliminated on-site testing.

RECENT REGULATIONS, RULES, AND PROPOSED RULES BY THE FOURTH BRANCH OF GOVERNMENT THAT AFFECT SOME ANDROLOGY LABORATORIES

Many cellular and tissue products are regulated by the Food and Drug Administration (FDA) under the auspices of the Public Health Service Act and the Federal Food, Drug, and Cosmetic Act. Because many andrology laboratories process semen for insemination, cryopreserve it for future use, or cryopreserve donor sperm, they fall under this authority. Most human tissues are regulated under the FDA's authority to prevent the transmission of communicable disease. In 1993, the FDA announced interim regulations that affected both andrology laboratories and tissue banks in the United States (21 CFR Part 1270). These rules stated that sperm and tissue banks perform serological tests for donors of tissue or cells for evidence of relevant communicable disease agents and diseases. This would require tissue banks and those facilities providing donor sperm to screen donors for viruses, such as hepatitis and human immunodeficiency disease. This rule authorized the FDA to inspect facilities that recovered, processed, or distributed tissues for transplant. The importation of tissues from outside the United States was prohibited unless the facility met the new FDA rules. The final rules were published in the Federal Register on July 29, 1997.

Since then, the FDA has proposed three regulations governing human cells, tissues, and tissue-based products: (1) Human Cells, Tissues and Cellular and Tissue-Based Products (HCT/Ps); Establishment and Registration and Listing *(11)*; (2) Suitability Determination for Donors of Human Cellular and Tissue Based Products *(12)*; and (3) Current Good Tissue Practice for Manufacturers of Human Cellular and Tissue-Based Products, Inspection and Enforcement *(13)*.

The first rule established a registration and listing system for all facilities or labs that manufacture HCT/Ps. The final regulation was published in January 2001 *(11)*, to become effective January 2003 for an estimated 400 assisted reproductive technology (ART) facilities with approx 110 sperm banks that could be affected *(14)*. Semen is considered to be an example of these HCT/Ps (21 CFR 1271.3 (d) *(2)*. There are exemptions from this registration. The use of HCT/Ps for nonclinical or educational uses is exempted. Laboratories that only recover reproductive cells or tissues for transfer into a sexually intimate partner of the cell or tissue donor are also exempted. Facilities that receive or store HCT/Ps, e.g., donor semen for the purpose of transplantation, implantation, or transfer, are exempted as well. Based on 21 CFR 1271.15 (e), all intrauterine insemination (IUI) and intracervical insemination (ICI) would be exempted along with in vitro fertilization (IVF) as long as they are done with cells or tissues from sexually intimate partners.

The initial registration for facilities with nonexempted sperm use is by April 2003. This can be done using form 3356 or a Web-based submission that is still in development at the time of this writing. Questions and answers about this form are available at http://www.fda.gov/cber/tissue/docs.htm. A list of establishments publicly available can be found at http://www.fda.gov/cber/tissue/hctregestabl.htm. The majority of establishments registered at this time are predominately tissue banks.

The second proposed rule establishes the screening and testing requirements for donors of reproductive tissue *(12)*. In this document, the FDA proposes to require that donors of cells and tissues be screened and tested for communicable diseases. An earlier interim rule was established in 1993 that covered some of these issues. When part 1270 was issued, the FDA was concerned and wanted to counteract the transmission of HIV and hepatitis B and C. This current proposed regulation is a more extensive coverage. The proposed regulations would increase the number of products covered and the amount of screening. The proposed regulation would test for all "relevant" diseases. Examples of such diseases are syphilis and spongiform encephalopathy, including Creutzfeldt-Jakob disease. Donors of reproductive cells or tissues would be tested for *Neisseria gonorrhea* and *Chlamydia trachomatis*. One issue to be resolved is if oocyte and embryo quarantine is going to be required. Sexually intimate couples will not be required to be screened or tested. Another issue is the requirement (1271.80 [b]) that oocyte donors be tested within 7 d of tissue recovery.

The third proposed regulation on good tissue practice (GTP) is intended to ensure that donors of human cellular and tissue-based products are free of communicable diseases *(13)*. During the "manufacturing" process, it aims to ensure cells and tissues are not contaminated and maintain their integrity and function. The key elements of this proposed regulation are: (1) establishment of a quality control (QC) program and recordkeeping; (2) establishment of standard operating procedures; (3) maintenance of facilities and an organizational structure to do the work; (4) appropriate storage for tissues; (5) maintenance of a complaint file; and (6) procedures for tracking the product from donor to recipient. The proposed regulations refer to all human cells and tissues as "products." Personnel who process, package, store, or handle products are termed "manufacturers."

The ASRM in a meeting with the FDA raised several potential issues concerning this third proposed rule *(15)*. First, the ASRM made the point that reproductive medicine is unique, and provisions of this proposed regulation may not apply. The ASRM requested some flexibility in this area related to reproductive practices. The ASRM expressed some concern regarding the retention, recall, and destruction pertaining to embryos, expressing that the patients "owned" the embryos, not the clinics. When there is potential contamination of embryos in storage, the clinics can only recommend disposal. There was also some concern about validation of processes. The ASRM pointed out that the use of embryos to validate a procedure is generally not acceptable. The FDA indicated that validation should apply to the procedures used in cryopreservation (as an example). The ASRM also questioned how adverse reactions would apply to reproductive tissues. For instance, would oocytes that did not fertilize constitute an adverse reaction? The FDA has stated that they would look into these issues.

OCCUPATIONAL SAFETY AND HEALTH ADMINISTRATION

The Occupational Safety and Health Administration (OSHA) implemented rules in 1992 (CFR 29:1910.1030; Bloodborne Pathogens) that were to protect health care workers from bloodborne pathogens. This applies to all occupational exposure to blood or other infectious materials. Employers have to set up a control plan with universal precautions to reduce or eliminate the possibility of contamination. This plan includes the use of handwashing, protective equipment (masks and gloves), banning food and drink in the laboratory, disposal of sharps, and so on. As part of training and orientation, employees must be taught in the use of protective equipment and handling hazardous waste materials. Employers must make available hepatitis B vaccination to all employees at no cost to the employee. Vaccination is important because health care workers are at substantial risk of hepatitis B infection. About 1% of health care workers in a hospital setting are positive for hepatitis B surface antigen *(16)*. The long-term risks of hepatitis B infection in workers with blood contact is between 15 and 30% *(17)*.

Further governmental regulations that affect andrology laboratories can be foreseen. The advent of any new communicable disease or virus is bound to attract the attention of regulatory agencies. The latest example is the workshop on donor screening for the West Nile Virus *(18)*, which is a virus that currently does not have a screening assay available. Preliminary recommendations would be that a donor should not be used until 14 d after the condition is considered to be resolved and at least 28 d from the onset of symptoms.

HEALTH INSURANCE PORTABILITY AND ACCOUNTABILITY ACT PRIVACY RULE

The Health Insurance Portability and Accountability Act of 1996 (HIPAA) creates a new set of privacy rules for the protection of patient health information. Although not all health information needs to be protected, most patient health information should be considered as Protected Health Information (PHI) and is accountable to HIPAA requirements.

Health care facilities must be in compliance with these regulations by April 14, 2003. Any laboratory inspected by an accrediting agency is required to have an agreement with the accrediting agency that protects the privacy and security of patient health information. The CAP is developing a model agreement to be used to meet HIPAA and will be posted on the CAP website.

BECOMING ACCREDITED

All US laboratories are subject to federal licensure under CLIA 88. In addition, there may be state licensure requirements, such as in California, Florida, and Tennessee. Semen analysis is considered to be a high-complexity test. Because of this, the laboratory director must meet stringent requirements. All doctors who direct laboratories must be licensed to practice in the state where the laboratory is located. Foreign doctors not licensed to practice cannot direct laboratories. Individuals with an MD must also be board-certified in anatomical or clinical pathology or have at least 1 yr of laboratory training during residency or have at least 2 yr experience supervising or directing a laboratory. An MD or DO degree cannot be considered to be an earned doctoral degree according to CMS. In CLIA 88, any doctoral laboratory director had to be board-certified. In practice, this particular requirement was moved to a future date several times by the CMS. A grandfather clause that affects directors with doctoral degrees has come from the CMS. After February 24, 2003, all directors of high-complexity laboratories with earned doctoral degrees will have to be board-certified. However, individuals with a doctoral degree with at least 4 yr of experience and at least 2 yr supervising or directing prior to February 24, 2003 do not have to be board-certified. Board certification must come from an organization recognized by CLIA 88, e.g., American Association of Bioanalysis, American Board of Medical Microbiology, American Board of Clinical Chemistry, American Board of Medical Laboratory Immunology, American Board of Medical Genetics, or American Board of Histocompatibility and Immunogenetics. The American Board of Bioanalysis is the only board that offers certification in andrology.

ISSUES COMMON TO ALL LABORATORIES

1. Each laboratory must have a program in place to evaluate the quality of its patient care services, using a method to identify problems, and ensure the program is implemented throughout. The laboratory must be able to evaluate the effectiveness of its policies and procedures. It is important to realize that the laboratory is responsible for the preanalytical, analytical, and postanalytical phases of testing. Indeed, of the errors that occur in analytical testing, only about 7% occur in the analytical stage of the procedure *(19)*. Simply put, this is the quality assurance plan.
   a. During the preanalytical phase, the physician should select the tests to be performed. All test specimens must be accompanied by a written requisition, which should be provided to the patient to explain how to collect a specimen or an ejaculate. There must be a chain of custody established to identify the specimen and the person handling or analyzing the specimen. The specimen needs to be delivered to the laboratory in a timely fashion for analysis.
   b. During the analytical phase, the specimen is prepared and analyzed.
   c. In the postanalytical phase, accurate results for the correct patient are reported. Interpretative analysis is provided so that the physician may read the report. The laboratory is responsible for the turnaround time of the specimen. There must be an ongoing procedure to determine if any errors have occurred during the reporting of results.
2. The laboratory must use a QC program to evaluate the performance of the laboratory. This is a surveillance system in which people, assays, and equipment are monitored in a systematic fashion and provides a record of the consistency of results. Pre-existing benchmarks or standards must exist in the laboratory, and when the limits for QC are beyond tolerance, corrective action must be taken. Examples of internal QC would be control samples run with endocrine assay, maintenance checks of machinery, determination of sperm count using known concentrations of beads, or calibration checks of machinery to ensure they are running properly. Most of the QC programs are centered on the training of the technical staff that perform the various tests. It is particularly important in the andrology laboratory for training to be thorough and ongoing because with any living, biological material, there is no immediate QC mechanism in place. Variation exists between technicians and among laboratories. Efforts must be made to reduce variation within the laboratory. The use of external PT provides the laboratory with an idea of how its' assays compare to other laboratories. But even here, evidence suggests that there is a lack of standardization in semen analysis in US laboratories and abroad *(20,21)*.

3. A general safety program and safety training must be included in the laboratory.
4. Procedures should be in place in cases of emergencies.
5. The laboratory should have rules for all required maintenance and the frequency of maintenance.
6. Complete procedure manuals must exist that cover all aspects of specimen acquisition, testing, and reporting.
7. Participation in an approved PT program is essential.

Why are these issues important? A good example is a report by Hurst et al. *(22)* in which they compared Physician Office Labs (POLs) to larger accredited laboratories. When they compared the PT data, the failure rate for POLs was three times higher than non-POLs (21.5 vs 8.1%). Stull et al. *(23)* also found that hospital and independent laboratories scored higher than other testing sites when they reviewed PT performance. This difference could be owing to several factors. One factor is probably a reflection of the training of laboratory professionals in the non-POL group. Ultimately, it is the responsibility of the laboratory director to recognize and minimize errors and increase the accuracy and reliability of the tests offered.

Yet, analytical testing only covers one area. The pre- and postanalytical handling of specimens is also important. In a study of one hospital's quality assurance program, Ross and Boone *(24)* indicated that 90% of the reported errors occurred before or after the actual analytical test. Nutting et al. *(25)* found similar evidence when looking at office-based, primary care practices, with more than 93% of laboratory errors during the pre- and postanalytical phases. Notably, PT does not measure either pre- or postanalytical errors. PT is a limited measure of daily function sample analysis, and the true relationship between PT and overall laboratory performance is unknown *(26)*. Indeed, many authors have suggested that PT specimens receive "special" handling owing to the pressure to report correct results *(27–29)*. Special handling may involve multiple assays of the same analyte, exchanging data with other laboratories, or use of another method to analyze the specimen. Other techniques to improve PT testing include using the most qualified technician to run the results or running the test sample immediately after controls to improve performance *(26)*. Simply, the only laboratories to be identified by PT as substandard are those with sustained systematic error, which is indicated by sustained unsatisfactory PT results.

The real question is if the analytical performance of the laboratory falls within the clinically useful results. The CAP quality assurance program demonstrated that about 96% of all results fell within medically useful limits *(26)*. In some cases, the accuracy and precision needed for a clinical assay may not be reflected in the PT results.

HOW TO PREPARE LABORATORIES FOR INSPECTION

The model developed by the CAP is used because their accredited laboratories must meet or exceed the requirements of CLIA 88, and the majority of andrology laboratories are accredited by the CAP. A participating laboratory is expected to be in compliance with the *Standards for Laboratory Accreditation*. The are four standards that specify: (1) qualifications of the director; (2) physical facility and safety; (3) quality control and performance improvement; and (4) inspection. To determine if the laboratory meets the standards, an inspection is conducted using checklists. The CAP has 21 checklists that cover different laboratory subspecialties. An andrology laboratory that also performs endocrine testing would be inspected with the General checklist (1), the Reproductive checklist (90), and part of the Special Chemistry checklist. The General checklist covers the responsibilities of the director, overall quality improvement plan, computer system, and other common areas. Each checklist has a list of questions that are followed by a "yes," "no," or "not applicable."

These checklists were developed by resource committees within the CAP, who are made up of individuals with an expertise in that particular discipline. On a periodic basis, these checklist questions are reviewed and revised and are available to anyone and can be obtained on a disk or downloaded from the website at www.cap.org.

These checklists are used during the on-site inspection of the laboratory. Any question that is marked "no" must be corrected within 30 d of the inspection. These are referred to as "deficiencies." Phase I deficiencies do not seriously affect the quality of patient care or endanger the safety of a laboratory worker. Phase II deficiencies may affect the patient care quality or the health and safety of laboratory personnel. After a review of the corrections by the technical staff at the CAP, each inspection summary, questions, and responses are forwarded to a commissioner for review. The commissioner reviews the packet and then can either recommend for or against accreditation. The commissioner can also recommend a reinspection of the laboratory if there are sufficient problems. The standard cycle of inspections is 2 yr between physical inspections and a self-inspection in the first year following inspection. The laboratory has the right to appeal a deficiency. If sufficient documentation exists to back up their appeal, then the deficiency will be expunged. This decision comes from the regional commissioner or special commissioner. The final accreditation decision is made by COLA, which is made up of all of the commissioners.

Prerequisites

Each laboratory must participate in a CAP-approved PT program for each patient reported analyte whenever there is an available program. Each laboratory must also have a current CLIA number prior to applying. In those with multiple CLIA numbers, each laboratory must be accredited separately.

Preinspection Phase

Each laboratory must complete the application forms, which consist of general background information about the laboratory, including demographics, personnel, licensure, and certification. A master activity menu designates all activities performed in the laboratory, and there are personnel forms for all directors and supervisors. Curriculum vitae for the director, an organizational chart, and a floor plan complete the application. The activity menu determines what checklists are appropriate for the inspection. An andrology laboratory would get General Laboratory checklist 1 and the section of Reproductive Laboratory checklist 90 that is appropriate to the andrology laboratory. If the laboratory has other disciplines, it receives customized checklists relevant to those disciplines. Now the laboratory should go through the checklist to ensure that they can answer every appropriate question with "yes." This is an "open book" inspection. The inspector cannot go beyond what is in the checklist.

Once the packet is complete, the commissioner or deputy commissioner appoints an inspector or inspection team, depending on the size of the laboratory. Most only require one inspector.

Inspection

After an inspector is assigned to the laboratory, they must contact the laboratory and set up an inspection date. Generally, the CAP does not believe that inspectors in competition with another laboratory have a conflict of interest. The inspector should act in a professional manner and judge each laboratory fairly. The commissioner has the ability to overturn deficiencies if the laboratory appeals. However, if the laboratory has strong objections, they can ask for a reassignment of inspector(s).

During the inspection, it is up to the inspector and director to work out a schedule of what they want to do. Most inspectors follow specimens through the laboratory to address preanalytical, analytic, and postanalytic processes in the laboratory. This is usually followed by document review. During this process, deficiencies may be found. Some may be corrected on site; others may take longer. It is useful for both the inspector and the laboratory to remain nonconfrontational. This experience should be educational. Disagreements can be brought up with the CAP and eventually the commissioner.

The inspector reviews physical documentation of events that occur in the laboratory. There must be procedure manuals established. Evidence of a QC program and PT must be complete. One has to have an ongoing quality assurance program and a quality improvement program, and there must be documentation of both. One part of the quality improvement program is an attempt to identify all sources of variation that might impact patient care. Remember: "If it hasn't been written, it hasn't been done." There should be evidence of troubleshooting and error resolution. Keep physical records for 2 yr, as the inspector looks for safety issues in the laboratory.

The Summation Conference

The summation conference is the final interaction of the inspectors and laboratory personnel. This is the last chance to correct on-site deficiencies. In addition to laboratory personnel, the laboratory can invite administrators or medical staff to the meeting. The inspectors then explain what deficiencies were noted, their level, and the response time that the laboratory has to correct these deficiencies.

Postinspection

The CAP provides forms to address any deficiencies. Once assembled, the corrections to the deficiencies can be forwarded to the CAP. In the case that a laboratory believes it has been unfairly cited with a deficiency, it may appeal it. This information is filed, and the reviewing commissioner can decide to either expunge the deficiency or require it be answered.

Resources/Contact Information

LAP checklists: These inspection checklists can be accessed at www.cap.org. If you do not have access to the Internet, then call the Laboratory Accreditation Program at 800-323-4040, extension 6055, and obtain a disk or hard copy of the checklist.

Laboratory accreditation questions: Any questions about the preinspection process or technical concerns can be answered at 800-323-4040, extension 6055. When you reach this extension, listen to the options to reach the correct person. Questions can also be sent via email to accred@cap.org.

LAP inspector training: Seminars, audio conferences and on-line inspector education are available at no cost and with continuing medical evaluation and continuing education credits. Numerous other CAP resources can be found at www.cap.org.

Tissue eegistration eegulation questions: Martha Wells (301-827-6106) at wells@cber.fda.gov or tissue registration questions at Vicky Carter (301-827-6176) at carterv@cber.fda.gov.

Joint commission on accreditation of healthcare organization: Contact Laboratory Services Accreditation Program at 630-792-5785.

Commission on laboratory accreditation: Contact Program information at 800-981-9883 or info@cola.org.

CONCLUSION

Ongoing debate exists concerning the improvement in laboratory quality attributed to federal and state regulation. However, government regulations are here to stay, regulations are in place, and a laboratory must be accredited to perform moderate- and high-complexity testing. Government regulation is never going to improve overall laboratory quality because regulations and rules are directed at finding fault. Striving for quality is an internal process of self-improvement within the laboratory with guidance from peer review professional organizations. Instead of focusing on government regulation, the laboratory should be concerned with quality of the services it provides. Quality improvement should be an ongoing process that is not dependent on some regulatory agency. If carried out, this process will transcend any regulatory issues and provide better patient care.

REFERENCES

1. Belk WP, Sunderman FW. A Survey of the Accuracy of Chemical Analysis in Clinical Laboratories. Am J Clin Pathol 1947;17:853–861.
2. Sunderman W. The history of proficiency testing/quality control. Clin Chem 1992:38:1205–1209.
3. Hamlin WB, Duckworth JK. The College of American Pathologists, 1946-1996, Laboratory Accreditation. Arch Pathol Lab Med 1997;121:745–753.
4. Rabinovitch A. The College of American Pathologists laboratory accreditation program. Accred Qual Assur 2002;7:473–476.
5. Federal Register. Clinical Laboratory Improvement Act. Clinical Laboratory Improvement Amendment. Final rules and regulations. Fed Reg 1992;57:7002–7288.
6. Bogdanich W. Medical labs, trusted as largely error-free are far from infallible. Wall Street Journal, February 2, 1987.
7. Bogdanich W. Risk Factor: inaccuracy in testing cholesterol hampers war on heart disease. Wall Street Journal, Feb. 3, 1987
8. Bogdanich W. The Pap test misses much cervical cancer through labs' errors. Wall Street Journal, November 2, 1987.
9. Clinical Laboratory Improvement Amendments of 1988. Publication Number 100-578, 42 US 201, 1988.
10. Born PH, Thran SL. The influence of CLIA '88 on physician office laboratories. J Fam Practice 1998;46:319–327.
11. Federal Register. Human cells, tissues and cellular and tissue-based products; Establishment Registration and Product Listing, Final Rule. Fed Reg 2001;66:5447–5469.
12. Federal Register. Suitability determinations for donors of human and cellular and tissue-based products. Proposed rule. Fed Reg 1999;64:52,696–652,723.
13. Federal Register. Current good tissue practice for manufacturers of human cellular and tissue-based products; inspection and enforcement. Proposed rule. Fed Reg 2001;66:1507–1559.

14. Wells M. Update on the implementation of FDA's registration and product listing regulation, human tissue establishment inspections training course. FDA, June 3, 2002.
15. FDA. Minutes meeting between FDA and ASRM Regarding current good tissue practice issues. FDA, April 16, 2001.
16. Dienstag JL, Ryan DM. Occupational exposure to hepatitis B virus in hospital personnel: infection or immunization. Am J Epidemiol 1982;115:26–38.
17. Chin J. The use of hepatitis B virus vaccine. N Engl J Med 1982;307:678–679.
18. Workshop on development of donor screening assays for West Nile Virus. FDA, November 5, 2002.
19. Sainato D. Proficiency testing: friend or foe? Clin Lab News 1997;24:1–5.
20. Matson PL. External quality assessment for semen analysis and sperm antibody detection: results of a pilot scheme. Hum Reprod 1995;10:620–625.
21. Keel BA, Stembridge TW, Peneda G, Serafy NT, Sr. Lack of standardization in performance of the semen analysis among laboratories in the United States. Fertil Steril 2002;78:603–608.
22. Hurst J, Karen N, Hilborne LH. Are physicians' office laboratory results of comparable quality to those produced in other laboratory settings? JAMA 1998;279:468–471.
23. Stull TM, Hearn TL, Hancock JS, et al. Variation in proficiency testing performance by testing site. JAMA 1998;279:463–467.
24. Ross JW, Boone KJ. Assessing the effect of mistakes in total testing process on the quality of patient care. In: Wilmington DE, ed. Proceedings of the 1989 Institute on Critical Issues in Health Laboratory Practice Improving the Quality of Health management Through Clinician and Laboratorian Teamwork. El Dupont de Nemours Co. Inc., El Paso, IL, 1991, p. 173.
25. Nutting PA, Main DS, Fischer PM, et al. Problems in laboratory testing in primary care. JAMA 1996;275:635–639.
26. Boone DJ. Literature review of research related to the Clinical Laboratory Improvement Amendments of 1988. Arch Pathol Lab Med 1992;116:681–693.
27. Gilbert RD. Progress and analytical goals in clinical chemistry. Am J Clin Pathol 1975;63:960–973.
28. Cembrowski GS, Vanderlinde RE. Survey of special practices associated with College of American Pathologists proficiency testing in the Commonwealth of Pennsylvania. Arch Pathol Lab Med 1988;122:374–376.
29. Lott JA, Manning NR, Kyler MK. Proficiency testing in a medical needs context. Clin Chem 1989;35:347–335.

9 Office Evaluaton of Male Infertility

Darius A. Paduch, MD, PhD
and Eugene F. Fuchs, MD

Contents

Infertility in the male should be considered as a sign and symptom...

INTRODUCTION

Until recently, male investigation has been marginalized secondary to the publication of uncontrolled studies with conflicting results and recommendations, along with underlying social prejudice relating male infertility to sexual dysfunction. To many, this evaluation begins and ends with a single test—the semen analysis. The explosion of molecular biology and basic and clinical knowledge of mechanisms involved in spermatogenesis and fertilization are leading factors in the emergence of andrology as a subspecialty of urology that focuses on male sexual and reproductive health *(1,2)*.

Modern andrology combines male reproductive endocrinology, molecular and clinical genetics, epidemiology, and statistics with the artistry of clinical medicine and urological surgery *(3)*. Initial evaluation and decisions to refer are based on the primary care practitioner, gynecologist, and reproductive endocrinologist. Many excellent articles and chapters discuss evaluation and treatment of male infertility and are written by senior experts in the field *(4–6)*. The goal

From: *Contemporary Endocrinology: Office Andrology*
Edited by: P. E. Patton and D. E. Battaglia

of this chapter is to provide a basic understanding of andrology for health care professionals who treat infertile couples.

EPIDEMIOLOGY OF MALE INFERTILITY

Infertility is defined as the inability to conceive after 12 mo of unprotected intercourse, affecting 10 to 15% of couples worldwide *(7–10)*. Generally, the evaluation of the infertile couple is initiated at this time. However, there exists a well-substantiated age-dependent decline in fertility potential in women and possibly men *(11–13)*; therefore, an earlier investigation is advocated, particularly in older couples. In tertiary infertility centers, the most common diagnoses in men after evaluation are: varicocele (16–38%), idiopathic infertility (23–31%), obstruction (1.7–13%), normal evaluation (9%), and cryptorchidism (3–8%) *(2,3,14)*.

CLASSIFICATION OF MALE INFERTILITY

There is no perfect classification system for male infertility. The following represents our efforts to assist in organization and decision making.

Male causes of infertility can be classified into anatomical categories, including pretesticular (mostly hormonal), testicular (varicocele, cryptorchidism, mumps, and injury), posttesticular (obstruction, retrograde ejaculation, and erectile dysfunction), and postcoital (Fig. 1).

HISTORY AND PHYSICAL EXAMINATION

History

1. *Fertility and sexual history.* The initial step is to establish a diagnosis of primary versus secondary infertility. A patient who has never fathered a child despite unprotected sexual intercourse suffers from primary infertility. Secondary infertility applies to men with proven paternity; however, up to 30% of paternity tests exclude the proband as the biological father of a child *(15)*. Primary infertility usually indicates a more complex set of problems (chromosomal and genetic abnormalities, primary endocrinopathy), whereas secondary infertility may be a result of correctable problems, e.g., varicocele, infection, and ejaculation problems. Proven live deliveries in the past by a female partner make male factor infertility more likely. The age of both partners should be noted because the highest fertility rates are achieved in younger women.
2. *Change in sexual drive.* Occurs in patients with hypogonadism, but sexual drive and performance depends on a complex interplay of hormonal, social, cultural, and psychological factors. Although a decreased libido should be further evaluated by measuring morning testosterone, a low libido is not pathognomic for

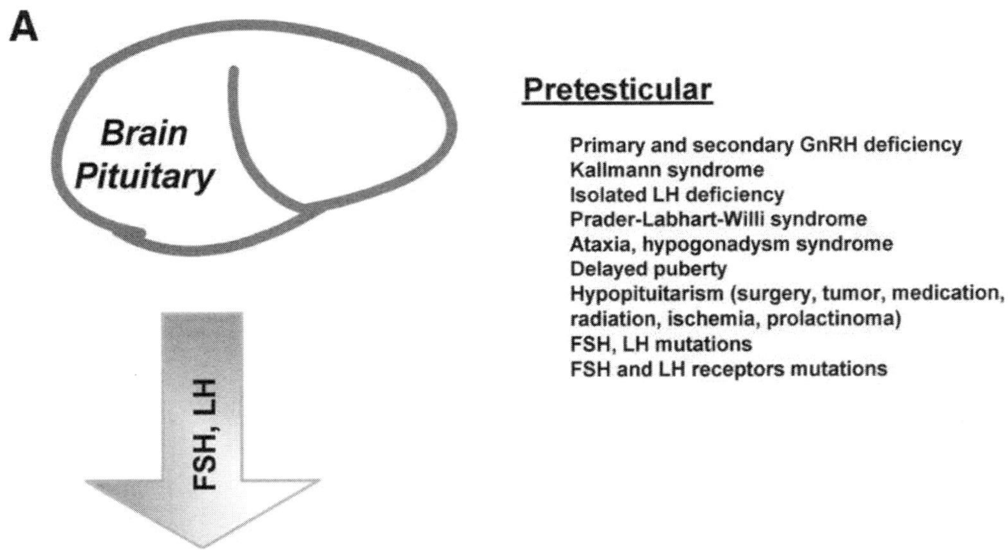

Fig. 1. Classification of male infertility. Classification system can also be based on the underlying physiological defect, including the diagnostic categories overlapped by endocrinopathies, developmental and inborn defects (cryptorchidism), genetic aberrations (y chromosome microdeletion and Klinefelter syndrome), vascular insults (varicocele and testicular torsion), infections and their complications (orchitis and urethritis), iatrogenic causes (medications), recreational drugs use, and trauma. All of these mechanisms can affect spermatogenesis, the sperm deposition, or both.

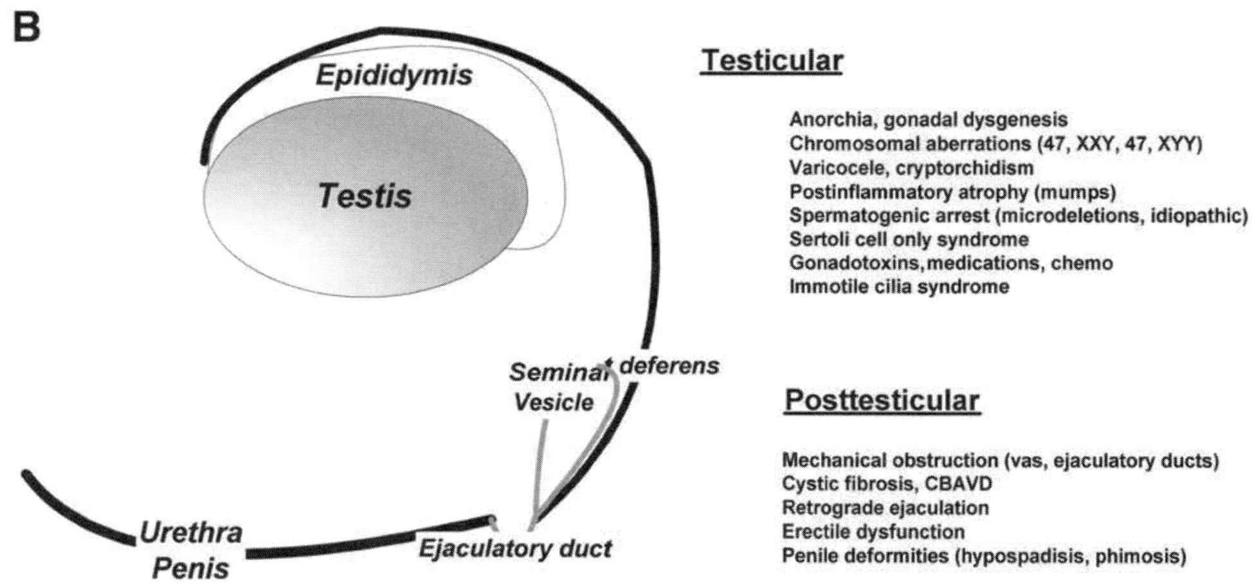

Fig. 1. *(continued)*

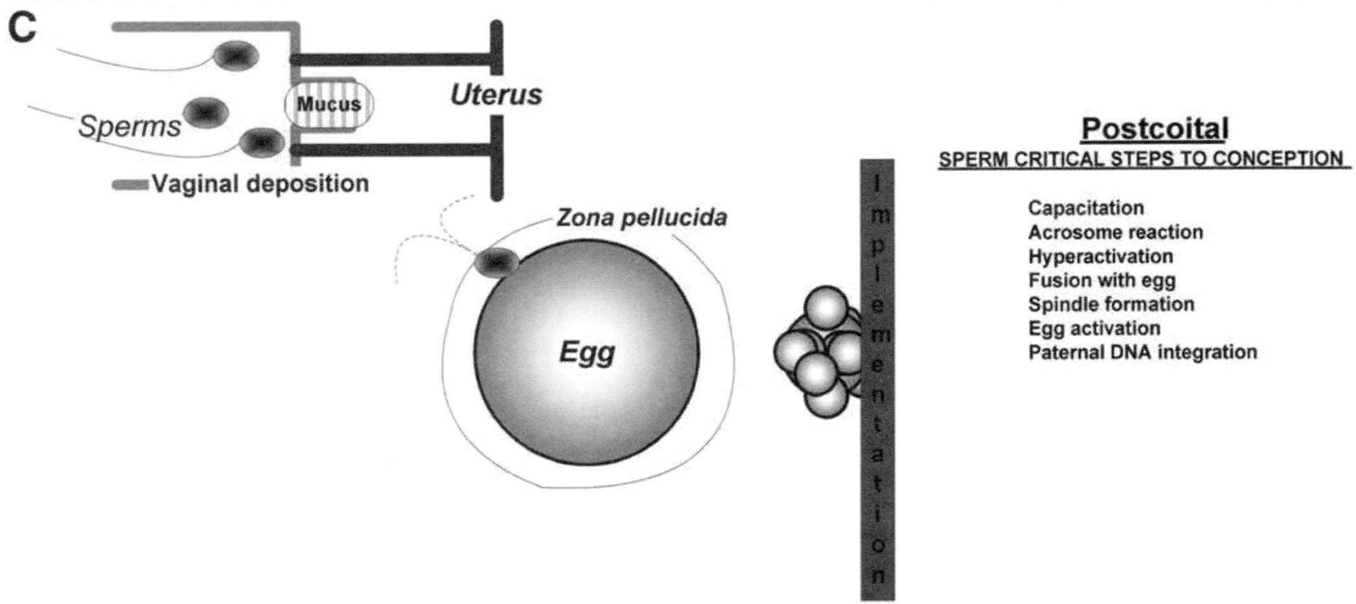

Fig. 1. *(continued)*

hypogonadism. Normal sexual performance does not exclude hypogonadism either, but a normal testosterone excludes hypogonadism as a cause of infertility.

3. *Frequency and timing of sexual intercourse, use of lubricants*, and any *difficulties during intercourse* should be noted. Although intercourse two to three times a week is often advocated, the majority of fertilization events occur with sexual intercourse within an interval of 6 d before and on the day of ovulation *(16)*. In severely obese women or women with an intact hymen, semen deposition may be an issue. Commercially available lubricants are often spermicidal, but in limited amounts, raw egg whites, peanut, and safflower oils have no known adverse effect on semen quality.
4. *Semen volume*. Low-semen volume can be a result of ejaculatory ducts or seminal vesicle obstruction and relative hypogonadism. Men with hypogonadism also report low-semen volume because testosterone is needed for normal prostate function. α-Blockers and serotonine uptake inhibitors can cause retrograde ejaculation and anejaculation. 5-α-reductase inhibitors can decrease semen volume *(16a)*.
5. *Puberty*. The initiation of puberty requires the integrated action of hypothalamus (processing signals from cortex and subcortical areas), pituitary gland, testes, and normal target tissues response elements. Thus, normal and timely progression of puberty excludes major inborn deficits in hormonal axis and can streamline further evaluation. An increase in testicular volume of more than 2.5 mL heralds onset of puberty and occurs between 10 and 14 yr of age *(17)*. Delayed puberty is present if there are no signs of testicular or genital development by age 14. Although delayed puberty is most commonly constitutional (1:40 adolescents), peer pressure and the concern of overt pathology warrants an investigation *(18)*.
6. A history of *recurrent bronchial infections or sinusitis* is seen in cystic fibrosis, Kartagener's syndrome, and Young's syndrome. Patients suffering from Young's syndrome present with azoospermia, but they have normal semen volume and a seminal fructose level *(19)*. A common feature of both Young's and Kartagener's syndromes is an abnormality in sperm tail structure and immotility *(20)*. The defect is ubiquitous and can be a part of immotile cillia syndrome *(21)*. Documentation of bilateral vas deferens ducts, normal testicular size and consistency, together with semen analysis, should aid in diagnosis.
7. *Mumps orchitis* after puberty, *trauma* to the testis, *testicular torsion*, and *cryptorchidism* can all affect spermatogenesis and contribute to infertility *(22)*.
8. *Genitourinary infections* (chronic prostatitis or chlamydial urethritis) may promote infertility by the production of free radicals (byproducts of inflammatory reaction) that affect sperm integrity *(23–25)*.
9. *Bilateral inguinal hernia repair* (especially done in the first year of life or later in life with the mesh) can result in vas deferens transsection or obstruction *(26)*.

10. *Bladder neck reconstruction, retroperitoneal surgery, spinal trauma,* or *surgery* can damage sympathetic chains or injure the bladder neck, thus contributing to retrograde ejaculation.
11. *Family history* of male infertility should prompt discussion about genetic testing because germinal microdeletions of Y chromosome can be transmitted to offspring *(27)*.
12. *Medication* and *recreational drug* use, *smoking*, *alcohol abuse*, and *heat exposure* can affect erectile function, libido, ejaculations, and spermatogenesis.

Physical Examination

General Appearance, Anthropometric Characteristics, and Body Habitus

Anthropometric measurements have a less important role in the era of molecular biology, but specific syndromes have quite characteristic phenotypic presentations. Klinefelter syndrome is associated with eunuchoid stature (arm span exceeds body length) secondary to delayed puberty and closure of epiphyseal plates in long bones *(28)*. Prader-Labhart-Willi (deletion of chromosomal region 15q11-13) syndrome is characterized by short stature, severe obesity, hypopigmentation, and muscular hypotonia *(29)*. Obesity, progressive retinal dystrophy, and mental retardation are common in Bardet-Biedl and Laurence-Moon syndrome. However, Bardet-Biedl syndrome is associated with hexadactyly, whereas Laurance-Moon syndrome displays spastic paraplegia and ataxia *(30,31)*. Patients with cerebrallar ataxia and hypogonadism syndromes often have normal intelligence and body habitus, but progressive neurological deterioration with hypogonadism leads to accurate diagnosis *(32)*. Scarce facial, pubic, and auxiliary hair are common signs of hypogonadism and may be seen in Klinefelter syndrome.

Eyes, Ears, and Nose

Visual field changes or new onset of blurred vision may indicate intracranial and pituitary tumors. Patients with Kallmann syndrome may suffer from hyposmia and anosmia, together with midline craniofacial deformities.

Chest and Abdomen

Bronchitis and recurrent sinusitis is seen in cystic fibrosis, but the diagnosis is usually established during childhood. Patients with immotile cilia syndrome also suffer from respiratory tract infections and are also infertile (Young syndrome or "9 + 0" syndrome). Diagnosis is confirmed by electron microscopy showing a missing central pair of microtubules in sperm tails. Young syndrome associated with situs invertus and bronchiectasis is the Kartagener syndrome. Hence, palpation of the liver and percussion of the chest should be performed.

Gynecomastia is common in adolescents and young obese males, but gynecomastia suddenly developing may indicate hormonally active testicular tumors *(33)*. Klinefelter syndrome is one of the predisposing factors for male breast cancer; hence, a breast exam is indicated *(34)*.

Testicular Size

Testicular tissue is primarily made of germinal epithelium (80%), and the volume ranges between 12 and 30 mL. During an exam, testicular size and consistency are noted, and volume is assessed (Prader orchidometer, ultrasound, or calipers). Any suspicious mass in the testis should be further evaluated with a scrotal ultrasound because testicular cancer can present in men with infertility *(35)*. Some practitioners advocate ultrasound of the scrotum for every infertile man, but the majority of tumors are palpable and benign *(36,37)*. The presence, location, and size of the epididymis, as well as any tenderness, are also recorded. The epididymis should be less than 1 cm in width, positioned on the posterior aspect of testis along the longitudinal axis. An enlarged epididymis may indicate an epididymal or vasal obstruction. A tender, enlarged epididymis with irritative voiding symptoms is consistent with epididymitis and should be treated with antibiotics. Smooth masses in the epididymis are common and include benign spermatoceles and epididymal cysts. A scrotal ultrasound confirms the cystic nature of the lesion and excludes extremely rare epididymal tumors. Small and hard testicles are typically found in end-stage testicular failure, particularly Klinefelter syndrome. Small and soft testicles are often seen in hypogonadotropic hypogonadism, anabolic androgen abuse, and spermatogenic failure after radiation or chemotherapy.

Varicocele

Dilated veins of pampiniform plexus (varicocele) are seen much more commonly in patients evaluated for infertility than in the general population, and are considered to be the leading cause of male infertility *(4)*. The diagnosis of a varicocele can be established by physical examination (Fig. 2).

Vas Deferens

The vas deferens should be palpable on both sides. Congenital bilateral aplasia (absence) of the vas deferens is the most common genetic cause of obstructive azoospermia and can be associated with pulmonary and gastrointestinal cystic fibrosis. More than 500 mutations and single-nucleotide polymorphisms in the cystic fibrosis transmembrane regulator (*CFTR*) gene are identified with variable phenotype and penetration. Unilateral absence of vas deferens can be either caused by mutation in the *CFTR* gene or as a result of Wolffian duct malformation. In the latter case, renal agenesis can be expected. Unilateral absence of vas

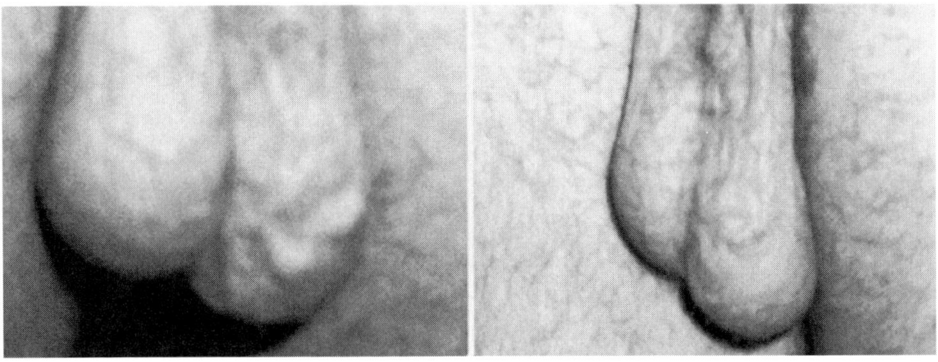

Fig. 2. Grade III varicocele—dilated veins of pampiniform plexus can be easily seen during physical examination.

deferens should prompt a renal ultrasound, and confirmed renal agenesis makes CFTR mutation less likely.

Penis

Fertilization requires deposition of semen in the fornix of the vagina. Normal penile function and anatomy is important from a fertility standpoint. During the physical examination, assess pubic hair distribution, penile length, presence of plaques in tunica albuginea, and the localization and configuration of the meatus. In uncircumcised men, the foreskin should be retracted to expose the glans and urethral meatus. Sparse pubic hair or a lack of male escutcheon should prompt testosterone measures. The penile size should be measured using a stretched penile-length technique by applying mild traction at the glans. Such measurement correlates well with penile length during erection. Micropenis is defined as a penile length below 2 standard deviations for local population. Presence of palpable plaques may be associated with penile curvature during erection, which in extreme cases can preclude deposition of semen in the fornix of the vagina. The meatus should be easily visible and present at the tip of the glans. Hypospadiasis is defined as the transposition of urethral meatus on the ventral aspect of the penile shaft. Proximal and mid-shaft hypospadiasis interferes with semen deposition, but the defect is usually repaired in early childhood in a majority of patients.

Prostate and Seminal Vesicles

A tender, doughy, soft prostate with positive-expressed prostatic secretions points to prostatitis. Expressed prostatic secretions can be stained with QuickDiff, which allows the differentiation of polymorphonuclears from lymphocytes and

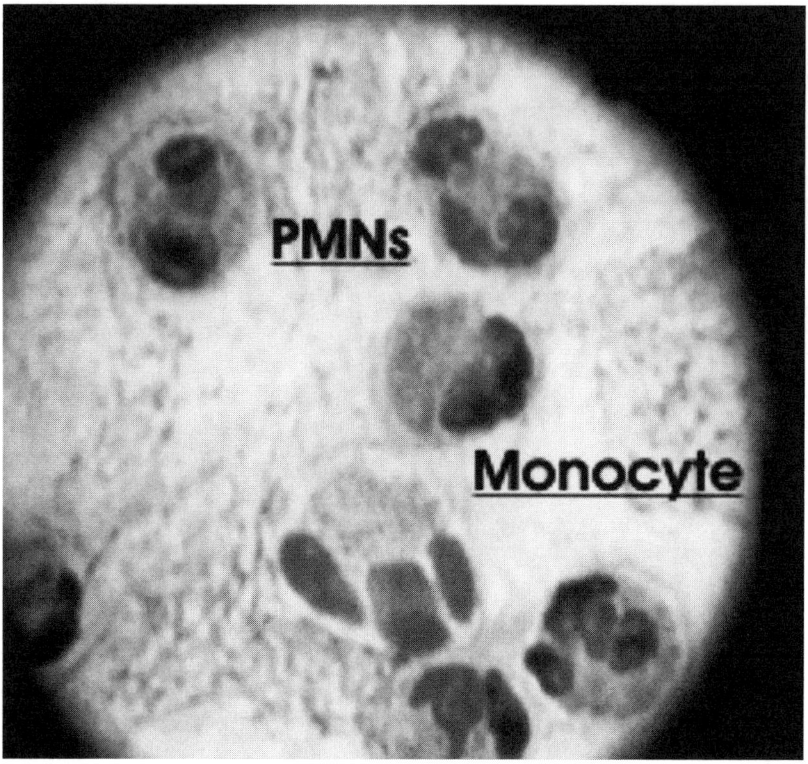

Fig. 3. QuickDiff staining of expressed prostatic secretions. Multiple polymorphonuclear cells (PMNs).

monocytes. Patients with more than 20 polymorphonuclears per high-power field respond much better to antibiotics in this author's (DP) experience (Fig. 3). Routinely, seminal vesicles are not palpable, but unless ejaculatory duct obstruction is present.

ADDITIONAL STUDIES

In men with an abnormal semen analysis, endocrine, genetic, and specialized sperm tests may be indicated, and these topics are covered elsewhere within this text (*see* Chapters 1, 2, and 5). In selected cases, imaging studies of the male reproductive system may provide important insights in infertile men.

Imaging

Scrotal Ultrasound

Scrotal ultrasound is a relatively inexpensive, easy to perform, and safe procedure to measure and compare the size of the testis (Fig. 4). It is a clinically

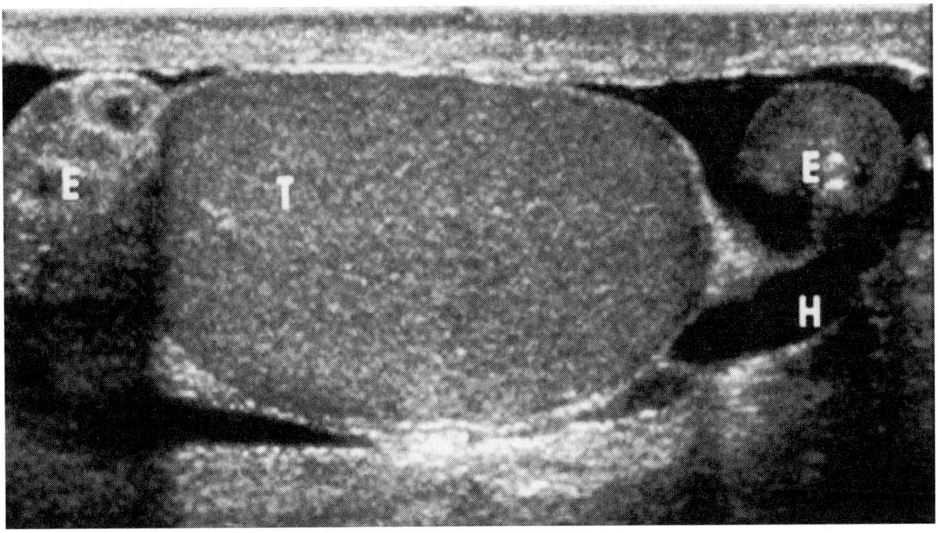

Fig. 4. Normal scrotal ultrasound. E, epididymis; H, small hydrocele; T, testis.

useful tool in the evaluation of a varicocele, especially in young adults and adolescents. A dilated pampinirom plexus vein greater than 1.8 mm is consistent with varicocele, and size differences over 2 mL are considered by some an indication of varicocele repair. Ultrasound findings correlate well with the clinical grade of varicocele. Varicoceles can be further confirmed by the presence of venous reflux (flow reversal) with a valsalva maneuver. Although venous reflux is diagnostic in some men, reflux is sometimes absent even in men with a grade III varicocele. A color-enhanced Doppler study may assess arterial perfusion, and a diminished or absent perfusion is seen in testicular torsion or subtorsin.

Scrotal ultrasound is invaluable in evaluating masses. A solid mass on ultrasound is most likely a testicular cancer, and a urological consultation is required. Epididymal size and blood flow can be assessed, and an epididymal head with more than 1 cm of increased perfusion is consistent with epididymitis.

Scrotal ultrasound is not indicated as a screening test in every patient with infertility to exclude malignancy. In 3518 consecutive patients with infertility, testicular cysts were found in 0.7% and solid masses in 0.4% of patients. It is unknown whether these testicular solid masses would be missed on a subsequent physical examination.

Continuous wave Doppler sonography (portable Doppler) can confirm the presence of reflux in patients with a varicocele. Although it is a fast and cost-efficient method, a physical examination is still the gold standard to diagnose varicocele.

Transrectal ultrasound (TRUS) can be used to measure the size of seminal vesicles and diameter of ejaculatory duct. When midline cysts or bilaterally dilated ejaculatory ducts are visible and the semen analysis reveals azoospermia, additional studies are necessary to exclude obstructive azoospermia. TRUS with ultrasound-guided seminal vesicles aspiration provides a reliable method to diagnose ejaculatory duct obstruction. In men with azoospermia and no evidence of retrograde ejaculation, the detection of sperm in the aspirite confirms ejaculatory duct obstruction. Ejaculatory duct obstruction can be treated with a transurethral resection of ejaculatory ducts or unroofing of the midline cyst.

Venography and Arteriography

Invasive radiological studies are rarely used; however, venography is done if and when retrograde embolization of spermatic veins is performed for treatment of a varicocele.

Magnetic Resonance Imaging and Computed Tomography

Imaging studies of the head and pituitary gland should be ordered when an intracranial or pituitary tumor is suspected. An elevated prolactin should be further evaluated with magnetic resonance imaging to exclude macroprolactinoma of the pituitary, but microadenoma may not be visible.

CONCLUSIONS

There are more questions than answers in andrology, but the field will expand and introduce more treatment options and diagnostic tools based on a better understanding of sperm physiology and regulation. We hope that this chapter will help other practitioners to better evaluate and treat the infertile male.

REFERENCES

1. Burrows PJ, Schrepferman CG, Lipshultz LI. Comprehensive office evaluation in the new millennium. Urol Clin North Am 2002;29:873–894.
2. Sigman M, Jarow JP. Male Infertility. In: Walsh PC, ed. Campbell's Urology, 8th ed. Saunders, Philadelphia, PA, 2002, p. 4, v.
3. Nieschlag E, Behre HM, Ahlen HV. Andrology: Male Reproductive Health and Dysfunction, 2nd ed. Springer, New York, 2001.
4. Brugh VM, III, Matschke HM, Lipshultz LI. Male factor infertility. Endocrinol Metab Clin North Am 2003;32:689–707.
5. Jarow JP, Sharlip ID, Belker AM, et al. Best practice policies for male infertility. J Urol 2002;167:2138–2144.
6. Sharlip ID, Jarow JP, Belker AM, et al. Best practice policies for male infertility. Fertil Steril 2002;77:873–882.
7. Gunnell DJ, Ewings P. Infertility prevalence, needs assessment and purchasing. J Public Health Med 1994;16:29–35.

8. Page H. Estimation of the prevalence and incidence of infertility in a population: a pilot study. Fertil Steril 1989;51:571–577.
9. Philippov OS, Radionchenko AA, Bolotova VP, et al. Estimation of the prevalence and causes of infertility in western Siberia. Bull World Health Organ 1998;76:183–187.
10. Ikechebelu JI, Adinma JI, Orie EF, Ikegwuonu SO. High prevalence of male infertility in southeastern Nigeria. J Obstet Gynaecol 2003;23:657–659.
11. Wright VC, Schieve LA, Reynolds MA, Jeng G. Assisted reproductive technology surveillance—United States, 2000. MMWR Surveill Summ 2003;52:1–16.
12. Williams RS, Vensel T, Sistrom CL, et al. Pregnancy rates in varying age groups after in vitro fertilization: a comparison of follitropin alfa (Gonal F) and follitropin beta (Follistim). Am J Obstet Gynecol 2003;189:342–347.
13. De La Rochebrochard E, McElreavey K, Thonneau P. Paternal age over 40 years: the "Amber Light" in the reproductive life of men? J Androl 2003;24:459–465.
14. Rolf C, Kenkel S, Nieschlag E. Age-related disease pattern in infertile men: increasing incidence of infections in older patients. Andrologia 2002;34:209–217.
15. Valentin J. Exclusions and attributions of paternity: practical experiences of forensic genetics and statistics. Am J Hum Genet 1980;32:420–431.
16. Dunson DB, Baird DD, Wilcox AJ, Weinberg CR. Day-specific probabilities of clinical pregnancy based on two studies with imperfect measures of ovulation. Hum Reprod 1999;14:1835–1839.
16a. Sirinarumitr K, Johnston SD, Kustritz MV, Johnston GR, Sarkar DK, Memon MA. Effects of finasteride on size of the prostate gland and semen quality in dogs with benign prostatic hypertrophy. J Am Vet Med Assoc 2001;218:1721–1722.
17. Kaplan SA 1982 Clinical pediatric and adolescent endocrinology. In: Saunders, Philadelphia, PA, 1982, pp. 307,308.
18. Albanese A, Stanhope R. Investigation of delayed puberty. Clin Endocrinol (Oxford) 1995;43:105–110.
19. Handelsman DJ, Conway AJ, Boylan LM, Turtle JR. Young's syndrome. Obstructive azoospermia and chronic sinopulmonary infections. N Engl J Med 1984;310:3–9.
20. Casey B. Two rights make a wrong: human left-right malformations. Hum Mol Genet 1998;7:1565–1571.
21. Afzelius BA. Genetical and ultrastructural aspects of the immotile-cilia syndrome. Am J Hum Genet 1981;33:852–864.
22. Kukadia AN, Ercole CJ, Gleich P, et al. Testicular trauma: potential impact on reproductive function. J Urol 1996;156:1643–1646.
23. Berger RE. Infection of the male reproductive tract. Curr Ther Endocrinol Metab 1994;5:305–309.
24. Sikka SC. Relative impact of oxidative stress on male reproductive function. Curr Med Chem 2001;8:851–862.
25. Pasqualotto FF, Sharma RK, Nelson DR, et al. Relationship between oxidative stress, semen characteristics, and clinical diagnosis in men undergoing infertility investigation. Fertil Steril 2000;73:459–464.
26. Seifman BD, Ohl DA, Jarow JP, Menge AC. Unilateral obstruction of the vas deferens diagnosed by seminal vesicle aspiration. Tech Urol 1999;5:113–115.
27. Cram DS, Ma K, Bhasin S, et al. Y chromosome analysis of infertile men and their sons conceived through intracytoplasmic sperm injection: vertical transmission of deletions and rarity of de novo deletions. Fertil Steril 2000;74:909–915.
28. Manning MA, Hoyme HE. Diagnosis and management of the adolescent boy with Klinefelter syndrome. Adolesc Med 2002;13:367–374.

29. Cassidy SB. Prader-Willi syndrome. J Med Genet 1997;34:917–923.
30. Beales PL, Elcioglu N, Woolf AS, et al. New criteria for improved diagnosis of Bardet-Biedl syndrome: results of a population survey. J Med Genet 1999;36:437–446.
31. Green JS, Parfrey PS, Harnett JD, et al. The cardinal manifestations of Bardet-Biedl syndrome, a form of Laurence-Moon-Biedl syndrome. N Engl J Med 1989;321:1002–1009.
32. Koeppen AH. The hereditary ataxias. J Neuropathol Exp Neurol 1998;57:531–543.
33. Daniels IR, Layer GT. Testicular tumours presenting as gynaecomastia. Eur J Surg Oncol 2003;29:437–439.
34. Giordano SH, Buzdar AU, Hortobagyi GN. Breast cancer in men. Ann Intern Med 2002;137:678–687.
35. Simon SD, Lee RD, Mulhall JP. Should all infertile males undergo urologic evaluation before assisted reproductive technologies? Two cases of testicular cancer presenting with infertility. Fertil Steril 2001;75:1226,1227.
36. Nashan D, Behre HM, Grunert JH, Nieschlag E. Diagnostic value of scrotal sonography in infertile men: report on 658 cases. Andrologia 1990;22:387–395.
37. Carmignani L, Gadda F, Gazzano G, et al. High incidence of benign testicular neoplasms diagnosed by ultrasound. J Urol 2003;170:1783–1786.

10 Varicocele and Infertility

Ulrike Zenke, MD *and Paul Turek,* MD

Contents

CASE STUDY

A 33-yr-old man has been trying to conceive for 1.5 yr with his 30-yr-old female partner. She is medically healthy, with a history of a terminated pregnancy 3 yr prior, has regular ovulatory cycles and a normal hysterosalpingogram. He has been evaluated by a urologist, which revealed that he is also medically healthy, with a grade III left varicocele and normal follicle-stimulating hormone (FSH) and testosterone levels. His semen analysis (repeated) consistently shows a normal ejaculate volume, a low-sperm concentration (16 million sperm/mL), low sperm motility (33% active), and poor strict morphology (5%). How should this couple be counseled regarding cost-effective treatment options? How would recommendations differ concerning varicocele repair if he had no sperm in the ejaculate?

Recognition that the varicocele may be a factor in male infertility dates back to the first-century AD. Celsus, a Greek physician, described these findings in *De Medicina*: " The veins are swollen and twisted over the testicle, which becomes smaller than its fellow, in as much as nutrition has become defective" *(1)*. The first evidence of semen quality improvement and pregnancy after varicocele repair were reported by Barwell in 1885 and Bennett in 1889 *(2,3)*. As the litera-

From: *Contemporary Endocrinology: Office Andrology*
Edited by: P. E. Patton and D. E. Battaglia © Humana Press Inc., Totowa, NJ

ture on varicocele has expanded, so does the confusion about its relevance to male fertility. Although the existence of this lesion is not controversial, its management certainly is. This chapter provides a basic review of varicoceles along with a discussion of its pathophysiology, diagnosis, and management in male infertility.

DEFINITION AND INCIDENCE

A varicocele is a vascular abnormality of the scrotum, consisting of elongated, dilated, and tortuous spermatic veins within the pampiniform plexus (Fig. 1). The veins most commonly involved are the internal spermatic veins, but the external spermatic (cremasteric) veins have also been implicated in varicocele development. The deferential veins are not involved in the genesis of this lesion *(4)*. Studies suggest that 78 to 93% of varicoceles are on the left side, and the remainder are bilateral. A unilateral right varicocele is rare and can indicate obstruction of the internal spermatic vein by retroperitoneal tumor or result from situs inversus *(5)*.

The importance of the varicocele stems from its common presentation in both healthy and infertile men. Varicoceles are found in approx 15% of the general male population *(6)*. Steeno et al. showed that the incidence of varicocele detection gradually increases in boys age 10 to 15 yr to approx 15%, whereas the incidence of varicoceles is constant in males older than 15 yr old *(7)*. This finding indicates that varicoceles are primarily acquired during puberty. In men with primary infertility, 35% have varicoceles; in cases of secondary infertility, 80% will harbor a varicocele without racial preponderance *(8)*. This prevalence data supports the contention that varicoceles can affect testis function, and this effect may be progressive with time.

ETIOLOGY

Varicoceles are presumably an evolutionary consequence of men's upright posture and are virtually absent in other species *(9)*. Among proposed theories that attempt to explain the genesis of varicocele, the following are most widely accepted:

- A varicocele is a result of anatomical differences in venous drainage between the left and right testicle. The right spermatic vein inserts into the inferior vena cava at an oblique angle (a natural valve), whereas the left spermatic vein inserts directly and at right angles (no natural valve) into the left renal vein. This difference in insertion angle and the added Venturi effect of enhanced venous drainage on the right side owing to higher blood flow within the vena cava than the renal vein, is believed to result in increased transmission of hydrostatic to the left when compared to the right pampiniform plexus *(10)*.

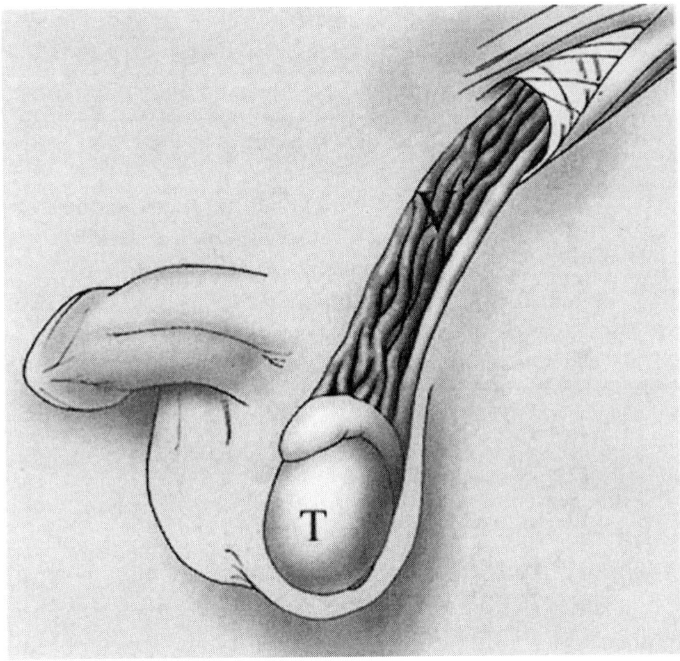

Fig. 1. Illustration of scrotal anatomy showing testis (T) and varicocele (V) within the spermatic cord.

- An absence (or incompetence) of venous valves results in the reflux of venous blood and a varicocele. Early studies suggested that the left spermatic veins harbored no valves to protect against venous reflux. More recently, Braedel et al. showed that 73% of men with varicocele had absent venous valves on venography, but 27% of men actually had intact valves *(11)*. It is now thought that valvular defects may contribute to, but are not the cause of, scrotal varicocele.
- Partial obstruction of the left spermatic vein causes increased hydrostatic pressure in the pampiniform plexus. One demonstrated mechanism of partial venous obstruction is the compression of the left renal vein between the aorta posteriorly and the superior mesenteric artery anteriorly. This so-called "nutcracker effect" could increase the venous pressure in the left renal vein and consequently in the internal spermatic veins that drain into the renal vein. In the study by Braedel et al., this finding occurred in 0.7% of patients, suggesting that, although present, it is not a common cause of varicocele *(11)*.

The etiology of varicocele formation most likely is multifactorial. Although the relative contributions of increased hydrostatic pressure and venous reflux to the development of varicoceles remains unclear, sufficient anatomic and physiologic evidence exists to support both as causative in this lesion.

Table 1
Pathophysiology of Varicoceles

Organ/parameter	*Possible effects*
Testis	Atrophy, histologic abnormalities
Epididymis	Decreased function
Sperm	Oligospermia (low-sperm concentration); Asthenospermia (low-sperm motility), Teratozoospermia ("stress" pattern morphology with increase in pyriform shapes)
Fertility	Impaired sperm-fertilizing ability
	Increased DNA/chromatin damage
Endocrine profile	Hypothalamic-pituitary-gonadal hormonal dysfunction

PATHOPHYSIOLOGIC EFFECTS

To date, the mechanism responsible for the pathologic effects of varicoceles is unknown. Human studies that try to address the issue of varicocele-related infertility generally measure semen parameters in men with and without varicoceles, as well as in men before and after varicocelectomy. Such observational data is subject to wide biological variability and routinely fail to reliably explain the effect of varicocele on the testis. The roles of hyperthermia, hormonal dysfunction, oxidative stress, and metabolite reflux have all been implicated from human or animals studies and is discussed. We suspect that the etiology may be multifactorial and possibly includes a genetic predisposition. A list of probable effects of varicocele on reproductive function is listed in Table 1.

Hyperthermia

Scrotal temperature is physiologically lower than body temperature. This temperature difference is maintained by (1) an important countercurrent heat-exchange system in the pampiniform plexus, and (2) the thermoregulatory effects of the scrotum with its highly variable surface area. Inflowing warm internal spermatic arterial blood is cooled by the more tepid venous outflow from the pampiniform plexus. By changing surface area, the scrotum likely also contributes to testis cooling, acting as a natural radiator. The dilated veins in a varicocele may decrease the effectiveness of these physiologic-cooling mechanisms.

The effect of heat on the testis has been shown to be clinically important. Macleod and Hotchkiss were the first to demonstrate that semen quality profoundly decreased in healthy men for 2 mo following a single episode of "fever treatment" (41ºC) *(12)*. Increased scrotal temperature has also been implicated in the pathophysiology of varicoceles. In adolescents with a palpable (grade II or III) varicocele, significant bilateral elevation of scrotal temperature is found relative to unaffected controls *(13)*. These findings have been confirmed with needle thermistor studies that directly measure intratesticular temperature, demonstrating significant temperature elevations bilaterally in association with the unilateral varicocele *(14)*. Exactly how heat affects spermatogenesis is the current the subject of much study. Direct thermal injury-causing apoptosis and damage to nuclear RNA-binding proteins and DNA within seminiferous tubules are likely explanations for this pathologic response *(15–17)*.

Hormonal Dysfunction

A World Health Organization (WHO) multicenter study on the influence of varicocele on fertility parameters demonstrated that in men with varicoceles, the mean testosterone levels decreased significantly with age, whereas this trend was not observed in men without varicoceles *(18)*. Furthermore, lower concentrations of circulating free testosterone, higher estradiol, and higher steroid-binding globulin levels have been observed in men with varicoceles *(19)*. Taken together, these findings implicate a subtle, intrinsic, and time-dependant detrimental effect of varicoceles on the testes and Leydig cell function. However, despite the observation of statistically significant reduction in testosterone levels, actual reported values were all within normal limits. In contrast, other investigators reported no significant difference in FSH, luteining hormone, testosterone, and estradiol in men with and without varicoceles *(20,21)*. There is also evidence to implicate a varicocele effect on the hypothalamic-pituitary-gonadal axis, as suggested by an increased gonadotropin response to gonadotropin-releasing hormone administration in affected men *(22,23)*. Even more controversial are reports regarding the reversibility of the hormonal dysfunction by varicocelectomy *(22–24)*. In summary, it is unclear whether an endocrinopathy is actually associated with varicoceles. If indeed there is an association, it is also unclear whether an endocrinopathy is the cause or effect of decreased spermatogenesis.

Oxidative Stress

Reactive oxygen species (ROS) production by sperm is a normal physiological process that helps mediate signal transduction, sperm hyperactivation, acrosome reaction, and sperm–oocyte attachment *(25)*. In normal healthy men, excessive ROS production is neutralized by antioxidants in the seminal plasma. However, if ROS production overwhelms the antioxidant capacity of semen, then oxidative stress occurs. ROS may cause defective sperm function, alter sperm morphology, and lead to decreased motility and ineffective spermatozoon–oocyte fusion *(6)*.

Increased oxidative stress has been implicated in the reduced fertility of varicocele patients. Elevated ROS concentrations have been observed in 80% of infertile varicocele patients, 77% with incidental varicocele, and 20% of normal sperm donors *(26,27)*. In addition to an increased incidence of elevated seminal

ROS levels in men with varicoceles, the degree of ROS elevation observed is statistically much higher than in men without varicoceles *(27)*. However, the physiologic mechanism that underlies this relationship is unexplained.

Metabolite Reflux

An early theory of varicocele effect stems from anatomic work that demonstrated internal spermatic vein reflux in varicocele patients *(28)*. From this observation, the hypothesis that reflux of metabolic products from the kidney or adrenal gland (e.g., catecholamines) might damage the testicle was proposed. This idea has not been confirmed and has been abandoned as an explanation for varicocele effect.

Molecular and Genetic Effects

As molecular biology is applied to the study of varicoceles, several interesting findings have been reported. Literature indicates that testis Topoisomerase I and DNA polymerase activities are altered with this lesion, suggesting that changes in testicular temperature from a varicocele may induce alterations in enzymatic activity *(29,30)*. Furthermore, there is increased testicular germ cell apoptosis observed with varicoceles *(15)*. More recent research shows that the increased delivery of gonadotoxin cadmium to the testis with varicocele may induce the process of apoptosis within the testis and reduce spermatogenesis *(31)*.

In men with impaired spermatogenesis and varicoceles, it is also possible that genetic abnormalities unrelated to the varicocele coexist. Data from one study suggests that varicocele repair in men with coexisting Y chromosome microdeletions, or a karyotype abnormality is not likely to improve spermatogenesis or infertility *(32)*. On the contrary, repair of varicocele in men with no definable genetic infertility demonstrated significant improvements in semen quality and fertility.

DIAGNOSIS

The vast majority of varicoceles are diagnosed by physical examination through palpation of the spermatic cord before and during a Valsalva maneuver with the patient in a standing position. Exercise and prolonged standing may also demonstrate a varicocele. The examination requires an adept clinician, a warm room, and a cooperative patient. Difficulties arise with the ability to palpate a varicocele through a thickened scrotal wall or contracted scrotum. The differential diagnosis of this lesion includes lipoma of the cord and hernia. The examiner should evaluate for epididymal and testicular pathology and should also assess testicular volume because varicoceles are associated with testis atrophy. Varicoceles have been arbitrarily divided into three grades based on physical examination findings as outlined in Table 2. Because this grading system is not

Table 2
Varicocele Grading

Subclinical	Varicocele not detected on physical exam, found by radiologic or other imaging study.
Grade I	Varicocele only palpable during or after Valsalva maneuver on physical exam.
Grade II	Varicocele palpable on routine physical exam without the need for the Valsalva maneuver.
Grade III	Varicocele visible to the eye and palpable on physical exam.

validated, accurate assessment of treatment outcomes is difficult. Subclinical varicoceles are lesions undetected by routine physical examination but are instead by radiologic or other imaging methods. Such lesions are generally smaller than clinical varicoceles, and the utility of varicocele repair of these lesions is unknown.

Diagnosis can also be made with ultrasound, thermography, scintigraphy and computed tomography, or magnetic resonance imaging (MRI). Among these techniques, venography is considered to be the best diagnostic test, but it is invasive. Conveniently, venography can be combined with embolization with balloons or coils to ablate the lesion after detection. Doppler ultrasound is less invasive than, and correlates well with, venography and relies on the detection of venous flow within the varicocele. Because of its increased sensitivity, Doppler ultrasound is more likely to detect subclinical varicoceles. However, it can be valuable to confirm varicocele presence in cases of clinically suspicious, but not overtly palpable, lesions. Thermography, scintography, and MRI are of limited clinical utility mostly because of increased cost and lack of controlled studies surrounding their use.

PREDICTION OF RESPONSE TO TREATMENT

Various clinical parameters have been examined to find features of varicocele presentation that may predict a successful outcome after treatment *(33)*. A list of these parameters is found in Table 3.

MANAGEMENT

Most men with varicoceles are able to conceive without intervention. However, varicocele in the setting of impaired semen quality constitutes the most common and correctable cause of male infertility. Therefore, among the majority of male infertility specialists, the crucial question is not *if* a varicocele should be treated, but *when* it should be treated. The goals of varicocele repair are to

Table 3
Features of Varicocele Presentation Predictive of Treatment Response

Normal testis volume without atrophy
Preoperative total motile sperm count >5 million sperm
Preoperative normal sperm motility (>60%)
Large grade III varicocele
Normal serum follicle-stimulating hormone levels

Source: ref. *33*.

improve testis function, semen quality, and chances of conception. Another goal is to shift the care of infertility treatment from more expensive and invasive options, such as in vitro fertilization (IVF) and intracytoplasmic sperm injection (ICSI) to less involved treatments, e.g., intrauterine insemination (IUI) *(34)*.

Indications for Varicocelectomy

Varicocelectomy is indicated in the following clinical situations:

- Adolescents with large varicocele and evidence of testis hypotrophy.
- In the presence of varicocele-induced orchialgia.
- Correction of male factor infertility (with adequate maternal reproductive potential).

Varicocelectomy may *not* be indicated in the following situations:

- Male factor infertility with coexisting genetic factors (e.g., Klinefelter Syndrome).
- Male factor infertility with a partner requiring assisted reproductive technology (ART) to conceive.
- Male factor infertility with age-related, diminished female reproductive potential.

Although there is a clear indication to treat patients with varicocele-induced orchialgia, whether or not to repair a varicocele in the context of male factor infertility is a more complex decision. When a varicocele coexists with impaired semen quality, varicocelectomy can potentially restore spermatogenesis and fertility. However, other contributing factors to male factor infertility should be ruled out, including infection, obstruction, and gonadotoxin exposure to heat, tobacco, or medications. The female partner should also be investigated to ensure that ovarian function and female reproductive tract anatomy is normal before proceeding with varicocelectomy. In addition, because the average time to spontaneous pregnancy after varicocele repair is 7 to 9 mo *(34)*, clinicians should make sure there is at least 9 to 12 mo of adequate maternal reproductive potential before varicocelectomy. Increasing the semen quality through this procedure may not be beneficial to the couple if the female partner requires IVF with donor eggs because of diminished ovarian reserve owing to age or other reasons.

More recently, genetic issues, including chromosomal abnormalities and Y chromosome microdeletions, have been recognized as increasingly important causes of male infertility. In oligospermic men, the likelihood of having an abnormal karyotype is 2%, and the risk of Y chromosome microdeletions is 6 to 8%. These risks increase to 15% and 13%, respectively, in men with azoospermia from testis failure. Generally, the lower the sperm concentration, the higher the chance that a genetic cause will be identified. Although genetic risk can be difficult to assess, there is now evidence that oligospermic men with varicocele might not respond as well to repair (in terms of improved semen quality and pregnancies achieved) in the presence of coexisting genetic factors when compared to men without coexisting genetic issues *(32)*.

Treatment Options for Varicoceles

Several modalities are available for varicocele treatment, such as incisional ligation of the veins through retroperitoneal, inguinal, or subinguinal approaches, percutaneus transvenous embolisation, and laparoscopic varicocelectomy (Table 4). All approaches usually give similar results; their differences mainly stem from potential complication rates. The overall complication rate ranges from 1% for the incisional approach to 4% for laparoscopy. The most significant complication with radiologic occlusion is the 10 to 15% chance that the culprit veins cannot be accessed or occluded (technical failure rate). Figure 2 demonstrates the incision and ligation of veins typical of the subinguinal varicocelectomy technique.

Varicocelectomy: Clinical Improvement and Pregnancy

Varicocelectomy improves sperm concentration, motility, and sperm morphology in 51 to 78% of patients and is associated with spontaneous pregnancy rates of 24 to 60% in recent series *(35)*. However, most of these data are derived from retrospective and poorly controlled studies. Only three randomized prospective-controlled trials in infertile men have been performed that examine outcomes in palpable varicoceles *(36,37)*, and the results of these trials are outlined in Table 5. The WHO trial was the largest randomized clinical trial ever conducted, but the results have not been formally published to date. Excluding this study, the most convincing evidence of a cause–effect relationship between varicocele and infertility was reported in a prospective, randomized, crossover study by Madgar et al. in which 60% of men conceived within 1 yr after varicocele repair ($n = 20$) in comparison to 10% in an untreated control group ($n = 25$) *(36)*. During the second year of the study, the control group underwent varicocele repair, and 44% of this group conceived. In azoospermic men, varicocelectomy can result in sperm in the ejaculate in 20 to 50% of men *(33)*.

Several meta-analyses have also examined outcomes of varicocele treatment *(38,39)*. In general, these studies have not supported varicocele repair as effec-

Table 4
Varicocele Treatment Options: Comparison of Outcomes

Outcome parameter	*Incisional*	*Laparoscopic*	*Radiologic*
Semen improvement	66%	50–70%	60%
Pregnancy rate	35%	12–32%	10–50%
Technical failure rate	<1%	<1%	10–15%
Recurrence	0–15%	5–25%	0–10%
Cost	X	2X	X
Pain pills	9.4	11	Minimal
Days to work	5.0	5.3	1

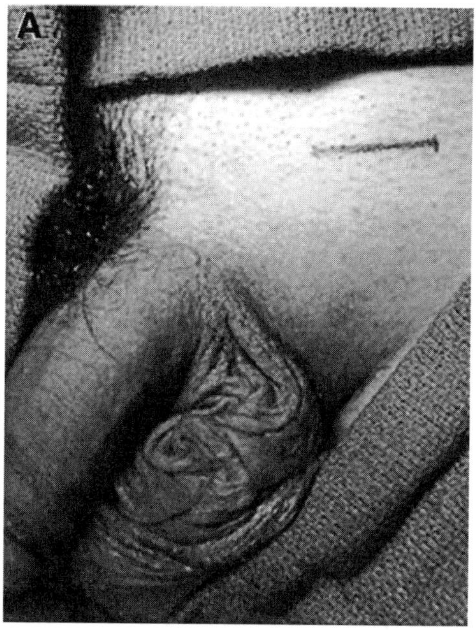

Fig. 2. Placement of incision **(A)** and ligation of internal spermatic veins **(B)** in a subinguinal microscopic varicocelectomy.

tive treatment for male infertility. Yet, even the more rigorous of these studies, in which only randomized controlled clinical trials were examined, shows significant design flaws *(39)*. Of the seven trials examined in this meta-analysis, four included men with only subclinical varicoceles, the clinical relevance of which are completely unclear. Furthermore, the study by Madgar et al. *(36)* that showed a relative benefit of 6.0 for varicocele repair was actually considered an "outlier" in the study, leaving only a single trial evaluable for clinical varicocele. Finally, the large WHO trial (238 patients) was excluded from the analysis. This

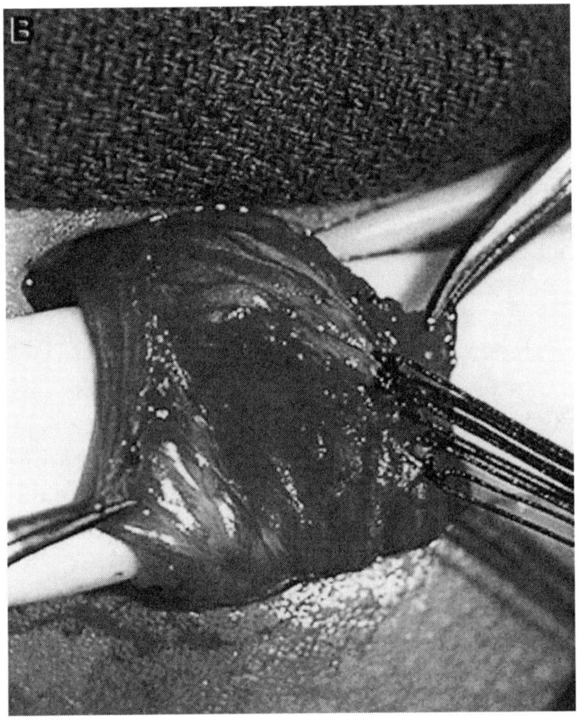

Fig. 2. *(continued)*

Table 5
Results of Randomized Controlled Clinical Trials for Treatment of Palpable Varicoceles in Male Subfertility

Study	*No. of patients/arm*		*Pregnancy rate*	
	Control	*Treatment*	*Control*	*Treatment*
WHO*	109	129	16.7%	34.8%
Nieschlag et al. *(37)*	63	62	25.4%	29.7%
Madgar et al. *(36)*	25	20	10%	60%
Unweighted Mean			*17%*	*41%*

*This study was conducted but never published. *See* ref. *37* for details.

points out that more and larger prospective trials are needed to prove that varicocelectomy improves fertility.

Varicocelectomy: Cost-Effectiveness

In addition to clinical care arguments that suggest varicocele repair is beneficial for infertility, economic analyses also support this concept. Cost–benefit

Table 6
Shift of Infertility Care Analysis After Varicocelectomy

Preoperative semen quality	*No. of patients*	*Preoperative IUI candidates*	*Postoperative IUI candidates*	*% of natural pregnancies*
ICSI	154	0%	20%	17%
IVF	79	0%	55%	31%

IUI, intrauterine insemination; ICSI, intracytoplasmic sperm injection; IVF, in vitro fertilization.

arguments have shown that varicocelectomy is more cost-effective than ART procedures *(40)*. In fact, the delivery rate achieved with varicocele treatment (30%) is actually higher than that obtained with a single cycle of IVF and ICSI (IVF ICSI). More recently, it has been demonstrated in "shift of care" analyses that as many as 50% of couples who would only be candidates for ART procedures owing to low-semen quality can be "rescued" from such procedures and conceive naturally or with IUI after varicocelectomy *(34)*. A summary of this data is outlined in Table 6.

SUMMARY

The varicocele is a common, yet complex, vascular lesion that has highly variable and individualized effects on men and male fertility. Despite numerous studies on this lesion, many controversies remain concerning its diagnosis and management. Based on currently available data, the following conclusions are well-supported concerning varicoceles:

- Varicoceles exert a deleterious and bilateral effect on testis function.
- Varicocele repair in the setting of genetic infertility is not likely to improve semen quality or fertility potential.
- There are different approaches for varicocele repair, both surgical and nonsurgical, that generate similar outcomes.
- Repair of larger varicoceles is likely to result in larger improvements in semen quality.

REFERENCES

1. Saypol DC. Varicocele. J Androl 1981;2:61–65.
2. Barwell R. One hundred cases of varicocele treated by the subcutaneous wire loop. Lancet 1885;1:978–980.
3. Bennet WH. Varicocele, particular with reference to its radical cure. Lancet 1889;1:261–262.
4. Jarrow JP. Effects of varicocele on male fertility. Hum Reprod Update 2001;7:59–64.
5. Grillo-Lopez AJ. Primary right varicocele. J Urol 1971;105:540–543.
6. Naughton CK, Nangia AK, Agarwal A, et al. Varicocele and male infertility: Part II. Pathophysiology of varicoceles in male infertility. Hum Reprod Update 2001;7:473–481.

7. Steeno O, Knops J, Declerck L, et al. Prevention of fertility disorders by detection and treatment of varicocele at school and college age. Andrologia 1976;8:47–53.
8. Cozzolino DJ, Lipshultz LI. Varicocele as a progressive lesion: positive effect of varicocele repair. Hum Reprod Update 2001;7:55–58.
9. Turner TT. Varicocele: Still an enigma. J Urol 1983;129:695–699.
10. Shafik A, Moftah A, Olfat S, et al. Testicular veins: anatomy and role in varicocelogenesis and other pathologic conditions. Urology 1990;35:175–182.
11. Braedel HU, Steffens J, Ziegler M, et al. A possible ontogenic etiology for idiopathic left varicocele. J Urol 1994;151:62-66.
12. Macleod J, Hotchkiss RS. The effect of hyperpyrexia upon spermatozoa counts in men. Endokrinologie 1941;28:780–782.
13. Zorgniotti AW, Macleod J. Studies in temperature, human semen quality, and varicocele. Fertil Steril 1973;24:854–863.
14. Goldstein M, Eid J. Elevation of intratesticular and scrotal skin surface temperature in men with varicoceles. J Urol 1989;142:743–745.
15. Yin Y, Hawkins KL, deWolf WC, et al. Heat causes stress testicular germ cell apoptosis in adult mice. J Androl 1997;18:159–165.
16. Fujisawa M, Yoshida S, Kojima K, et al. Biochemical changes in testicular varicocele. Arch Androl 1989;22:149–159.
17. Nishiyama H, Danno S, Kanneko Y, et al. Decreased expression of cold induced RNA-binding proteins (CIRP) in male germ cells at elevated temperature. Am J Pathol 1998;152: 289–296.
18. World Health Organization. The influence of varicocele on parameters of fertility in a large group of men presenting to infertility clinics. Fertil Steril 1992;74:1298–1202.
19. Hudson RW. Free sex steroid and sex hormone-binding globulin levels in oligospermic men with varicoceles. Fertil Steril 1996;66:299–304.
20. Swerdloff RS, Walsh PC. Pituitary and gonadal hormones in patients with varicoceles. Fertil Steril 1975;26:1006–1012.
21. Hudson RW, Crawford VA, McKay DE, et al. The gonadotropin response of men with varicoceles to a 4 hour infusion of gonadotropin-releasing hormone. Fertil Steril 1981;36:633–637.
22. Hudson RW, Perez-Murrero RA, Crawford VA, et al. Hormonal parameters of men with varicoceles before and after varicocelectomy. Fertil Steril 1985;43:905–910.
23. Segenreich E, Shnuley H, Singer R, et al. Andrological parameters in patients with varicoceles and fertility disorders treated by high ligation of the left spermatic vein. Int J Fertil 1986;31:200–203.
24. Su L, Goldstein M, Schlegel PN. The effects of varicocelectomy on serum testosterone levels in infertile men with varicoceles. J Urol 1995;154:1752–1755.
25. Schreck R, Rieber P, Baeuerle PA. Reactive oxygen intermediates as apparently widely used messengers in the activation of NF-kappa β transcription factor and HIV-1. EMBO J 1991; 10:2247–2258.
26. Sharma RK, Pasqualotto FF, Nelson DR. The reactive oxygen species-total antioxidant capacity (ROS-TAC) score is a new measure of oxidative stress to predict male infertility. Hum Reprod 1999;14:2801–2807.
27. Hendin BN, Kollettis PN, Sharma RK, et al. Varicocele is associated with elevated spermatozoal reactive oxygen species production and diminished seminal plasma antioxidant capacity. J Urol 1999;161:1831–1834.
28. Ahlberg NE, Bartley O, Chideckel N. Retrograde contrast filling of the left gonadal vein. ACTA Radid Diag 1965;3:385–392.

29. Fujisawa M, Yoshida S, Matsumoto O, et al. Decrease of topisomerase I activity in the testis of infertile men with varicocele. Arch Androl 1988;21:45–50.
30. Fujisawa M, Matsumoto O, Kamidono S, et al. Changes of enzymes involved in DNA synthesis in the testis of cryptorchid rats. J Reprod Fertil 1988;84:123–130.
31. Benoff S, Hurley IR, Barcia M, et al. A potential role for cadmium in the etiology of varicocele-associated infertility. Fertil Steril 1997;67:336–347.
32. Cayan S, Lee D, Black LD, et al. Response to varicocelectomy in oligospermic men with and without defined genetic infertility. Urology 2001;57:530–535.
33. Fretz PC, Sandlow JI. Varicocele: Current concepts and pathophysiology, diagnosis and treatment. Urol Clin N Am 2002;29:921–937.
34. Cayan S, Erdemir F, Ozbey I, et al. Can varicocelectomy significantly change the way couples use assisted reproductive technologies? J Urol 2002;167:1749–1756.
35. Pryor JL, Howards SS. Varicocele. Urol Clin North Am. 1987;14:499–513.
36. Madgar I, Korasik A, Weissenberg R, et al. Controlled trial of high spermatic vein ligation for varicocele in infertile men. Fertil Steril 1995;63:120–124.
37. Nieschlag E, Hertle L, Fischedick A, et al. Update on treatment of varicocele: counseling as effective as occlusion of the vena spermatica. Hum Reprod 1998;13:2147–2150.
38. Kamischke A, Nieschlag E. Varicocele treatment in the light of evidence-based andrology. Hum Reprod Update 2001;7:65–69.
39. Evers JLH, Collins JA. Assessment of efficacy of varicocele repair for male subfertility: a systematic review. Lancet 2003;361:1849–1852.
40. Schlegel PN. Is assisted reproduction the optimal treatment for varicocele-associated male infertility? A cost-effectiveness analysis. Urology 1997;49:83–90.

11 Strategic Therapies for Ejaculatory Disorders and Erectile Dysfunction in the Infertile Man

Mustafa F. Usta, MD
and Wayne J. G. Hellstrom, MD, FACS

CONTENTS

INTRODUCTION

Although ejaculatory disorders and erectile dysfunction (ED) are rare causes of male infertility, these conditions may challenge both the couples' determination and physicians' ingenuity. Dubin and Amelar reported that 2% of men presenting for infertility evaluation are diagnosed with ejaculatory dysfunction *(1)*, many of which require specialized treatment *(2,3)*. The spectrum of clinical presentations includes premature ejaculation, retarded ejaculation, anejaculation, and retrograde ejaculation. Premature ejaculation is the most common ejaculatory dysfunction, affecting up to 70% of normal men at some point in their active sexual life *(2,3)*. ED, defined as the inability to attain or maintain penile erection for satisfactory sexual intercourse, is a global health problem with increasing recognition *(4)*. Men who suffer from ED and infertility can be more difficult to treat than men who suffer from either condition alone.

This chapter reviews the normal anatomy and physiology of ejaculation, categorization of ejaculatory dysfunction, and treatment options. Additionally, options for patients with infertility and ED are presented.

From: *Contemporary Endocrinology: Office Andrology*
Edited by: P. E. Patton and D. E. Battaglia © Humana Press Inc., Totowa, NJ

EJACULATORY DISORDERS

Physiology of Ejaculation

Normal antegrade ejaculation involves three basic, distinct, and coordinated events identified as: (1) emission of sperm, (2) forceful ejaculation of semen through urethra, and (3) orgasm *(3)*.

Although the same sympathetic nerves principally control these three different phases, they are distinct from each other *(5)*. Seminal emission consists of two actions: (1) reflex activity from the thoracolumbar sympathetic nerves, causing the simultaneous contraction of smooth muscle cells in the testicular tubules, efferent ducts, epididymis, and vas deferens; and (2) seminal fluid deposition into the posterior urethra by rhythmic contractions of the seminal vesicles and prostate.

At the time of emission, the bladder neck closes simultaneously to prevent retrograde ejaculation of seminal fluid into the bladder *(3,4)*. After seminal fluid is deposited into the posterior urethra, reflex pathways stimulate the pelvic floor (bulbospongiosus and ischiocavernous somatic muscles, smooth muscles of the vas deferens, ejaculatory ducts, proximal urethra, and bladder neck) to collaborate actively in producing an ejaculation *(3,4)*. The subjective, perceptual-cognitive event of pleasure, defined as orgasm, occurs concomitantly but is distinct from ejaculation *(3)*.

Diagnosis and Evaluation of Ejaculatory Dysfunction

An accurate history is vitally important in making the diagnosis of an ejaculatory disorder. History details the chief complaint, as many patients cannot differentiate ejaculatory disorders from ED. Various genitourinary surgeries and traumas, such as spinal cord injury (SCI), retroperitoneal lymph node dissection (RPLND), and Y-V plasty of the bladder neck, are directly responsible for ejaculatory disorders *(6)*. Additionally, history of genitourinary infections and all medications associated with ejaculatory disorders need to be carefully tabulated. An astute physician carefully distinguishes information regarding sexual function, ejaculation, and orgasm. Some men have never experienced orgasm, whereas others may relate a progressive loss in the amount of ejaculate that leads to a dry ejaculate. Cloudy urine after a sensation of orgasm suggests retrograde ejaculation. Reviewing systems may provide important clues. For example, the development of peripheral neuropathy or vasculopathy in a diabetic patient will increase the suspicion of an ejaculatory disorder as the cause for male factor infertility.

The physical examination naturally measures the size and consistency of the testicles, epididymidis, and presence of vas deferens. Rare presentations include sparse body and facial hair. Semen analysis is a cornerstone in the diagnosis of ejaculatory dysfunction, and semen volume is the most important initial implication to the existence of an ejaculatory disorder. Although a low-semen volume can be caused by inadequate abstinence, it usually suggests some form of pathology, e.g., aplasia or obstruction of the seminal vesicles. A fructose-negative or low-pH semen sample further supports this suspicion. Levels of serum testosterone, follicle-stimulating hormone (FSH), and luteinizing hormone (LH) are obtained in these cases as some instances of hypogonadism have low-volume ejaculates. A centrifuged postejaculatory urine sample easily differentiates retrograde ejaculation from anejaculation.

If ejaculatory duct obstruction is suspected, transrectal ultrasonography can identify seminal vesicle and ejaculatory duct dilatation, Wolfian or Mullerian duct cysts, prostatic stones, and calcifications *(6)*.

Causes and Treatment of Ejaculatory Disorders

Premature Ejaculation. Premature ejaculation (PE) is the most common male sexual disorder with an estimated prevalence of 30 to 70% *(2)*. Historically, PE was believed to be psychogenic in origin, originating from performance anxiety, fear, psychological trauma, or marital discord *(3)*. Recent data suggest an organic basis *(7)*. Metz and Pryor distinguished several subtypes of biogenic and psychogenic PE. Physiological PE derives from: (1) abnormal neurological constitution, (2) acute physical illness, (3) physical injury, and (4) pharmacological-based side effects. Psychological PE is caused by: (1) altered psychological constitution, (2) acute psychological distress, (3) relationship discord, and (4) deficit in psychosexual skills *(8)*. Although active research and development in this area are ongoing, the exact cause and definition of this condition have yet to be established.

Historically, Masters and Johnson described PE according to qualitative descriptions, such as female partner satisfaction and male voluntary control *(9,10)*. They defined PE as the inability of the male partner to inhibit ejaculation long enough for the female partner to reach orgasm in 50% of intercourse attempts *(9,10)*. Others have defined PE by quantitative measures, specifically the intravaginal latency time or number of thrusts before ejaculation. The literature varies in defining the normal time between vaginal entry and ejaculation from 1 to 7 min *(11–14)*. Other researchers have focused on the number of thrusts as a criterion for PE, with anywhere between 8 to 15 thrusts before ejaculation regarded as normal *(15)*. The difficulty in establishing a uniform definition has hindered progress in this area of sexual medicine. Nevertheless, a good history and physician intuition can easily identify PE as an etiology of infertility.

Treatment Interventions. Early treatments for PE were behavioral in nature and included the "pause squeeze" technique and "stop–start" method *(3)*. Fein reported successful intercourse (100%) using intracavernosal self-injections with vasoactive agents in eight patients suffering from PE and with an underlying psychogenic origin of performance anxiety *(16)*. This method can be especially effective in the 5% of PE men who ejaculate prior to vaginal entry.

Various drugs can delay or eliminate ejaculation and affect orgasm as well. These include antiandrogens, monoamine oxidase inhibitors, tricyclic and serotoninergic antidepressants. Double-blind placebo-controlled studies with clomipramine and other selective serotonin reuptake inhibitors have demonstrated efficacy *(17)*. Waldinger et al. compared fluoxetine, fluvoxamine, paroxetine, and sertraline in treating rapid ejaculation and reported that paroxetine caused the longest delay in ejaculation *(18)*.

In 46 potent men with PE, McMahon showed that sertraline hydrochloride in doses of 25, 50, and 100 mg increased the mean ejaculatory interval to 7.6, 13.1, and 16.4 min, respectively. The most commonly encountered side effect of this treatment was anejaculation, which occurred in 4 (50 mg) and 10 patients (100 mg), respectively *(19)*.

Chen et al. recently demonstrated the efficacy of sildenafil as an adjuvant therapy to paroxetine in patients with PE. Sildenafil in combination with paroxetine and psychological counseling alleviated PE in patients in whom other modalities had failed *(20)*. Another study showed that paroxetine combined with sildenafil provided better results in terms of ejaculatory latency time and intercourse satisfaction than paroxetine alone in patients with PE *(21)*. Althof reported that clomipramine was highly effective in increasing the ejaculation latency periods and improving the sexual and relationship satisfaction in men with PE *(22)* (Table 1).

Sexual satisfaction (SS)-cream is an Asian topical agent made from the extracts of nine natural products. The cream is applied to the glans penis 1 h before sexual intercourse and has been shown in controlled double-blind studies to delay ejaculatory latency and improve sexual satisfaction. However, mild local pain and burning were noted side effects *(23,24)*. More importantly, the concern over possible teratogenic effects of such agents on the gametes of these infertile patients makes this option less favorable.

Idiopathic Anejaculation. Idiopathic anorgasmia is defined as the inhibition of the ejaculatory reflex, with absent or reduced seminal emission, impaired ejaculatory contractions, and lost orgasm *(3)*. This condition is not common and thought to have a psychological basis. History usually makes the diagnosis obvious. Important issues include medical history, neurological pathologies, and the use of specific medications. Psychological etiologies range from strict religious background, lack of spousal attraction, psychologic trauma, and underlying homosexuality *(3)*. In men with a psychological etiology, ejaculation during masturbation is often normal. Treatment of psychogenic anejaculation is centered on psychotherapy. If this option fails, collection of the ejaculate for assisted reproductive technology (ART) purposes can be obtained using a condom, some-

Table 1
Oral Medical Therapies for Premature/Rapid Ejaculation

Nonselective Serotonin Reuptake Inhibitor		
Clomipramine	Anafranil	25–50 mg/d or 25 mg 4–24 h prior
Selective Serotonin Reuptake Inhibitors		
Fluoxetine	Prozac, Sarafem	5–20 mg/d
Paroxetine	Paxil	10, 20, 40 mg/d or 20 mg 3–4 h prior
Setraline	Zoloft	10, 20, 40 mg/d or 20 mg 3–4 h prior

Table 2
Drugs Affecting Ejaculation

Antiandrogens	Fluvoxamine	Parglyline
Alprozolam	Guanedrel	Paroxetine
Aminocaproicacid	Guanethidine	Perphenazine
Amitriptiline	Haloperidol	Phenelzine
Amoxapine	Imipramine	Phenoxibenzamine
Alcohol	Iproniazid	Prazosin
Butaperazine	Izocarboxazid	Phentolamine
Baclofen	Labethanol	Reserpine
Chlorpromazine	Lorazepam	Sertraline
Chlorprothixine	Mebanizine	Thiroidazine
Clomipramine	Mesoridazine	Trazodone
Chlordiazepoxide	Methyldopa	Trifluoperazine
Citalopram	Methadone	Terazosin
Desmethylimipramine	Naproxen	Thiazides
Fluoxetine		

Source: refs. *3* and *34*.

times with the assistance of penile vibratory stimulation or electroejaculation *(25–28)*.

Primary anejaculation with intact orgasm can be caused by congenital abnormalities, such as Mullerian duct cyst, Wolfian duct abnormalities, bladder neck incompetence, or hypogonadism *(29)*. Secondary anejaculation is often related to drug therapy (Table 2), neurological disease, surgery, congenital abnormalities, psychological problems, and complications from infections or stones in the genitourinary tract. Local inflammation from chronic urinary tract catheterization can cause scarring and ejaculatory duct obstruction *(6)*.

Congenital ejaculatory duct cysts can be remedied by transurethral resection *(30)*. With bilateral absence of the vas deferens in men with Wolfian duct abnormalities, sperm retrieval from the epididymis or testis is an option *(6)*. If hypogonadism is the cause, testosterone replacement therapy can be administered. In cases with anejaculation secondary to medications, the drug dose can be reduced or withdrawn. Anejaculation cases that do not respond to medical therapy are also candidates for ejaculation induction procedures, e.g., penile vibratory stimulation and/or electroejaculation.

Retrograde Ejaculation. The inability of the bladder neck to close during the ejaculation process causes retrograde ejaculation (RE). Transurethral or open prostatectomy and Y-V plasty of the bladder are well-recognized surgical causes of RE *(31,32)*. Medical causes of RE include α-blockers, such as doxazosin, terazosin, and tamsulosin, which are used for the treatment of benign prostatic hyperplasia *(33)*. Discontinuation of these drugs will resolve the ejaculatory disorder.

RE can be converted to antegrade using medical options. Initial treatments include sympathomimetic agents. Drugs commonly used are ephedrine, phenylpropanolamine, and tricyclic antidepressants. Men who do not respond to medical intervention must be considered for sperm retrieval and ART. Catheterization empties the bladder and filled with a sperm-friendly medium (e.g., HAMS-F-10). The patient then masturbates to climax, and the sperm is harvested for ART—artificial insemination, in vitro fertilization (IVF), or intracytoplasmic sperm injection (ICSI).

Absence of Seminal Emission. Absence of seminal emission is commonly seen in patients who have SCI, diabetic neuropathy, or history of retroperitoneal lymph node dissection for testis cancer. Although diabetic patients have concurrent anorgasmia, orgasm is usually maintained in patients with a previous history of retroperitoneal surgery. Other conditions that can cause complete or partial absence of emission include abdominal vascular surgery, pelvic or colorectal surgeries, sympathectomies, and neurologic diseases, such as multiple sclerosis *(34)*. Patients should undergo a trial of α-sympathomimetic drug therapy before moving to surgical retrieval and more advanced ART procedures, such as IVF and/or ICSI therapies *(34)*.

ERECTILE DYSFUNCTION

ED, the inability to attain or maintain sufficient penile erection for satisfactory sexual intercourse, is estimated to affect 20 to 30 million men in the United States *(4)*. A few decades ago, ED was believed to be caused by nonspecific psychological causes. However, extensive research has demonstrated that organic etiologies are present in 50 to 80% of affected men *(35)*. The treatment algorithm for patients with ED is the same as those for men who have concomitant infertility. A step-care approach to ED treatment ranges from the least invasive methods to more invasive surgical management.

Physiology of Erection

Recent studies using molecular biological techniques have given researchers many insights into erectile physiology. Most research has focused on the peripheral mechanism of corpus cavernosum smooth muscle relaxation *(36–38)*. The principal neurotransmitter mediating the relaxation of cavernosal smooth muscle and penile erection is nitric oxide (NO). NO is synthesized from the substrate L-arginine by the catalytic activity of the enzyme nitric oxide synthase. NO interacts with the soluble form of guanylate cyclase to increase intracellular cyclic guanosine monophosphate (cGMP) levels. The increase in cGMP induces smooth muscle relaxation, primarily through the activation of cGMP-dependent protein kinase, which increases K^+ channel activity and decreases intracellular Ca^{2+} concentrations *(39,40)*.

Diagnosis and Evaluation of Erectile Dysfunction

Clinical evaluation of ED includes a detailed sexual history with special attention to recognized comorbidities, a thorough physical examination, and a limited number of laboratory tests. Attention should be given to the man's sexual desire and ejaculatory function. The onset and duration of ED, surrounding events, frequency of sexual intercourse, and the complete inventory of sexual partners need to be carefully assessed.

Therapy of Erectile Dysfunction

Therapeutic options for ED have changed dramatically in the last three decades. In the 1960s, psychotherapy was the primary treatment modality. Surgery introduced many urologists to the field of sexual medicine in the 1970s *(41,42)*. Evolution to effective medical therapies has involved many clinical subspecialties and primary care physicians into the treatment of ED *(43)*.

First-Line Therapy

PDE5 Inhibitors. First-line treatment of ED is a phosphodiesterase type 5 (PDE5) inhibitor, such as sildenafil (Viagra; US Pharmaceutical Group, New York, NY) *(44)*. Sildenafil is an orally active and selective inhibitor of cGMP-specific PDE5. Sildenafil increases cavernosal cGMP levels, which enhances smooth muscle relaxation, and penile erection *(45)*. Sildenafil potentiates the hypotensive effects of nitrates and, for this reason, is contraindicated in patients who use organic nitrates *(46)*. Since 1998, more than 20 million men have been prescribed sildenafil *(47)*. In long-term follow-up studies at 1 yr ($n = 2482$), 2 yr ($n = 900$), and 3 yr ($n = 245$), more than 95% of men had improved their erections and ability to engage in sexual activity *(42)*. The most commonly reported side effects with sildenafil include headache, flushing, nasal congestion, dyspepsia, abnormal vision, diarrhea, and dizziness *(48)*.

Second-Line Therapy

When first-line therapies fail or are contraindicated, intracavernosal and intraurethral vasoactive medications are important second-line treatment options. In this area, the use of topical vasoactive agents continues to evolve *(49)*. For thoroughness, vacuum constriction devices (VCD) are considered as another first- or second-line treatment options, but semen is trapped by the constricting penile ring, making its use in infertility cases somewhat problematic.

Drugs for Intracavernosal Injection

Papaverine. Papaverine hydrochloride was the first vasoactive agent used for intracavernosal self-injection. It is a nonspecific phosphodiesterase inhibitor, which causes an increase in intracellular cyclic adenosine monophosphate (cAMP) and cGMP, resulting in excellent smooth muscle relaxation and penile erection *(49)*. Side effects included prolonged erections in 14% of patients, priapism in 4%, and corporal fibrosis *(50)*.

Papaverine and Phentolamine. Combination of papaverine hydrochloride and phentolamine mesylate increased success rates for intracavernosal pharmacologic erections *(50)*. Several studies have documented that papaverine/phentolamine combination therapy has high success rates with fewer side effects *(49)*.

Prostaglandin E1. In the penile tissue, PGE1 increases cAMP levels by modulating adenyl cyclase. This causes a decrease in intracellular-free calcium, which induces cavernosal smooth muscle relaxation and penile erection *(42)*. The clinical investigation by the Alprostadil Study Group demonstrated that 87% of injections in 683 men resulted in an erection suitable for sexual intercourse *(51)*. Prolonged erections occurred in 5%, priapism occurred in 1%, and penile fibrosis developed in 2% of participants.

"Trimix" Combinations. Combination therapy using a mixture of papaverine, phentolamine, and PGE1 is a popular modality because of its high efficacy, low incidence of pain, and relatively low cost. In a crossover study, McMahon compared PGE1 alone with the three-drug mixture in 228 ED patients. Trimix treatment is particularly valuable in men with severe ED, such as combined arterial insufficiency and venous leak *(52)*.

Drugs for Intraurethral Therapy

Although intracavernosal injection of vasoactive agents is a very beneficial treatment modality for ED, long-term follow-up reveals a high dropout rate *(51)*. Transurethral drug administration allows for the transfer of vasoactive agents directly into the corpora cavernosa via vascular communications from the spongiosa to the cavernosa. Intraurethral alprostadil has been developed and marketed by VIVUS (Menlo Park, CA). The medicated transurethral system for erection, is available in four dosage strengths: 125, 250, 500, and 1000 μg *(49)*.

The most common side effects of intraurethral alprostadil are local pain (29–41%), urethral bleeding (4–5.5%), dizziness (1.9–14%), and urinary tract infection (0–0.2%) *(49)*.

Effects of Drugs Used for Erectile Dysfunction on Human Sperm Function

Several drugs can enter into the seminal fluid, where they may theoretically have direct effects on sperm function. Because sperm motility is associated with fertilization, drugs that affect motility may affect fertility. It has been reported that PDE inhibitors have the potential to increase sperm motility. Lefievre et al. reported that sildenafil triggers human sperm motility and capacitation, likely via the inhibition of PDE activity other than PDE5, resulting in increased cAMP levels *(52)*. However, Burger et al. reported that sildenafil (125, 250, and 750 ng/mL) had no significant effect on sperm motility, viability, membrane integrity, or sperm penetration characteristics in human spermatozoa from normal and infertile men *(53)*.

Although the 200 μg/mL dose of sildenafil had no effect on sperm motility, Andrade et al. demonstrated that 2000 μg/mL significantly reduced sperm motility by approximately 50%. Similarly, these authors reported that phentolamine had no effect on sperm motility at a low dose of 20 μg/mL, whereas a higher dose of 200 μg/mL caused a significant reduction in sperm motility *(54)*. Recent randomized placebo-controlled studies in 421 men showed that chronic daily administration of tadalafil at doses of 10 and 20 mg for 6 mo had no adverse effects on spermatogenesis or reproductive hormones (serum testosterone, LH, and FSH) *(55)*.

Another study demonstrated that neither alprostadil nor prazosin at doses used in transurethral therapy of ED had any effect on sperm motility, viability, or membrane integrity *(56)*.

Vacuum Constriction Devices

VCDs have been used for the nonsurgical treatment of ED. Numerous authors have reported their results in patients suffering from a variety of medical conditions. VCD therapy is appropriate for nearly all patients with ED *(57,58)*, with the exception of those with bleeding disorders, on anticoagulant therapy, or with a history of priapism. VCD treatment is especially beneficial in patients who partially respond to intracavernosal injection therapy. Oral medications are highly effective, but the VCD still remains a preferred treatment option for a significant number of patients with ED. In a recent study, 52 patients with ED achieving satisfactory erectile function with VCDs were switched to sildenafil treatment. At the completion of this study, 33.3% of patients who had satisfactory erections with both VCD and sildenafil preferred to continue with VCD treatment *(59)*.

Third-Line Therapy

Penile Prosthesis. Whereas first- and second-line treatment options for ED have significantly improved, men who fail to respond to these approaches may be considered for surgical treatment. Patients with severe ED, especially with comorbidities, such as diabetes, hypertension, hyperlipidemia or history of radical pelvic surgery, are the most common candidates for penile prosthesis implantation *(42)*. In a recent study, Rajpurkar and Dhabuwala reported that at a mean follow-up of 19 mo patients who underwent penile implant surgery had significantly better erectile function and treatment satisfaction than those receiving sildenafil citrate and intracavernous PGE1 therapy *(44)*.

SUMMARY

Ejaculation is a complex and integrated process that involves the coordination of neurologic, anatomic, and psychologic events. Ejaculatory dysfunction is a rare cause of infertility. To properly evaluate and manage such patients, the normal ejaculatory mechanism must be well-understood by treating clinicians. Stepwise assessment allows for the identification of the source of ejaculatory dysfunction in most cases. In certain circumstances, ejaculation induction procedures combined with ART can provide successful conception.

PE is the most common ejaculatory dysfunction. Over the last decade, neurobiological research has provided new insights into the mechanisms responsible for PE. Although cognitive and emotional factors can influence ejaculation, most current approaches involve pharmaceutical agents. Both paroxetine and clomipramine have proven to be valuable in the treatment of PE. Further research and development of new drugs will bring further benefit to patients afflicted with this common problem.

The treatment algorithm of the infertile man with concomitant ED is similar to those with ED alone. Oral treatment with PDE5 inhibitors (that have shown no deleterious effects on semen parameters) remains to be first-line therapy for men with both infertility and ED. More severe ED cases require more invasive methods. Creative approaches are sometimes needed in extreme cases of infertility, ejaculatory dysfunction, and ED. Newer technologies can provide many alternatives for success.

REFERENCES

1. Dubin L, Amelar RD. Etiologic factors in 1294 consecutive cases of male infertility. Fertil Steril 1971;22:469–474.
2. McMahon CG, Samali R. Pharmacological treatment of premature ejaculation. Curr Opin Urol 1999;9:553–561.
3. Jannini EA, Simonelli C, Lenzi A. Disorders of ejaculation. J Endocrinol Invest 2002;25:1006–1019.

4. Feldman HA, Goldstein I, Hatzichristou DG, et al. Impotence and its medical psychosocial correlates: results of the Massachusetts male aging study. J Urol 1994;151:54–61.
5. Newman HF, Reiss H, Northrup JD. Physical basis of emission, ejaculation, and orgasm in the male. Urology 1991;19:341–350.
6. Schuster TG, Ohl DA. Diagnosis and treatment of ejaculatory dysfunction. Urol Clin N Am 2002;29:939–948.
7. Screponi E, Carosa E, DrStasi SM, et al. Prevalence of chronic prostatitis in men with premature ejaculation. Urology 2001;58:198–202.
8. Metz ME, Pryor JL. Premature ejaculation: a psychophysiological approach for assessment and management. J Sex Marital Ther 2000;26:293–320.
9. Masters WH, Johnson VE. Human sexual inadequacy. Little, Brown & Co., Boston, MA, 1970.
10. Waldinger MD. The neurobiological approach to premature ejaculation. J Urol 2002;168: 2359–2367.
11. Cooper A, Magnus R. A clinical trial of the beta blocker propranolol in premature ejaculation. J Psychsom Res 1984;28:331–336.
12. Spiess WF, Geer JH, O'Donohue WT. Premature ejaculation: investigation of factors in ejaculatory latency. J Abnorm Psychol 1984;93:242–245.
13. Strassberg GS, Mahoney JM, Schaugaard M, Hale VE. The role of anxiety in premature ejaculation: a psychophysiological model. Arch Sex Behav 1990;19:251–258.
14. Shover LR, Friedman JM, Weiler SJ, et al. Multiaxial problem-oriented system for sexual dysfunction. Arch Gen Psych 1982;39:614–619.
15. Colpi GM, Fanciulacci F, Beratta G, et al. Evoked sacral potentials in subjects with true premature ejaculation. Andrologia 1986;18:583–586.
16. Fein RL. Intracavernous medication for treatment of premature ejaculation. Urology 1990;35: 301–303.
17. Seftel AD, Althof SE. Rapid ejaculation. Curr Urol Rep 2000;1:302–306.
18. Waldinger MD, Hengeveld MW, Zwinderman AH, Olivier B. Effect of SSRI antidepressants on ejaculation: a double-blind, randomized, placebo-controlled study with fluoxetine, fluvoxamine, paroxetine, and sertraline. J Clin Psychopharmacol 1998;18:274–281.
19. McMahon CG. Treatment of premature ejaculation with sertraline hydrochloride. Int J Imp Res 1998;10:181–184.
20. Chen J, Mabjeesh NJ, Matzkin H, et al. Efficacy of sildenafil as adjuvant therapy to selective serotonine reuptake inhibitor in alleviating premature ejaculation. Urology 2003;61:197–200.
21. Salonia A, Maga T, Colombo R, et al. A prospective study comparing paroxetine alone versus paroxetine plus sildenafil in patients with premature ejaculation. J Urol 2002;168:2486–2489.
22. Althof SE, Levine EB, Corty EW, et al. A double-blind crossover trial of clomipramine for rapid ejaculation in 15 couples. J Clin Psychiatry 1995;56:402–407.
23. Choi HK, Jung GW, Moon KH, et al. Clinical study of SS-cream in patients with lifelong premature ejaculation. Urology 2000;55:257–261.
24. Choi HK, Xin ZC, Choi YD, et al. Safety and efficacy study with various doses of SS-cream in patients with premature ejaculation in a double-blind, randomized, placebo controlled clinical study. Int J Imp Res 1999;11:261–264.
25. Hovav Y, Kafka I, Horenstein E, et al. Prostaticmassage as a method for obtaining spermatozoa in men with psychogenic anejaculation. Fertil Steril 2000;74:184,185.
26. Okada H, Fujisawa M, Koshida M, et al. Ampullary, seminal vesicular, and prostatic massage for obtaining spermatozoa from patients with anejaculation. Fertil Steril 2001;75:1236,1237.
27. Wheeler Jr JS, Walter JS, Culkin DJ, et al. Idiopathic anejaculation treated by vibratory stimulation. Fertil Steril 1998;50:377–379.

28. Denil J, Kupker W, Al-Hasani S, et al. Succesful combination of transrectal ejaculation and intracytoplasmic sperm injection in the treatment of anejaculation. Hum Reprod 1996;11: 1247–1249.
29. Thompson S, Honig S, Lipschultz LI. Sexual and ejaculatory dysfunction as a cause of male infertility. In: Infertility Evaluation and Treatment. Keye W, Rebar R, Chang R, Soules M, eds. WB Saunders, Philadelphia, PA, 1995, pp. 671–685.
30. Pryor JP, Hendry WF. Ejaculatory duct obstruction in subfertile males: analysis of 87 patients. Fertil Steril 1991;56:725–730.
31. Dunsmir WD, Emberton. There is a significant sexual dysfunction following TURP. Br J Urol 1999;22(Suppl. 1):39,40.
32. Ochsner MG, Burns E, Henry HH. Incidence of retrograde ejaculation following bladder neck revision as a child. J Urol 1970;104;596–597.
33. Debruyne FM. Alpha blockers: are all created equal? Urology 2000;56(Suppl):20–22.
34. McCullough AR. Ejaculatory disorders. In: Mulcahy JJ, ed. Male Sexual Function. Humana Press Inc., Totowa, New Jersey, 2001, pp. 351–370.
35. Bivalacqua TJ, Champion HC, Hellstrom WJG, Kadowitz PJ. Pharmacotherapy for erectile dysfunction. Trends Pharmacol Sci 2000;21:484–489.
36. Nehra A. Intracavernosal therapy: when oral agents fail. Curr Urol Rep 2001;2:468–472.
37. Saenz de Tejada I. In the physiology of erection, signposts to impotence. Contemp Urol 1992; 7:52–68.
38. Andersson KE, Wagner G. Physiology of erection. Physiol Rev 1995;75:191–236.
39. Burnett AL, Lowenstein CJ, Bredt DS, et al. Nitric oxide: a physiologic mediator of penile erection. Science 1992;257:401–403.
40. Rajfer J, Aronson WJ, Bush PA, et al. Nitric oxide as a mediator of relaxation of the corpus cavernosum in response to nonadrenergic, noncholinergic neurotransmission. N Engl J Med 1992;326:90–94.
41. Mulhall JP. Deciphering erectile dysfunction drug trials. J Urol 2003;170:353–358.
42. Rajpurkar A, Dhabuwala CB. Comparison of satisfaction rates and erectile function in patients treated with sildenafil, intracavernous prostaglandin E1 and penile implant surgery for erectile dysfunction in urology practice. J Urol 2003;170:159–163.
43. Kloner RA. Erectile dysfunction and cardiovascular risk factors. Hosp Prac 2001;36:41–51.
44. Padma-Nathan H, Giuliano F. Oral drug therapy for erectile dysfunction. Urol Clin North Am 2001;28:321–334.
45. Wysowski DK, Swann J. Use of medications for erectile dysfunction in the United States, 1986 through 2001. J Urol 2003;169:1040–1042.
46. Shabsigh R, Anastasiadis G. Erectile dysfunction. Annu Rev Med 2003;54:153–168.
47. Morales A, Gingell C, Collins M, et al. Clinical safety of oral sildenafil citrate (VIAGRA) in the treatment of erectile dysfunction. Int J Imp Res 1998;10:69–73.
48. Leugwattanakij S, Flynn V, Hellstrom WJG. Intracavernosal injection and intraurethral therapy for erectile dysfunction. Urol Clin North Am 2001;28:343–354.
49. Buvat J, Lemaire A, Marcolin G, et al. Intracavernous injection of papaverine: assessment of its diagnostic and therapeutic value in 100 impotent patients. World J Urol 1987;5:150.
50. Porst H. The rationale for prostaglandin E1 in erectile failure: a survey of worldwide experience. J Urol 1996;155:802–815.
51. McMahon CG. A comparison of the response to the intracavernosal injection of a combination of papaverine and phentolamine, prostaglandin E1, and a combination of all three agents in the management of impotence. Int J Imp Res 1991;3:113.

52. Lefievre L, De Lamirande E, Gagnon C. The cyclic GMP-specific phosphodiesterase inhibitor, sildenafil, stimulates human sperm motility and capacitation but not acrosome reaction. J Androl 2000;21:929–937.
53. Burger M, Sikka SC, Bivalacqua TJ, et al. The effect of sildenafil on human sperm motion and function from normal and infertile men. Int J Imp Res 2000;12:229–234.
54. Andrade JR, Traboulsi A, Hussain A, Dubin N. In vitro effects of sildenafil and phentolamine, drugs used for erectile dysfunction, on human sperm motility. Am J Obstet Gynecol 2000;182: 1093–1095.
55. Hellstrom WJG, Overstreet JW, Yu A, et al. Tadalafil has no detrimental effect on human spermatogenesis or reproductive hormones. J Urol 2003, in press.
56. Hellstrom WJG, Wang R, Peterson CA, et al. Effects of alprostadil and prazosin on motility, viability and membrane integrity of human sperm. J Urol 1998;159:1559–1562.
57. Cookson MS, Nadig PW. Long term results with vacuum constriction device. J Urol 1993; 149:290–294.
58. Vrijhof HJEJ, Delaere KPJ. Vacom constriction devices in erectile dysfunction: acceptance and effectiveness in patients with impotence of organic and mixed etiology. Br J Urol 1994;74: 102–105.
59. Chen J, Mabjeesh NJ, Greenstein A. Sildenafil versus the vacuum erection device: patient preference. J Urol 2001;166:1779–1781.

12 Vasectomy Reversal

Eugene F. Fuchs, MD
and Darius A. Paduch, MD PhD

Contents

1. INTRODUCTION

Every year in the United States, approx 500,000 men undergo vasectomy as a form of permanent birth control. Although this may seem a large number, in the early 1970s, more than 700,000 men had the procedure annually *(1)*. The vast majority of men choose vasectomy to limit the size of their families because when compared to a tubal ligation, it is an easier procedure and less expensive. A small fraction of this population will choose vasectomy while still single and before ever having children. Another subset will select vasectomy after marriage but before having children because the couple never intends to have children. It is estimated that as many as 3 to 5% of men who have had a vasectomy will later seek consultation to consider a vasectomy reversal for procreation. A few men will consider a vasectomy reversal to treat chronic postvasectomy pain.

In 1830, Sir Ashley Cooper reported that transection of the vas deferens of the dog would not, as then believed, result in testicular atrophy but would interrupt the flow of spermatozoa into the ejaculate *(2)*. His observations set the stage for the future use of vasectomy as a form of permanent birth control.

Human vasectomy as practiced today evolved from the Eugenics movement of the late 1800s and early to mid-1900s. The first report of vasectomy in humans appeared in US literature in 1899 when Ochnser reported performing vasectomy on two male inmates at the Indiana Institute for the Criminally Insane *(3)*. His purpose was to prevent procreation by the mentally ill of what was then thought

From: *Contemporary Endocrinology: Office Andrology*
Edited by: P. E. Patton and D. E. Battaglia © Humana Press Inc., Totowa, NJ

to be a genetically transmitted illness. In 1909, Sharp expanded the concept and concluded that vasectomy also induced better behavior among the inmates *(4)*. Thousands of men were involuntarily subjected to vasectomy by the time all Eugenics sterilization laws were repealed in the early 1970s *(2)*.

V. J. O'Conor reported the first significant series of vasectomy reversals by vasovasostomy in 1948. He surveyed 750 North American urologists and found that 135 of them had performed 420 cases. The operation was considered a success in 160 men *(5)*. It is not clear in the study whether success was determined by pregnancy or the presence of sperm in the postoperative ejaculate. The work of O'Conor and others provided the foundation from which evolved modern microsurgical vasovasostomy.

In 1967, Phadke and Phadke reported a pregnancy rate of 55% in 73 patients who had undergone a macrosurgical vasovasostomy *(6)*. Other significant early series by Middleton and Schmidt reported pregnancy rates of 39% in 72 patients *(7)*, and 31% in 64 patients *(8)*, respectively. Pregnancy rates were not correlated to the interval of time from vasectomy or spousal/partner age—two factors now considered important in predicting success. The largest reported series by Amelar and Dubin using loupe magnification for vasovasostomy observed that 38% of 119 men achieved pregnancy *(9)*.

The modern era of microsurgical vasectomy reversal began in the mid-1970s with reports from Silber *(10)* and Owens *(11)* and others who found pregnancy rates as high as 71 and 79%, respectively. Silber's contributions cannot be overstated. He perfected the technique and popularized the procedure among male infertility specialists in the United States and even worldwide. His reported patency results were superior and set the standard to which we all aspire. Microsurgeons throughout the world recognize his commitment to perfecting the basic surgical technique that we all now use. He has also contributed significantly to the understanding of how the back pressure of the occluded vas deferens may adversely affect the patency and physiological function of the epididymis. Those observations led to the development of microsurgical epdidymovasostomy to bypass epididymal obstruction, which is caused by the back pressure changes in the epididymis *(12)*.

Most men seek consultation for vasectomy reversal because they are divorced and considering having another family with a new spouse/partner. They depend on their family physician or their spouse/partner's gynecologist for referral to a urologist. Perhaps just as frequently if not more, is using the Internet to research various aspects of vasectomy reversal and locate an experienced microsurgeon.

The demographic evaluation of more than 2200 vasectomy reversals performed by the senior author (EFF) indicates that the typical surgical candidate is 36 yr old and has had his vasectomy for 8.5 yr at the time of his vasectomy reversal. His spouse/partner is 5 yr younger (31 yr old) and as a rule has not had children. Roughly, 90% of men will have their vasectomy reversal before 10 yr has elapsed since vasectomy. Interestingly, 23% of our male cohort remained married to the same spouse when reversal was contemplated, and about 2% of men never had children prior to their vasectomy *(13)*.

A detailed description of the technical aspects of vasectomy reversal is beyond the scope of this text. Most experienced male fertility specialists use either a single- or double-layer microsurgical technique. Urological surgery literature and textbooks are replete with descriptions of the various surgical techniques for those interested. It is important to recognize that the need for more technically complicated epididymal bypass procedures increases as the elapsed time from vasectomy increases. In our series of more than 2200 procedures, we showed that only 3% of men required the epididymal bypass when the reversal was done within 4 yr of vasectomy. At 10 yr elapsed time, 40% required the bypass procedure, and at 20 yr, almost 70%. It can be argued that no surgeon should attempt a vasovasotomy when they are unable to perform an epididymal bypass.

All vasectomy reversals can be performed at an ambulatory surgical center as an outpatient procedure. Substantial cost can be saved by performing the procedure under moderate sedation and cord block anesthesia without the services of an anesthesiologist as we have done for many years *(14)*.

Postoperative recovery generally requires 1 wk off work. We ask our patients to wear an athletic supporter for 2 wk or longer when needed for comfort. Sexual activity is discouraged for 2 wk. There have been only few complications in our series of more than 2200 men. All men are started on a first-generation cephalosporin preoperatively and continued for 3 d postoperatively. Scrotal hematomas are the most frequent postoperative complication, but they rarely cause a significant problem other than persistent swelling for a few weeks.

We typically recommend a postoperative semen analysis at about 3 mo. When the sperm count and sperm motility are normal, we do not repeat the analysis unless the couple has not achieved pregnancy within 6 mo postoperatively. A repeat semen analysis a few months after the first is recommended when the initial sample is abnormal in any way. Pregnancy typically occurs within 6 to 8 mo but as early as 4 wk in rare cases. Overall, the pregnancy rate for this cohort was 61%.

About 8% of the men in our series never attempted to achieve pregnancy after the vasectomy reversal for a variety of reasons. Some men divorced and never attempted to sire a child or decided against having a child. Also included in this group are couples in which the female partner was found to be infertile. The time to pregnancy after vasectomy reversal is typically about 8 mo. Pregnancy does seem to occur more rapidly in couples that have had pregnancy together before the vasectomy reversal.

The increasing availability and success of sperm surgically extracted form the testicle for use with in vitro fertilization (IVF) and intracytoplasmic sperm injection (ICSI) for obstructive azoospermia provides additional options and, in many cases, more confusion for these couples. Many couples now inquire about what option will provide them with the best chance of conception. In most cases, but not all, cost is a major factor in their decision. The National Vasovasostomy Study Group in 1993 reported that the pregnancy rate after vasovasostomy declined as the elapsed time from vasectomy increased *(15)*. A pregnancy rate of 44% was achieved when the elapsed time since vasectomy was over 9 yr and 30% when longer than 15 yr. The study serves as the benchmark of success after vasectomy reversal because it represents the combined results of several experienced surgeons who represent a cohort of over 1469 patients who underwent vasectomy reversal by the 5 participants over the study period. Based on this report, and the assumption that IVF results were superior, some IVF centers began recommending IVF with ICSI with vasectomy-induced obstructive azoospermia when the male had a vasectomy for longer than 10 yr.

In 2001, we reported our series of vasectomy reversals in men who had their vasectomy for longer than 15 yr *(16)*. We correlated our pregnancy results to spousal/partner age and elapsed time since vasectomy. Overall, 66% of men achieved pregnancy when their spouse/partner was less than 30 yr old. When the spouse/partner was 40 or older, pregnancy was achieved in 20% of cases. Vasectomy was superior to IVF with ICSI for all groups except when the spouse was 40 or older, in which case IVF with ICSI and vasectomy reversal had comparable results. My personal experience with vasectomy reversal has shown that pregnancy typically occurs 6 to 8 or more months after vasectomy. This delay may be an important factor in determining which option to exercise, particularly when the female partner is older.

The significance of antisperm antibodies is controversial. In 1983, we published our findings that high levels of serum antisperm antibody were a significant deterrent to pregnancy *(17)*. The direct immunobead test (IBT) performed on freshly ejaculated sperm has now replaced serum testing. It is not known whether our previous findings (1983) using serum would carry over to men who test positive by the IBT. Subsequent reports by Kay et al. *(18)* and Meinerty et al. *(19)* have confirmed that finding antisperm antibody by IBT is associated with lower pregnancy probability after vasovasostomy. Although it is certain that some couples with high levels of immunoglobulin binding to sperm will have difficulty achieving pregnancy, it is not certain that this is universally true. We do test men with the IBT who have low-sperm motility and sperm clumping 3 mo postoperatively and/or when they have not achieved pregnancy within 1 yr of vasovasostomy and have an adequate sperm count.

CONCLUSIONS

Vasectomy continues to be used by about 500,000 men annually in the Unites States as a form of permanent birth control. It has been estimated that 3 to 5% of these men who have had a vasectomy may seek a vasectomy reversal to have more children. Vasectomy reversal by an experienced surgeon should allow 60% of these men to sire more children. Pregnancy rates after vasectomy reversal are superior to pregnancy rates for IVF with ICSI for obstructive azoospermia unless the female is age 40 or older, in which instance the two options for procreation have comparable results.

REFERENCES

1. Population Reports, Male Sterilization, Nov-Dec 1983. The Johns Hopkins University, Hampton House, Baltimore, MD.
2. Drake MJ, Mills IW, Cranston D. On the Chequered History Vasectomy. BJU International 1999;84:475.
3. Ochsner AJ. Surgical treatment of habitual criminals. JAMA 1899;33:1897.
4. Sharp HC. Vasectomy as a means of preventing procreation in defectives. JAMA 1909;53: 1897.
5. O'Conor VJ. Anastomosis of vas deferens after purposeful division for sterility. JAMA 1948;136:162.
6. Phadke GM, Phadke AG. Experience in the reanastamosis of the vas deferers. J Urol 1976;97:888.
7. Middleton RG, Henderson D. Vas deferens reanastamosis without splints and without magnification. J Urol 1978;119:763.
8. Schmidt SS. Vas reanastamosis: a return to simplicity. BJU 1975;110:309.
9. Amelar RD, Dubin L. Vasectomy Reversal. J Urol 1979;121:547.
10. Silber SJ. Microscopic technique for reversal of vasectomy. SG&O 1976;143:603.
11. Owen ER. Microsurgical Vasovasostomy: a reliable vasectomy reversal. Aust NZ J Surg 1977;47:305.
12. Silber SJ. Epididymal extravasation following vasectomy as a cause for failure of vasectomy reversal. Fertil Steril 1979;31:309.
13. Fuchs EF, Paduch DA. Single surgeon experience with more than 2200 vasectomy reversals. Fertil Steril 2004;80(Suppl 3):Abstract P-329.
14. Fuchs E. Cord block anesthesia for scrotal surgery. J Urol 1982;128:718.
15. Belker AM, Thomas AJ, Fuchs EF, et al. Results of 1469 microsurgical vasectomy reversal by the Vasovasostomy Study Group. J Urol 1991;145:505.
16. Fuchs EF, Burt RA. Vasectomy reversal performed 15 years of more after vasectomy: correlation of pregnancy outcome with partner age and with pregnancy results of in vitro fertilization with intracytoplasmic sperm injection. Fert Steril 2002;77.
17. Fuchs EF, Alexander NJ. Serum antisperm antibody before and after vasectomy reversal. Fert Steril 1983;49:497–499.
18. Kay DJ, Clifton V, Taylor JS, Boettcher B. Anti-sperm antibodies and semen profiles in reanastomosed men. Reprod Fertil Dev 1993;5:135–139.
19. Meinerty H, Linnert L, Fogh-AndersenP, Hjort T. Antisperm antibodies and fertility after vasovasostom: a follow up study of 216 men. Fert Steril 1993;54:315–321.

13 Infection and Male Infertility

Emmett F. Branigan, MD

CONTENTS

CASE STUDY

A 32-yr-old couple that had no problems conceiving their first child 3 yr ago had now been trying to conceive again for over 2 yr. The female work-up was normal and included a normal hysterosalpingogram, biphasic basal body temperature charts with adequate luteal phases, and ovulatory mid-luteal progesterone levels. The husband's basic semen analysis was normal with the exception of decreased progressive motility and leukocytospermia. He had no signs or symptoms of acute genitourinary tract infection. A diagnosis of subclinical chronic prostatitis was made, and he was prescribed doxycycline for 1 mo and told to frequently ejaculate during the treatment interval. On the second menstrual cycle after the antibiotic treatment, the couple conceived and had an uneventful pregnancy and delivery.

INTRODUCTION

The role of leukocytes in the male genital tract and seminal fluid is complex and dynamic. Leukocytes are found in virtually every ejaculate and function on multiple levels. Leukocytes have a positive impact in the immunosurveillance of

From: *Contemporary Endocrinology: Office Andrology*
Edited by: P. E. Patton and D. E. Battaglia © Humana Press Inc., Totowa, NJ

the male genital tract and clearance of abnormal sperm by phagocytosis *(1)*. High leukocyte concentrations in semen are important indicators of male genital tract infection or inflammation *(2)*. Leukocytospermia is a reliable finding in men with symptomatic genital tract infections but not in subclinical infections *(3)*.

In many studies, leukocytospermia is associated with male infertility. Decreased sperm concentrations and motility, as well as increased abnormal sperm morphology and immature germ cells, are reported in men with leukocytospermic samples *(4,5)*. Leukocyte products are also linked to reduction in sperm function and male infertility *(6)*. In men without genitourinary symptoms, leukocytospermia is a frequent finding of men who attend fertility clinics.

The differentiation of pathologic from nonpathologic leukocytes in the male genital tract is not clear secondary to multiple factors. Using conventional microscopy, it is difficult to accurately distinguish white blood cells (WBC) from immature germ cells in the semen which makes accurately counting leukocyte concentrations difficult. The subtype of leukocyte present may be as important as the overall concentrations of leukocytes. The site of origin leukocytes within the male genital tract is also important because of longer or shorter contact times to the sperm. Finally, the leukocyte activation status and any protective effect by seminal fluid must be taken into account.

DIAGNOSIS OF MALE GENITAL TRACT INFECTION/INFLAMMATION

Many studies link infection or inflammation of the male genitourinary tract with male infertility. However, there is frequent confusion about the clinical research associated with the various prostatitis syndromes and their effect on fertility. Different diagnostic criteria are used in various studies, which make the interpretation of treatment outcomes difficult. There are no well-designed prospective-controlled clinical trials with fertility as the outcome to serve as the gold standard. Lastly, the urologic and fertility literature are often referring to different syndromes that further complicates the problem.

UROLOGIC PERSPECTIVE ON PROSTATITIS

Urologic study is focused primarily on symptomatic prostatitis *(7,8)*. Three criteria are usually considered to differentiate the various prostatitis syndromes:

1. Patient symptoms.
2. Presence or absence of bacteruria.
3. Inflammation in expressed prostatic secretions.
4. Prostatitis syndromes can then be divided into four groups based on these criteria:

a. Acute bacterial prostatitis: bacteruria with associated acute lower genitourinary tract symptoms, a tender prostate, and symptoms of a systemic illness.
b. Chronic bacterial prostatitis: recurrent bacteruria associated with the same organism as the acute phase and inflammation in their expressed prostatic secretions.

The majority of urologic literature focuses on the first two syndromes. However, less than 10% of men with prostatitis have bacterial prostatitis *(9,10)*. Syndromes with symptomatic prostatitis but without bacteruria include:

c. Non-bacterial prostatitis: prostatic symptoms and inflammation in their expressed prostatic secretions but no bacteruria or bacterial pathogen that localizes to the prostate on cultures.
d. Prostadynia: prostatic symptoms but normal prostatic secretions.

MALE INFERTILITY LITERATURE

The diagnosis of prostatitis or male accessory gland infection in the fertility literature usually depends on the analysis of seminal fluid inflammation in asymptomatic men *(11,12)*. The presence of leukocytospermia in semen suggests prostatic or lower genital tract inflammation. Urologists often have problems with this approach, because these men are usually asymptomatic, and the site of leukocyte origin in the genital tract is not defined or identified. Although it is widely believed that leukocytospermia often reflects subclinical genital tract infection, most studies on bacterial pathogens in semen have failed to document an association between elevated levels of specific organisms and high seminal leukocyte counts. Thus, the relationship between infection and seminal fluid inflammation is controversial.

Symptoms of acute prostatitis syndromes are distinct and leave little doubt about diagnosis. However, only a small percentage (<10%) of the total number of prostatitis patients present with the acute phase of this disease. Occasionally, a history of dysuria—frequency or vague scrotal pain—may be given. A short course (<2 wk) of antibiotic treatment often treats the acute symptoms, but the infection continues in the chronic form. Most infertility patients have no acute episodes, which makes diagnosis even more difficult. Diagnosis is then dependent on findings of inflammation (leukocytospermia) in the seminal fluid analysis. As mentioned previously, the relationship between infection of the male genital tract and seminal fluid leukocytes is under debate *(13)*. Most studies show no correlation between the presence of WBC and bacteria in the semen. Furthermore, researchers have not found bacteria in semen to be associated with oligozoospermia, abnormal morphology *(14,15)*, or decreased sperm motility, but have linked WBC and their products to these problems.

LEUKOCYTOSPERMIA

Leukocytes are present throughout the entire male genital tract and found in every human ejaculate. The presence of abnormally high concentrations of leukocytes in semen is called "leukocytospermia." The World Health Organization *(16)* defines leukocytospermia as the presence of 1×10^6 WBC per milliliter of semen. However, there are methodological problems in how the WBC are differentiated from immature germ cells that are also present in the seminal fluid. Round-cell populations in human seminal fluid primarily consist of immature germ cells and leukocytes. They contribute usually less than 5% to the total cellular content of semen. Conventional staining techniques of semen do not reliably differentiate these cells. Spermatocytes are easily confused with lymphocytes and monocytes, as well as multinucleated spermatids with polymorphonuclear granulocytes. Studies on the effects of leukocytospermia on male fertility are based on the ability to accurately and precisely identify and quantify the leukocytes in the semen. The site of origin in the male genital tract and their activation status may be equally important to determine fertility effects.

Identification Methods of Leukocytes in Seminal Fluid

Conventional staining methods like Giemsa or Papanicolaou cannot reliably differentiate leukocytes from immature germ cells. The introduction of the Bryan-Leishmann stain *(17)* allows better differentiation of these round cells; however, it underestimates the granulocytes and overestimates the lymphocyte populations in the seminal fluid. The introduction of the peroxidase stain *(18,19)*—a cytochemical method for detecting polymorphonuclear granulocytes—provides a simple and accurate method for detecting leukocytes in semen. This test takes about 5 min to perform at a cost of cents per specimen. The peroxidase stain does not identify monocytes or lymphocytes in semen, but because polymorphonuclear granulocytes are the most prevalent WBC in semen, it is sufficient for clinical purposes. The gold standard for the identification of leukocytes in semen uses monoclonal antibodies and immunocytochemistry staining. Common leukocyte antigen monoclonal antibody *(20,21)* can accurately detect all granulocytes, macrophages, and lymphocytes in a single sample. Different monoclonal antibodies can be used to detect leukocyte subpopulations. However, the use of these agents to detect WBC in semen is a very expensive and labor-intensive procedure that limits its usefulness to the research area. In a laboratory that is set up to perform this procedure, it can cost several dollars per sample and take 6 h to complete. For clinical purposes, the peroxidase stain *(22,23)* is the most practical method of leukocyte detection in semen. Yet, the Bryan-Leishmann stain can also be useful in the clinical setting.

Etiology of Leukocytospermia

The assumption that leukocytospermia is only a result of a subclinical male genital tract infection is incorrect. Most studies on bacterial pathogens do not show a direct association between specific organisms and high-leukocyte counts in semen *(24)*. Infections, which damage or cause dysfunction in a particular organ, must be differentiated from harmless bacterial colonization of that organ. *Chlamydia trachomatis* and *Ureaplasma urealyticum (25)* can induce both prostatitis and urethritis, as well as acute epididymitis. However, these pathogens are rarely present in asymptomatic infertility patients. The number of microorganisms present may be more important in determining the degree of inflammation present than the specific organism. The presence of sexually transmitted viruses in the genital tract and their effect on leukocytospermia has not been studied.

Other possible etiologies of leukocytospermia besides infection need to be considered. Environmental factors, e.g., smoking, alcohol consumption, and marijuana use *(26)*, increase WBC in semen. Prolonged abstinence and certain sexual practices (use of vaginal products or anal intercourse) can produce leukocytospermia. Increased WBC in semen may be seen in men with abnormal spermatogenesis as a mechanism for the removal of defective sperm from the ejaculate. Finally, varicocele or vasovasostomy can result in a high number of leukocytes in semen. Regardless of the etiology, leukocytospermia can have deleterious effects on sperm and sperm function and can also contribute to male infertility.

Effect of Leukocytospermia on Fertility

To determine the effects of leukocytes on fertility, it is important to consider not only the leukocyte number or concentration but which leukocyte subtype is present, the site of origin in the male genital tract, activation status, and the presence of immunosuppressive factors. The complex and dynamic interaction of these factors determines the overall effect.

Considerable evidence now indicates that leukocytes and their products have significant effects on sperm and sperm function. Wolff *(4)* showed that leukocytespermia is associated with a decrease in the total number of sperm per ejaculate, decreased sperm motility and velocity, and quanitity of total motile sperm. Overall, an increased number of leukocytes in semen is associated with poor-semen quality.

Poor performance in the hamster egg sperm penetration assay is linked to leukocytes and leukocyte products. Berger showed significantly worse performance in the hamster egg sperm penetration assay with increasing WBC in semen *(27)*. Treatment of leukocytospermic men with doxycycline remarkably improves their hamster egg sperm penetration assay performance *(28)*. Furthermore, adding peripheral blood leukocytes or their products to previously fertile men with good hamster egg sperm penetration assay scores results in a significant decrease in penetration scores *(29)*. High numbers of WBC in semen show an inverse relationship to in vitro fertilization (IVF) success *(30,31)*.

Other studies postulate a positive role for seminal leukocytes *(32)*. Proven fertile men in control groups can have leukocytospermia, and many infertility patients with high seminal leukocyte counts have normal semen parameters. Studies using transmission electron microscopy *(33)* often find sperm and sperm fragments in seminal leukocytes, which suggests a phagocytic effect for these cells. Other studies using light microscopy observed similar results in men with normal semen parameters, suggesting a mechanism for the removal of abnormal sperm *(34)*. However, phagocytosis can only affect a limited number of sperm, but the process may represent an important positive influence for seminal leukocytes.

Activated leukocytes produce a variety of soluble immunologic by-products that can have toxic effects on sperm function. Granulocytes release large amounts of reactive oxygen species that can damage sperm *(35)*. Aitken *(36)* and Alvarez *(37)* showed that reactive species led to oxidative damage of the sperm membrane, which reduces fluidity of the membrane and disrupts the fusion events of the acrosome reaction. Sperm damaged by reactive oxygen species lose motility, especially progressive motility, and have decreased viability and diminished fertilizing ability in the hamster egg sperm penetration assay and in IVF *(38)*. Most oxidative bursts of granulocytes can be inhibited by the powerful antioxidative substances found in seminal plasma *(39)*. This fluid contains vitamin C, zinc, albumin, urate, superoxide dismutase, and other substances that can have large protective effects. However, large differences are prevalent in the protective properties of different men's seminal plasma *(40)*. Some men with leukocytespermia can have complete protection of their sperm from the adverse effects of leukocytes because of the antioxidative properties of their seminal plasma. Other men with a much lower number of leukocytes that are activated can have significant sperm function problems because of their limited protection from seminal plasma. This further complicates the relationship between WBC in semen and male infertility.

Cytokines—inducible immunologic mediators—have the potential to directly and indirectly affect sperm function *(41)*. The monokine tumor necrosis factor α and the lymphokine interferon γ considerably decreases sperm motility and fertilization in the hamster egg sperm penetration assay when added in high concentrations in vitro *(42)*. Eisermann showed that the physiologic levels of tumor necrosis factor α significantly inhibit sperm motility, and the addition of antitumor necrosis factor α monoclonal antibody completely reversed this effect *(43)*.

Many studies suggest that male genital tract inflammation may induce the formation of antisperm autoantibodies. Pashke *(44)* found that the incidence of leukocytospermia notably increased the chance of a man having autoantibodies against his own sperm. These antibodies can lead to agglutination and decreased fertilizing ability of the sperm. However, other authors *(45,46)* have not found this association. It is also theorized that the autoantibody response to inflammation may result from an imbalance of certain subsets of leukocytes in the male reproductive tract. Production of antibodies may be secondary to a decrease in the ratio of T suppressor to T helper cells. This allows the local recruitment of B lymphocytes and plasma cells that produce antibodies. However, it is not completely clear which is the cause and which is the effect. Does a hyperactive immune system cause both the leukocytospermia and the antibodies, or is the genital inflammation inducing the antibody formation? The inflammation site may play an important role in this interaction. Lymphocytes in the testes and epididymis are exposed to sperm for a much longer time than the prostate or upper tract glands, allowing for a more vigorous immune response. Whether or not the seminal plasma is present during the leukocyte contact with sperm is also very important because of its immunosuppressive and anti-inflammatory properties. Seminal plasma, as mentioned earlier, cannot only protect sperm from leukocyte products but can inhibit natural killer cells, T-cell function, and the complement system. This protective effect is highly variable, which may explain the variability of the immune response as well.

Poor-quality sperm chromatin characterized by damaged DNA has recently been shown to be indicative of decreased fertility potential. Alvarez *(47)* showed a significant increase in sperm DNA damage in samples from leukocytespermic men in comparison to fertile donors and leukocyte-free semen samples. They further showed that leukocyte concentrations in semen were directly correlated with immature germ cell concentrations and abnormal morphology sperm *(48)*, suggesting that leukocytospermia may be associated with an inflammatory process in the testes that could lead to alterations in the regulation of spermatogenesis. Sperm nuclear DNA damage has been linked to decreased embryo quality and lower IVF pregnancy rates. This damage may also result in lower fertilization rate in intracytoplasmic sperm injection (ICSI). Leukocytospermia has thus been linked to sperm nuclear chromatin damage with further impairment of fertility potential.

Distribution of Leukocytes in the Male Genital Tract

Leukocytes normally inhabit the male genital tract and are found in every ejaculate. These consist of granulocytes, macrophages, and lymphocytes that are distributed differently throughout the genital tract.

The blood–testes barrier effectively blocks leukocytes from the seminiferous tubules, but an occasional macrophage can be seen *(49)*. The interstitial tissue of the testes contains large numbers of macrophages and mast cells *(50)*. The rete testes is lined with T suppressor lymphocytes that most likely prevent immune response to sperm *(51)*.

In the epididymis, large numbers of macrophages and lymphocytes are present *(52)*, representing an active site of immune regulation to prevent antibody formation *(53)*. The majority of sperm phagocytic macrophages in semen originate from the epididymis—the primary site where dead and abnormally formed sperm are removed by macrophages *(54)*. The fact that the epididymis contributes substantial leukocytes is evident in postvasectomy samples. Anderson found only 16% of the median leukocyte numbers in vasectomized men when compared to nonvasectomized controls *(55)*.

The epithelium of the vas deferens has high concentrations of macrophages and T lymphocytes *(56)*. Their primary function appears to be in preventing ascending infections from progressing past the prostate and preventing residual sperm from ejaculates in producing an antibody response. It is unlikely that these leukocytes contribute to the WBC in semen.

Most granulocytes in semen originate in the prostate gland *(56)*—the primary leukocyte seen in vasectomized men. The prostate also contains T and B lymphocytes. It is doubtful that the urethra contributes significant leukocytes to the seminal fluid in the absence of urethritis.

The role of residual sperm in the prostate and seminal vesicles must be considered when discussing the distribution of leukocytes in the male genital tract *(57,58)*. Just as the female cervix mounts a strong leukocyte reaction to the presence of sperm, the residual sperm postejaculation may cause a similar leukocyte infiltration in the prostate *(59)*. These leukocytes could then be present in subsequent ejaculations.

Frequency of Leukocytospermia

The detection method used and population studied are the important variables to determine the prevalence of leukocytospermia. Studies have shown a wide range of frequencies, from 2 to 8% to as high as 35% in infertility patients *(60–62)*. The majority of studies with the greatest amount of patients estimate the prevalence of leukocytospermia to be between 12 and 20% of all infertility patients. This is a very common problem that is often overlooked in routine semen analyses.

Treatment of Leukocytospermia

The heterogeneity of etiologies of leukocytospermia makes it unlikely that any single therapy would be beneficial to treat all cases. However, when infection or inflammation secondary to chronic subacute infection is present, antibiotics are usually the first treatment option used. Doxcycline is an excellent antibiotic choice, because it has a broad antimicrobial spectrum and anti-inflammatory properties, which are independent of its antibiotic effect. In couples with otherwise unexplained infertility but with leukocytospermia present, doxcycline treatment can result in both resolution of the leukocytospermia and a significant improvement in pregnancy rates *(63,64)*. This same antibiotic has been shown to improve hamster egg sperm penetration assay scores of men with leukocytospermia *(28)*. In acute male genital tract infections caused by specific organisms, appropriate antibiotic treatment is clearly indicated. Using antibiotics to treat leukocytospermia should be continued for at least 4 wk instead of the standard 10 to 14 d treatment regimens.

If the leukocytospermia cannot be resolved by antibiotic treatment, then it is advisable to separate the leukocytes from the sperm as quickly as possible during sperm preparation for intrauterine insemination or IVF. Both density gradient and swim-up sperm preperations can be used to effectively separate sperm from WBC and limit the adverse effects of leukocytes and leukocyte products on the sperm *(65)*. Sperm washing techniques with high centrifugation should particularly be avoided, as these will accelerate sperm damage in leukocytospermic samples. The use of pentoxyfylline—a phosphodiesterase inhibitor—before sperm processing may further reduce or reverse the effects of leukocyte products on sperm function. The use of antioxidant vitamins C and E have been used to scavenge free oxygen radicals in men with high levels of free radicals *(66)*.

CONCLUSIONS

The impact of leukocytes in the male genital tract are complex and not completely understood. Low levels of WBC have important positive effects in phagocytosis of abnormal sperm and immunosurveillance. However, leukocytes in high concentrations can have adverse effects on sperm and sperm function and may result in male infertility.

Leukocytospermia is a common finding in the infertility population; identifying it should be part of a routine semen analysis. The peroxidase stain is a simple and low-cost method of identifying leukocytes in semen. Once identified, treatment with 1-mo course of antibiotic is the first therapy option. When leukocytospermia persists, a density gradient sperm preparation to rapidly separate the sperm from leukocytes and their byproducts is recommended.

When clinical research tools are developed to differentiate pathologic from nonpathologic leukocyte numbers, and the role of leukocytes in infertility are explored, improved methods of treatment or prevention will be found.

REFERENCES

1. Tomlinson MJ, White A, Barratt CL, et al. The removal of morphologically abnormal sperm forms by phagocytes: a positive role for seminal leukocytes. Hum Reprod 1992;7:517–522.

2. Comhaire F, Verschraegen G, Vermeulen L. Diagnosis of accessory gland infection and its possible role in male infertility. Int J Androl 1980;3:32–45.
3. Barratt CL, Robinson A, Spenser RC, et al. Seminal peroxidase positive cells are not an adequate indicator of asymptomatic urethral genital infection. Int J Androl 1990;13:361–368.
4. Wolff H, Politch JA, Martinez A, et al. Leukocytospermia is associated with poor semen quality. Fertil Steril 1990;53:528–536.
5. Sigman M, Lopes L. The correlation between round cells and white blood cells in the semen. J Urol 1993;149:1338–1340.
6. Hill JA, Haimovici F, Politch JA, Anderson DJ. Effects of soluble products of activated lymphocytes and macrophages (lymphokines and monokines) on human sperm motion parameters. Fertil Steril 1987;47:460–465.
7. Krieger JN, McGonagle IA. Diagnostic considerations and interpretation of microbiological findings for evaluation of chronic prostatitis. J Clin Microbiol 1989;27:2240–2244.
8. Wright ET, Chmiel JS, Grayhack JT, Schaeffer AJ. Prostatic fluid inflammation in prostatitis. J Urol 1994;152:2300–2303.
9. Keriger JN, Egan KJ. Comprehensive evaluation and treatment of 75 men referred to chronic prostatitis clinic. Urology 1991;38:11–19.
10. de la Rosette JJ, Hubregtse MR, Meuleman HJ, et al. Diagnosis and treatment of 409 patients with prostatitis syndromes. Urology 1993;41:301–307.
11. Toth A, Lesser ML. Asymptomatic bacteriospermia in fertile and in fertile men Fertil Steril 1981;36:85–91.
12. Aitken RJ, West K, Buckingham D. Leukocyte infiltration into human ejaculate and its association with semen quality, oxidative stress, and sperm function. J Androl 1994;15:343–352.
13. Purvis K, Christiansen E. Infection in the male reproductive tract. Impact, diagnosis and treatment in relation to male infertility. Int J Androl 1993;16:1–13.
14. Naessens A, Foulon W, Debrucker P, et al. Recovery of microorganisms in semen and the relationship to semen evaluation. Fertil Steril 1986;452:101–105.
15. Makler A, Urbach Y, Lefler E, Merzbach D. Factors affecting sperm motility. Sperm viability under the influence of bacterial growth in human ejaculates. Fertil Steril 1981;35:666–670.
16. World Health Organization. WHO Laboratory Manual for the Examination of Human Semen and Sperm-Cervical Mucus Interaction. Cambridge University Press, Cambridge, UK, 1992.
17. Couture M, Ulstein M, Leonard J, Paulsen JA. Improved staining method for differentiating immature germ cells from white blood cells in human seminal fluid. Andrologia 1976;8:61–66.
18. Endtz AW. A rapid staining method for differentiating granulocytes from "germinal cells" in Papanicolaou stained semen. Acta Cytol 1974;18:2–7.
19. Nahoum CRD, Cardozo D. Staining for volumetric count of leukocytes in semen and prostate-vescular fluid. Fertil Steril 1980;34:68,69.
20. Eggert-Kruse W, Bellmann A, Rohr G, et al. Differentiation of round cells by means of monoclonal antibodies and relationship with male infertility. Fertil Steril 1992;58:1046–1055.
21. Wolff H, Anderson DJ. Immunohistologic chacterization and quantitation of leukocyte subpopulations in human semen. Fertil Steril 1988;49:497–504.
22. Wolff H, Panhans A, Zebhauser M, Meurer M. Comparison of three methods to detect white blood cells in semen: leukocyte esterase dipstick test, granulocyte elastase enzymeimmunoassy and peroxidase cytochemistry. Fertil Steril 1992;58:1260–1262.
23. Politch JA, Wolff H, Hill JA, Anderson DJ. Comparison of methods to enumerate white blood cells in semen. Fertil Steril 1993;60:372–375.
24. Hillier SL, Rabe LK, Muller CH, et al. Relationship of bacteriologic characteristics to semen indices in men attending an infertility clinic. Obstet Gynecol 1990;75:800–804.

25. Brunner H, Weidner W, Schiefer HG. Studies on the role of Ureaplasma urealyticum and Mycoplasma hominis in prostatitis. J Infect Dis 1983;147:807–813.
26. Close CE, Roberts PL Berger RE. Cigarettes, alcohol and marijuana are related to pyospermia in infertile men. J Urol 1990;144:900–903.
27. Berger RE, Karp LE, Williamson RA, et al. The relationship of pyospermia and seminal fluid bacteriology to sperm function as reflected in the sperm penetration assay. Fertil Steril 1982;37:557–564.
28. Berger RE, Smith WD, Critchlow CW, et al. Improvement in the sperm penetration (hamster ova) assay (SPA) results after doxycycline treatment of infertile men. J Androl 1983;4:126–130.
29. Maruyama DK, Hale RW, Rogers BJ. Effects of white blood cells on the in vitro penetration of zona-free hamster eggs by human spermatozoa. J Androl 1985;6:127–135.
30. Talbert LM, Hammond MG, Halme J, et al. Semen parameters and fertilization of human oocytes in-vitro: a multivariable analysis. Fertil Steril 1987;48:270–277.
31. De Geyter C, De Geyter M, Behre HM, et al. Peroxidase-positive round cells and microorganisms in human semen together with antibiotic treatment adversely influence the outcome of in-vitro fertilization and embryo transfer. Int J Androl 1994;17:127–134.
32. Tomlinson MJ, Barratt CLR, Cooke ID. Prospective study of leukocytes and leukocyte subpopulations in semen suggests they are not a cause of male infertility. Fertil Steril 1993;60: 1069–1075.
33. Smith DC, Barratt CLR, Williams MA. The characterization of non-sperm cells in the ejaculates of fertile men using transmission electron microscopy. Andrologia 1989;21:319–333.
34. Phadke AM, Phadke GM. Occurrence of macrophage cells in the semen and in the epididymis in cases of male infertility. J Reprod Fertil 1961;2:400–403.
35. Weiss SJ. Tissue destruction by neutrophils. N Engl J Med 1989;320:365–376
36. Aitken RJ, Clarkson JS, Fishel S. Generation of reactive oxygen species, lipid peroxidation and human sperm function. Biol Reprod 1989;40:183–197.
37. Alvarez JG, Touchstone JC, Blasco L, Storey BT. Spontaneous lipid peroxidation and production of hydrogen peroxide and superoxide in human spermatozoa. Superoxide dismutase as major enzyme protectant against oxygen toxicity. J Androl 1987;8:338–348.
38. Krausz C, Mills C, Rogers S, et al. Stimulation of oxidant generation by human suspensions using phorbol esters and formyl peptides: relationships with motility and fertilization in vitro. Fertil Steril 1994;62:599–605.
39. Schopf RE, Schramm P, Benes P, Morsches B. Seminal plasma induced suppression of the respiratory burst of polymorphonuclear leukocytes and monocytes. Andrologia 1984;16:124–128.
40. Kovalski NN, de Lamirande E, Gagnon C. Reactive oxygen species generated by human neutrophils inhibit sperm motility: protective effect of seminal plasma scavengers. Fertil Steril 1992;58:809–816.
41. Comhaire F, Bosmans E, Omblet W, et al. Cytokines in semen of normal men and of patients with andrological diseases. Am J Reprod Immunol 1994;31:99–1103.
42. Hill JA, Cohen J, Anderson DJ. The effect of lymphokines and monokines on sperm fertilizing ability in the zona-free hamster egg penetration test. Am J Obstet Gynecol 1989;160:1154–1159.
43. Eisermann J, Register KB, Strickler RC, Collins JL. The effect of tumor necrosis factor on human sperm motility in vitro. J Androl 1989;10:270–274.
44. Paschke R, Schulze-Bertelsbeck D, Bahrs S, et al. Seminal sperm antibodies exhibit an unstable spontaneous course and an increased incidence of leukocytospermia. Int J Androl 1994;17:135–139.

45. Kortebani G, Gonzales GF, Barrera C, Mazzolli AB. Leukocyte populations in semen and male accessory gland function: relationship with antisperm antibodies and seminal quality. Andrologia 1992;24:197–204.
46. Fedder J, Askjaer SA, Hjort T. Nonspermatozoal cells in semen: relationship to other semen parameters and fertility status of the couple. Arch Androl 1993;31:95–103.
47. Alvarez JG, Sharma RK, Ollero M, et al. Increased DNA damage in sperm from leukocytospermic semen samples as determined by the sperm chromatin assay. Fertil Steril 2002; 78:319–329.
48. Thomas JF, Fishel SB, Hall JA, et al. Increased polymorphonuclear granulocytes in seminal plasma in relation to sperm morphology. Hum Reprod 1997;12:2418–2421.
49. Tjioe DY, Steinberger E. Spermiophages in human testes. Fertil Steril 1967;18:807–811.
50. Hermo L, Lalli M. Monocytes and mast cells in the limiting membrane of human seminiferous tubules. Biol Reprod 1978;19:92–100.
51. Pollanen P, Cooper TG. Immunology of the testicular excurrent ducts. J Reprod Immunol 1994;26:167–216.
52. Yeung CH, Nashan D, Sorg C, et al. Basal cells of the human epididymis-antigenic and ultrastructural similarities to tissue fixed macrophages. Biol Reprod 1994 50:917–926.
53. Ritchie AWS, Hargreave TB, James K, Chisholm GD. Intraepithelial lymphocytes in the normal epididymis: a mechanism for tolerance to sperm-autoantigens. Br J Urol 1984;56:79–84.
54. Phadke AM. Spermiophage cells in man. Fertil Steril 1975;26:760–764.
55. Olsen GP, Sheilds JW. Seminal lymphocytes, plasma and AIDS. Nature 1984;309:116,117.
56. El-Demiry MIM, Hargreave TB, Busutti A, et al. Lymphocyte sub-populations in the male genital tract. Br J Urol 1985;57:769–774.
57. McClinton S, Eremin O, Miller ID. Inflammatory infiltrate in prostatic hyperplasia evidence of a host response to intraprostatic spermatozoa? Br J Urol 1990;65:606–610.
58. Maroni MS, Symon DNK, Wilkinson PC. Chemotaxis of neutrophil leukocytes towards spermatozoa and seminal fluid. J Reprod Fertil 1972;28:359–368.
59. Pandya IJ, Cohen J. The leukocyte reaction of the human uterine cervix to spermatozoa. Fertil Steril 1985;43:417–421.
60. Wang AW, Politch J, Anderson DJ. Leukocytospermia in male infertility patients in China. Andrologia 1994;26:167–172.
61. Kung AWC, Ho PC, Wang C. Seminal leukocytes subpopulations and sperm function in fertile and infertile Chinese men. Int J Androl 1993;16:189–194.
62. Barratt CLR, Bolton AE, Cooke ID. Functional significance of white blood cells in the male and female reproductive tract. Hum Reprod 1990;5:433–451.
63. Branigan EF, Muller CH. Efficacy of treatment and recurrence rate of leukocytospermia in infertile men with prostatitis. Fertil Steril 1994;62:580–584.
64. Ng FL, Liu DY, Baker HWG. Comparison of Percoll, mini-Percoll, swim-up methods for sperm preparation from abnormal sperm. Hum Reprod 1992;7:261–266.
65. Baker HWG, Brindle J, Irvine DS, Aitken RJ. Protective effect of antioxidants on the impairment of sperm motility by activated polymorphonuclear leukocytes. Fertil Steril 1996;65: 411–419.

14 Obstructive and Nonobstructive Azoospermia

Kinloch Nelson, MD *and Peter Schlegel,* MD

CONTENTS

INTRODUCTION

Defined as the inability to conceive a pregnancy within 12 mo of unprotected regular intercourse, subfertility affects approx 15% of couples in the United States. Of these couples, 40 to 60% or less will have a particular male factor responsible for their difficulty conceiving. Recent advances in assisted reproductive technology have dramatically improved the chances of fatherhood for subfertile men, even those with azoospermia (the complete absence of sperm in the ejaculate). This chapter reviews the diagnosis and treatment of men with both obstructive and nonobstructive azoospermia.

Much of the diagnostic evaluation for azoospermia is focused on classifying the problem as obstructive or nonobstructive, as this largely determines the direction of treatment. Nonobstructive azoospermia is caused by failure of the testes to generate enough sperm to be detectable in the semen. Importantly, although the presence of nonobstructive azoospermia implies the complete absence of sperm production in the testes, focal areas of sperm production are

From: *Contemporary Endocrinology: Office Andrology*
Edited by: P. E. Patton and D. E. Battaglia © Humana Press Inc., Totowa, NJ

found in most men with nonobstructive azoospermia. Therefore, testicular sperm extraction (TESE) may succeed or fail to identify sperm production in patients with nonobstructive azoospermia. Despite the fact that no finding on preoperative evaluation can definitively predict whether sperm will be successfully retrieved, a thorough evaluation can nevertheless provide some guidance for a couple regarding their chances of conception.

Obstructive azoospermia is the absence of sperm in the ejaculate because of failure to deliver the sperm from the testis to the urethra. Obstruction can occur at any point from the epididymis through the vas deferens to the ejaculatory ducts. Obstructive azoospermia is most commonly a result of surgery—either a vasectomy or an unrecognized injury to the vas during groin or scrotal surgery. There are congenital causes for obstructive azoospermia. Men with obstructive azoospermia can be treated with either sperm retrieval or reconstruction of the reproductive tract.

EVALUATION OF THE AZOOSPERMIC MALE

To establish the presence of azoospermia, a centrifuged specimen of seminal fluid must be examined. To confirm the diagnosis, a semen analysis should be repeated at least three times over a period of several months, each time preceded by a 48-h period of abstinence. The initial step in the evaluation of a subfertile couple is a thorough and accurate history. Relevant issues for an azoospermic male are largely the same as those for any man presenting with subfertility. Has the man contributed to any pregnancies in the past, with his current partner or any prior partner? In cases of azoospermia, aspects relating to the timing and frequency of intercourse are less important. The man's developmental history can shed some light on the etiology of azoospermia. Men with congenital hypogonadism may relate a history of delayed puberty.

Any history of surgical procedures in the inguinal or scrotal regions should be noted. Childhood orchiopexies can lead to injury to the vas and epididymis or to the blood supply to the testis. In addition, men with undescended testicles tend to have sperm production problems bilaterally. Low-sperm density has been reported in 30% of adults with a history of unilateral cryptorchidism and 50% with bilateral cryptorchidism *(1)*. Other inguinal and scrotal surgeries, including hernia repairs, varicocelectomies, hydrocelectomies, and testis biopsies, can all lead to obstructive azoospermia through damage to the vas or epididymis. Transurethral procedures can also bring forth ejaculatory duct obstruction. Finally, any history of serious systemic illnesses should be noted. Post pubertal mumps orchitis is a rare cause of nonobstructive azoospermia. Cystic fibrosis (CF) is often associated with the congenital absence of the vas deferens. Other, more rare syndromes, such as the Kartagener and Young syndrome, present with a history of frequent respiratory infections and are associated with obstructive azoospermia. Prior malignancies with exposure to gonadotoxic chemotherapy agents or radiation are causes of nonobstructive azoospermia. Also, any serious illness or stress can temporarily diminish sperm production to very low levels. Spermatogenesis is a process that is several months long; thus, precedent illnesses should be especially noted. Any history of sexually transmitted disease should also be taken into account. Episodes of epididymitis in the past, regardless of etiology, can lead to epididymal obstruction. Lastly, exposure to gonadotoxic drugs should be documented. Agents that are known to impair sperm production include marijuana, alcohol, cimetidine, alkylating chemotherapeutic drugs, sulfa drugs, nitrofurantoin, calcium channel blockers, and cholesterol-regulating agents. Frequent use of saunas and hot tubs can raise intrascrotal temperature and should be discouraged. No evidence indicates that the kind of undergarment worn has any impact on sperm production or quality.

PHYSICAL EXAM

Initial physical examination should consider the body habitus and overall appearance. Men with congenital hypogonadism often have a body type that reflects delayed or absent puberty. Limbs are disproportionately long, suggesting delayed epiphyseal closure caused by a relative lack of testosterone in adolescence. Similarly, hair distribution may be less virilized than expected.

The examination of the genitals begins with checking for old incision sites. Penile conformation and the location of the meatus is noted. Any skin lesions suggestive of sexually transmitted disease should prompt further questioning for a history of epididymitis.

The testes are noted for size, consistency, masses, and symmetry. Normal testes are at least 16 cc in volume. Small and soft testes suggest a defect in sperm production. Very small (<5 cc) and firm testes suggest Klinefelter syndrome. Tumors of the testicle are found with much greater frequency in the infertile population than in the general population.

The epididymis is normally soft and flat. Induration and swelling implicate obstruction and perhaps prior infection. The vas deferens is always palpable within the scrotum as a firm "Venetian blind cord"-like structure. Inability to palpate the vas indicates congenital bilateral absence of the vas (CBAVD), which is often associated with cystic fibrosis. In patients with CBAVD and no CF gene abnormalities, renal anomalies often coexist. The spermatic cord should be checked for a varicocele. The patient is examined in the standing position with the scrotal skin warm and relaxed. In grade II and III varicoceles, the dilated scrotal vessels are either easily palpable or visible. To detect a grade I varicocele, the examiner palpates the cord with two fingers and asks the patient to perform a valsalva maneuver. In the presence of a varicocele, a distinct impulse will be felt, as the increase in abdominal pressure temporarily reverses venous flow back into the spermatic veins. The patient is also examined in the supine position to ensure the varicocele reduces, as a nonreducing varicocele raises the suspicion of a retroperitoneal mass.

Rectal examinations are routinely performed in men with azoospermia or abnormal semen volume. On occasion, dilated seminal vesicles can be palpated, indicating the presence of ejaculatory duct obstruction. An inflamed boggy prostate may indicate the presence of infection, which could lead to obstructive azoospermia.

LABORATORY EVALUATION

A semen analysis showing azoospermia must be repeated on three separate occasions to confirm the diagnosis as previously discussed. Absence of sperm in a centrifuged specimen confirms the diagnosis of azoospermia.

Other parameters of the semen analysis can help to distinguish between semen obstructive and nonobstructive azoospermia. The seminal vesicles are the primary contributors of semen volume, fructose, and alkalinity. Thus, low volume, absence of fructose, and acidic pH are all indicators of either ejaculatory duct obstruction or congenital absence of the seminal vesicles. Patients with vasal or epididymal obstruction typically have normal semen volume with an absence of sperm. Low-volume ejaculate can also herald androgen deficiency, which could lead to nonobstructive azoospermia

Urine analysis can be helpful to identify an infectious cause of obstructive azoospermia. Additionally, the presence of sperm on the microscopic analysis can reveal retrograde ejaculation as a cause for infertility, ruling out either obstructive or nonobstructive azoospermia.

Hormonal Studies

Sperm production is under the control of the hypothalamic-pituitary-gonadal axis. Gonadotropin-releasing hormone is released in a pulsatile fashion from the hypothalamus, stimulating the release of follicle-stimulating hormone (FSH) and luteinizing hormone (LH) from the pituitary. LH primarily induces the testicular production of testosterone (T), whereas FSH stimulates Sertoli cells to maintain sperm production. Inhibin is a Sertoli cell product that provides feedback inhibition of pituitary secretion of FSH. T causes feedback inhibition of LH release. Sperm production requires the presence of adequate amounts of FSH and very high local levels of testosterone in the testicle. Exogenous T, especially if administered at a dose sufficient to give supranormal serum levels, shuts down LH production, subsequently stopping testicular T production. Without endogenous T production, spermatogenesis is prevented.

We typically obtain testosterone and FSH levels on all patients with azoospermia. Hormonal studies can help to distinguish obstructive azoospermia from nonobstructive azoospermia. Men with pure obstructive azoospermia should have normal hormonal profiles. Many men with nonobstructive azoospermia have elevated levels of FSH, revealing the lack of feedback inhibition from the dysfunctional germinal epithelium. Men with primary testicular failure also have low T and a high LH. Hypothalamic hypogonadism, of which Kallman syndrome is one form, is a hypothalamic defect and therefore presents with low levels of FSH, LH, and T.

Elevated levels of prolactin, another pituitary hormone, can impair LH and FSH release and cause a secondary nonobstructive azoospermia. Headaches or visual field changes in an azoospermic man raise the suspicion of a prolactinoma.

Imaging Studies

Scrotal sonograms are frequently used in the evaluation of the subfertile male. In most cases, sonograms serve only to confirm impressions gathered during the history and physical exam. The presence and degree of varicoceles can be confirmed by sonogram and can also effectively characterize intratesticular masses. Sonography is not a beneficial test for CBAVD. Physical examination is more reliable in assessing the presence of the vas. A transrectal ultrasound can accurately assess dilatation of the seminal vesicles, which is an important finding in men with possible ejaculatory duct obstruction.

Testis Biopsy

Percutaneous testis biopsy has been performed frequently in the past partly to establish if sperm production is present in the testis. In addition, men who have normal sperm production and obstructive azoospermia have viable sperm reliably retrieved. Thus, testis biopsy has been advocated as a potentially diagnostic and therapeutic procedure. In fact, a thorough evaluation, as detailed previously, distinguishes between obstructive and nonobstructive azoospermia in all but very few cases. Also, trials of percutaneous techniques versus microsurgical epididymal aspiration have shown far greater numbers of viable sperm retrieved with the latter technique. In men with nonobstructive azoospermia, percutaneous testis biopsy is much less likely to identify the rare sites with viable sperm when compared with microsurgical retrieval techniques. Because percutaneous biopsy is rarely needed as a diagnostic measure and rarely the most effective therapeutic choice, its use should be reserved.

When a testis biopsy is performed, the results can help predict success rates of subsequent treatment for patients with nonobstructive azoospermia. The most advanced pattern of spermatogenesis (but not the predominant pattern) appears to predict the results of sperm retrieval. For men who had at least one area of hypospermatogenesis present on diagnostic testis biopsy, retrieval of spermatozoa was achieved in 79% of attempts; whereas for men with maturation arrest as the most advanced pattern, only 47% of men had sperm retrieved by TESE. If the entire diagnostic biopsy had a Sertoli cell-only pattern, then sperm were retrieved in 24% of TESE attempts. Although no finding absolutely determined sperm retrieval or negated the possibility of successful TESE, the results of diagnostic biopsy were helpful in evaluating the chance of success with TESE *(2)*. If this information would prevent a couple from going forth with in vitro fertilization-intracytoplasmic sperm injection (IVF-ICSI), then testis biopsy is justified.

GENETIC TESTING

Men with nonobstructive azoospermia have an increased incidence of genetic abnormalities that can affect prognosis for sperm retrieval. All men who are diagnosed with nonobstructive azoospermia should have a karyotype performed to assess for Klinefelter syndrome. In the author's experience, men with Klinefelter's actually have a better likelihood of successful sperm retrieval at TESE when compared with the nonobstructive azoospermia population at large *(3)*. Three different regions of microdeletions in the long arm of the Y chromosome have also been identified in 7% of infertile men. Of these regions, termed "azoospermic factor" (*AZF*) a, b, and c, deletions in the *AZF* a and b regions portend the worst prognosis. In our series, 0 of 22 men with deletions involving the entire *AZF* a or b regions had sperm retrieved at TESE. A contemporary series of men without *AZF* a or b deletions had a sperm retrieval rate of 67% (85/126). Men with CBAVD and idiopathic epididymal obstruction have a high incidence of abnormalities in the *CF* gene. These men and their partners should be tested for *CF* carrier status before proceeding with any infertility treatment. All men with detectable genetic abnormalities undergo counseling with a geneticist before proceeding with sperm retrieval. Couples are advised regarding the potential risk to offspring and the option of preimplantation selection to select unaffected embryos.

Treatment

Treatment of nonobstructive azoospermia and obstructive azoospermia are obviously quite different. The purpose of the extensive work-up detailed earlier is to avoid unnecessary diagnostic procedures and opt with the most effective treatment for the individual patient.

Nonobstructive Azoospermia

The mainstay of treatment for nonobstructive azoospermia is TESE combined with IVF, including ICSI. Before proceeding with costly and invasive therapies, the first step is to identify and correct factors that could inhibit spermatogenesis, with the hope of converting azoospermia into oligospermia, thus eliminating the need for surgical sperm retrieval. Even if azoospermia persists, rectifying correctable problems maximize the chances of successful sperm retrieval at TESE. The first step is to eliminate exposure to all potential gonadotoxins.

Hormonal Therapy

Men with hypogonadotropic hypogonadism, either idiopathic or from Kallman's syndrome, respond well to treatment with exogenous replacement of FSH and LH. We use a regimen of human chorionic gonadotropin (2500 U 3×/wk) until serum T levels are normalized. If no sperm appear in the ejaculate, then recombinant FSH (75 IU 3×/wk) can be added. This approach may take 1 or 2 yr until optimal sperm production is identified but results in naturally conceived pregnancies for over 50% of couples.

Azoospermic men with primary testicular failure, whether idiopathic or secondary to Klinefelter's syndrome, typically have elevated gonadotropin levels. Many of these men have a decreased T-to-estradol (E) ratio. Fertile men have T (ng/dL)/E_2 (pg/mL) ratios of 14.5 ± 1.2, whereas men with nonobstructive azoospermia have a T/E_2 of 6.9 ± 0.6, and men with Klinefelter syndrome have a ratio of 4.4 ± 0.5. Men with abnormal T/E_2 ratios benefit from the use of aromatase inhibitors, such as testolactone and anastrazole, to decrease the conversion of T and androstenedione to estradiol and estrone. Men with Klinefelter syndrome appear to benefit from the administration of testolactone instead of anastrazole. The effectiveness of aromatase inhibition suggests that aromatase activity from Leydig cell hyperplasia may be responsible for increased T-to-estradiol conversion and impaired semen parameters.

Aromatase inhibitor therapy is not likely to convert azoospermia to oligospermia, but we do believe that it optimizes sperm production prior to attempted TESE *(4)*. Our practice has been to start men who ultimately require TESE on an aromatase inhibitor 3 to 6 mo before planned sperm retrieval.

Many men with nonobstructive azoospermia are mistakenly placed on exogenous androgens in the aim to increase spermatogenesis, but this technique is always an error. Exogenous T rapidly produces normal or elevated levels of serum T, thus suppressing secretion of LH from the pituitary. Consequently, the testis produces no T. Very high levels of local T are needed at the testis to induce spermatogenesis, many times higher than the serum levels achieved with exogenous T therapy. Thus, exogenous T effectively shuts down spermatogenesis.

Varicocele Repair

Varicocele is an important cause of subfertility that is present in about 15% of all males. Typically, varicoceles produce a decline in all parameters of sperm activity on semen, including motility, morphology, count, and concentration. In some cases, the effect of a varicocele may produce azoospermia.

Treatment of varicoceles in men with nonobstructive azoospermia is controversial. Repairing large varicoceles markedly improves all semen analysis parameters in men with oligospermia. We extrapolate that varicocele repair could have a salutatory effect on sperm production in some azoospermic men as well. The approach for repair of varicoceles in infertile men should be microsurgical to lessen the chance of an arterial injury. Varicocele repair should be done at least 3 to 6 mo before TESE to allow for maximal potential benefit of the repair. Although the return of sperm in the ejaculate after varicocele repair in azoospermic men is only 7.5%, we continue to perform this procedure in selected cases to optimize intratesticular sperm production. When the female partner is more than 35 yr old, the delay in TESE-ICSI secondary to varicocele repair must be weighed against the age-related decline in fertility for these women.

Sperm Retrieval in Nonobstructive Azoospermia

Once all correctable factors are addressed, we proceed with sperm retrieval. The retrieval of testicular sperm is a remarkable step forward in the treatment of infertile men. Before the advent of sperm retrieval and ICSI, all men with testicular failure were considered irreversibly sterile. However, in the last decade, the prognosis has changed. Men with azoospermia usually have at least rare foci of sperm production within the testis, and these testicular sperm are able to successfully fertilize oocytes with the help of ICSI. There are several approaches available for sperm retrieval. Fine-needle aspiration (FNA) is proposed as a technique for mapping the testis in preparation for open surgical sperm extraction. Yet, as a primary technique for extracting sperm, FNA is inferior to open techniques in multiple-controlled trials *(5–7)*.

Several techniques of open sperm extraction procedures are available. A single open biopsy performed before ovarian stimulation has the advantage of avoiding unnecessary hyperstimulation when no sperm are found. Unfortunately, frozen spermatozoa from men with nonobstructive azoospermia often do not survive freeze-thaw and result in a lower pregnancy rate (in our experience) when used for ICSI. In addition, a single biopsy is often an insufficient sampling of the testis. We recently quantified our results with a multibiopsy technique and found that nearly one-half of men with sperm extractable from the testis would have been denied an opportunity for effective treatment if only one biopsy sample was taken *(8)*.

A multiple biopsy approach has been shown to be superior to the single biopsy in terms of frequency of sperm extraction. But multiple biopsies endanger the blood supply to the testis by injuring the major subtunical branches of the testicular artery, leading to testicular atrophy *(8)*. To minimize the chances of injury to testicular blood supply while providing the advantage of multiple biopsies, a microdissection TESE is performed. A large incision in the tunica albuginea is created under ×8 to ×15 magnification, avoiding large subtunical vessels and intratesticular vessels. In addition to preservation of blood supply, the microdissection technique carries a second substantial advantage. Direct high-power examination (×15 to ×25) of the individual tubules allows the surgeon to identify seminiferous tubules that contain sperm. The functional tubules are wider and more opaque than the fibrotic and Sertoli cell-only–containing tubules. Using the microscope, smaller volumes of testicular tissue are excised *(9)*.

Generally, TESE procedures should be performed on the day before or day of oocyte retrieval during a programmed IVF cycle. Couples are counseled that the chance of successful sperm retrieval is about 60%, and as such, should consider having donor sperm available as backup. Before beginning a TESE procedure, a semen sample is closely analyzed for the presence of sperm. Of men with sperm counts inadequate for ICSI, 10 to 20% have sufficient numbers of sperm in the ejaculate on the day of oocyte retrieval. We do not advocate the use of cryopreserved sperm retrieved at TESE for the initial IVF-ICSI cycle. Even those sperm that do survive have decreased motility and fertilizing capacity when compared with fresh sperm. Immotile sperm produce lower pregnancy rates, possibly because of poor embryo development.

TESE retrieval rates at Cornell have averaged about 58%. Of the patients in whom sperm were retrieved, 49% had clinical pregnancies and 39% produced live deliveries. Twins were delivered in 27% of cases, triplets in 1.8%.

Treatment of Obstructive Azoospermia

For men with obstructive azoospermia, the choice of treatment depends both on the etiology of the obstruction, and to some extent, on the preferences of the couple. Previously fertile men who have had an elective vasectomy can undergo a vaso-vasostomy (VV) or a vaso-epididymostomy (VE), depending on the obstruction level. With experienced surgeons, the patency rate for a VV is 99% when sperm are found in the vas before anastomosis, whereas VE patency is 50 to 80%. Patency does not equate to pregnancy, but the return of sperm to the ejaculate in any amount makes subsequent treatment for infertility much easier. Unassisted pregnancy rates after VV approach 63%. After a VE, unassisted pregnancy rates are 43%. Because sperm return to the ejaculate may take many months, the age of the female partner should be considered before proceeding to reconstruction.

Men with ejaculatory duct obstruction can often be treated with transurethral resection of the ejaculatory ducts. Our approach to these men is to aspirate the seminal vesicles under transurethral ultrasound guidance with injection indigo carmine. Aspiration can provide large numbers of motile sperm that can be cryopreserved. Once the dye has been instilled into the seminal vesicles, the opening of the ejaculatory ducts can be resected until blue dye is seen to flow freely into the urethra. Using this approach, the rate of sperm return to the ejaculate is 50%.

Men with CBAVD and some men with iatrogenic injuries to the vas cannot be reconstructed. In these men, the treatment of choice is surgical extraction of sperm. FNA of the testis, percutaneous epididymal aspiration, and percutaneous biopsy of the testis are all efficient methods of retrieving sperm. Of the three percutaneous techniques, FNA provides the fewest sperm with the poorest motility.

The most effective method of retrieving large numbers of motile sperm is microsurgical epididymal sperm aspiration (MESA). The testis is delivered through a scrotal incision, then the obstructed epididymis is aspirated under the microscope. Aspirated fluid is checked for the presence of motile sperm. If no viable sperm are viewed, the procedure is repeated all the way to the caput, and even to the efferent ducts if necessary. MESA has the disadvantage of being an open surgical procedure, but more than 100 million sperm can typically be retrieved and preserved. MESA should be strongly considered for couples that plan more than one pregnancy.

RESULTS

MESA results in sperm retrieval in almost 100% of cases. Because retrieved sperm have not passed fully through the epididymis, these sperm are not completely mature; consequently, motility of sperm is not as high as that observed with ejaculated sperm *(10)*. Recent improvements in ICSI techniques have shown the clinical pregnancy rates of 74% and delivery rates of 65%.

CASE PRESENTATIONS

Case 1

A 27-yr-old man and his 27-yr-old wife present with 12 mo of unsuccessful attempts at conception. Neither has contributed to a prior pregnancy. The wife has regular menses and no history of pelvic inflammatory disease. They have been having unprotected intercourse three to four times per week over the past year. Semen analysis reveals normal volume, normal pH, and no sperm.

On physical examination,the patient is tall, with disproportionately long limbs and sparse body hair. His testes are each 3 cc and firm. Hormonal studies reveal elevated FSH and T at the low end of normal.

A likely diagnosis in this man is Klinefelter syndrome (47,XXY). The body habitus and the small firm testes are highly suggestive of this diagnosis. His elevated FSH with relatively low T are indicators of primary testicular failure, of which Klinefelter syndrome is a possible etiology. He should have a karyotype performed. If the Klinefelter diagnosis is confirmed, the couple should undergo genetic counseling before proceeding with assisted reproduction. If they choose to go ahead, he should receive 3–6 mo of testolactone followed by TESE with ICSI. They should be counseled that the chances of sperm retrieval in patients with Klinefelter syndrome are equal to or better than those of the azoospermic population as a whole.

Case 2

An otherwise healthy 25-yr-old man has an 18-mo history of primary infertility. His wife's work-up has been completely normal. His history is unremarkable except for a cousin with frequent respiratory infections. Semen analysis reveals a low volume, pH of 6.5, and no sperm.

On physical examination, the patient is normally virilized. His testes are 20 cc with normal firm consistency. No vas is palpated. His hormonal profile shows a normal FSH and T.

The probable diagnosis in this patient is obstructive azoospermia from CBAVD. His normal testes, normal virilization, and normal hormonal studies all support obstructive azoospermia. The lack of a vas on physical exam allows the diagnosis of CBAVD. He should have ultrasonography to evaluate for renal anomalies. His wife should be screened for CF carrier status, as the patient is almost certain to be a carrier if no renal anomalies are found. Genetic counseling is recommended if the wife is a carrier. If they wish to proceed with assisted reproduction, he will likely have abundant amounts of motile sperm in the proximal epididymis that can be harvested via MESA and effectively used with ICSI.

Case 3

A 31-yr-old man presents with a year of primary infertility. The female partner has been evaluated and is apparently normal. He relates a history of childhood surgery in the inguinal region. Semen analysis reveals normal volume, normal pH, and no sperm.

He is normally virilized and has bilateral well-healed groin incisions. His spermatic cords are both normal. His left testis is 3 cc and soft; the right is 14 cc and also soft. His hormonal profile shows a normal FSH and normal T.

Here, the diagnosis is unclear. The patient may have had correction of undescended testicles or inguinal hernia repairs. The small left testis may reflect atrophy from interruption of blood supply, or it may be naturally small with impaired sperm-producing ability. The right testis is also small, but much larger than the left. The status of the vas deferens on either side is in question. A testis biopsy would be a reasonable next step to determine whether or not he has normal sperm production in the right testicle. If the testis biopsy is normal, he will likely be a good candidate for MESA or even a crossed microsurgical VV. If not, he will have to undergo TESE.

Case 4

A 52-yr-old man requests reversal of his vasectomy. He had the procedure 15 yr ago but now would like to father another child. His wife is 39. Semen analysis is normal except for azoospermia. Physical exam is normal except for a dilated epididymis bilaterally.

This patient can undergo reconstruction of his reproductive tracts, or he can proceed directly to MESA. This couple should be counseled closely regarding the relative success rates of each technique. Given the length of time that has passed since the vasectomy, he will likely require a VE, which gives him a 50 to 80% chance of having sperm in the ejaculate in the next 2 yr. Unfortunately, his wife will be over 40 by the time patency is achieved, and the chances of successful pregnancy progressively diminish for her with every passing month. With MESA and ICSI, the wife will have to undergo ovarian stimulation, but the potential of a successful pregnancy may be greater because they can initiate attempts at pregnancy immediately.

Case 5

A 31-yr-old man presents for infertility evaluation with his wife of 2 yr. They have been trying unsuccessfully to achieve pregnancy for 8 mo. She has been pregnant before, but he has never contributed to a pregnancy. Semen analysis shows normal volume and pH but no sperm. He is well-virilized. His testes are 15 cc with slightly soft consistency. FSH is high, T is normal, and T/E ratio is normal.

This patient likely has nonobstructive azoospermia. Other than azoospermia, his normal semen parameters suggest against ejaculatory duct obstruction, and he has no history to indicate vasal or epididymal obstruction. The high FSH also indicates diagnosis of nonobstructive azoospermia, but some men with nonobstructive azoospermia can have a normal FSH. He should have a karyotype performed and genetic testing for microdeletions of the long arm of the Y chromosome. If the patient is found to have deletions of the *AZF* a or b regions, he should be counseled against TESE, as the likelihood of finding sperm with TESE is very low. If not, this couple could be candidates for TESE with ICSI.

CONCLUSIONS

Current assisted reproduction techniques have markedly improved the outlook for men with azoospermia who wish to become fathers. Treatment choices range from reconstruction of the interrupted reproductive tract to microsurgical retrieval of isolated pockets of sperm production in the testis. Determining the etiology of azoospermia can be a valuable aid in guiding therapy and counseling couples about their prognosis.

REFERENCES

1. Kogan SJ. Cryptorchidism, In: Kelalis PP, King LR, Belman AB, eds. Clinical Pediatric Urology, W.B. Saunders, Philadelphia, PA, 1985, p. 876.
2. Turek PJ, Cha I, Ljung BM. Systematic fine-needle aspiration of the testis: correlation to biopsy and results of organ "mapping" for mature sperm in azoospermic men. Urology 1997;49:743–748.
3. Schiff JD, Palermo GD, et al. Success of TESE-ICSI in men with non-mosaic Klinefelter's syndrome. Abstract presented at ASRM, 2002.
4. Raman JD, Schlegel PN. Aromatase inhibitors for male infertility. J Urol 2002;167:624–629.
5. Girardi SK, Mielnik A, Schlegel PN. Submicroscopic deletions of the Y chromosome in infertile men. Hum Reprod 1997;12:1635–1641.
6. Rosenlund B, Kvist U, Ploen L, et al. A comparison between open and percutaneous needle biopsies in men with azoospermia. Hum Reprod 1998;13:1266–1271.
7. Rucker GB, Mielnik A, King P, et al. Preoperative screening for genetic abnormalities in men with non-obstructive azoospermia prior to testicular sperm extraction. J Urol 1998;160:2068–2071.
8. Sheynkin YR, Ye Z, Menendez, et al. Controlled comparison of percutaneous and microsurgical sperm retrieval in men with obstructive azoospermia. Hum Reprod 1998;13:3086–3089.
9. Schlegel PN, Palermo GD, Goldstein M, et al. Testicular sperm extraction with ICSI for non-obstructive azoospermia. Urology 1997;49:435–440.
10. Pavlovich CP, Schlegel PN. Fertility options after vasectomy: a cost-effectiveness analysis. Fertil Steril 1997;67:133–141.

15 Testis Biopsy and the Infertile Male

Sherman J. Silber, MD

Contents

INTRODUCTION

This chapter begins with the use of diagnostic testis biopsy to evaluate azoospermia. It then describes the basics of spermatogenesis in oligospermic and normospermic men, and the use of therapeutic testis biopsy for sperm retrieval and intracytoplasmic sperm injection (ICSI). Finally, it discusses the differences in embryo quality, chromosomal abnormalities, and pregnancy rates with testis sperm versus ejaculated sperm.

In the modern era, the only clinical indication for diagnostic testis biopsy is azoospermia. However, invaluable information on the basis of spermatogenesis has been obtained by testis biopsies performed (in the past) on men with a wide range of sperm counts, from severe oligospermia to more than 100 million sperm per cc.

From: *Contemporary Endocrinology: Office Andrology*
Edited by: P. E. Patton and D. E. Battaglia © Humana Press Inc., Totowa, NJ

AZOOSPERMIA

Approximately 1 out of every 200 men in any population (even excluding those who have had a vasectomy) is azoospermic. Approximately 20% of couples in the United States are infertile *(1,2)*, and 25% of all infertile couples have a low-sperm count *(3)*. About 2% of infertile couples have azoospermia *(3)*. Thus, azoospermia represents approx 8% of the cases of male infertility.

We classify azoospermia as obstructive and nonobstructive. Obstructive azoospermia can be secondary to a vasectomy, congenital absence of the vas deferens (CBAVD), accidental surgical interruption of the vas or epididymis during a hernia or hydrocele operation, or primary epididymal blockage from previous infections. In all of these cases there is normal spermatogenesis in the testes. Most of these, with the exception of congenital absence of the vas (CAV), are amenable to microsurgical repair *(4–16)*. For obstructive azoospermia, ICSI simply adds a secondary alternative following failed reconstructive attempts or in cases of CAV (which is not reconstructable) *(17–19)*. In fact, because of ICSI, virtually any man with obstructive azoospermia can now father his own child, with the only limitation being the fertility of the wife *(18)*.

Evaluation of the Azoospermic Man

The diagnosis of obstructive versus nonobstructive azoospermia should really be quite simple. However, it is sometimes approached in a confusing way that can lead to misjudgments, such as performing a vasoepididymostomy on a patient who has no obstruction or a sperm retrieval blindly for nonobstructive azoospermia when the problem is actually obstruction. If the diagnosis is obstructive azoospermia, the management is quite different than for nonobstructive azoospermia.

A few simple principles avoid these difficulties and allow a proper preoperative decision to be made: (1) If a testicle biopsy shows normal spermatogenesis (and azoospermic), then obstruction is the cause of the azoospermia. Everything else is superfluous. (2) If in addition, the vas deferens is palpable on physical examination, then the patient is a candidate for surgical exploration and probable vasoepididymostomy. All other data are irrelevant. (3) If the vas deferens is not palpable on physical examination, then the obstruction is nonreparable, and sperm retrieval with ICSI is required. In this case, no diagnostic testis biopsy is warranted.

A vasogram should be performed only as part of an operative procedure for correcting obstruction. It should not be used to make a diagnosis or to determine the need for surgery. Performing a vasogram as an isolated diagnostic procedure creates many problems. First, a scrotal exploration is not needed to ascertain that the vas is present; that should be easily discernible by physical examination. Second, unless performed as part of a careful microsurgical procedure, any injection or transection of the vas in performing a vasogram could result in obstruction where originally there was none. Third, the vasogram data are not necessary for preoperative planning. Most important, the test tells nothing about the epididymis, which is the location of the usual site of obstruction. If the diagnosis is obstruction, and a vas is present, then the most logical time to perform a vasogram is at the time of a planned scrotal exploration and vasoepididymostomy (to confirm that the vas empties distally into the ejaculatory duct and prostatic urethra). However, when the semen volume or fructose is normal, it is certain that the ejaculatory duct is not blocked.

A normal follicle-stimulating hormone (FSH) does not necessarily indicate normal spermatogenesis or obstruction. In fact, more commonly, a normal FSH indicates maturation arrest and nonobstructive azoospermia. The serum FSH level correlates most closely with the total number of spermatogonia, not with the number of mature spermatids or sperm count *(20–22)*. The most typical diagnosis for patients with azoospermia and a normal serum FSH level is maturation arrest, not obstruction. FSH is usually in the normal range in cases of nonobstructive azoospermia caused by maturation arrest because the total number of spermatogonia in these cases is normal. It is true that an elevated FSH level usually relates to reduced spermatogenesis because of an overall deficiency in the number of spermatogenic cells. This can be partial or complete Sertoli cell-only syndrome or can just be caused by a reduced number of seminiferous tubules. However, an elevated FSH can also be associated with only modest oligospermia and is definitely *not* predictive of whether an azoospermic man will or will not have sperm present in the testis or at a testicular sperm extraction procedure (TESE) *(23,24)*. Thus, endocrine evaluations are only modestly helpful in the diagnosis and management of azoospermia.

Semen volume and fructose are important to distinguish whether the seminal vesicles are present or whether the ejaculatory duct is blocked. A normal fructose or semen volume does *not* mean there is patency, but signifies that there is a seminal vesicle present with no ejaculatory duct blockage. Men with CAV usually have absent fructose and low-semen volume. However, this is only because in most cases, absence of the vas is accompanied also by absence of the seminal vesicle.

Physical examination of the epididymis and testes, along with a history (or lack thereof) of infection, can be very misleading. Testicles that produce a normal amount of sperm may be small, and those that produce no sperm (with maturation arrest) may often be quite large. Similarly, historical data can be confusing. At least half of our patients who were found to have epididymal obstruction from inflammatory causes had no prior history of clinical epididymitis. We assume that whatever infection caused their epididymal obstruction must have been subclinical.

In conclusion, most of the ancillary medical information that we routinely consider in male fertility evaluation is irrelevant regarding whether or not the patient has obstruction. The physical examination is only relevant in that if a vas deferens is not palpable (i.e., CAV), and the semen volume is less than 1.0 cc, then no surgical anastomosis can be planned. Furthermore, normal spermatogenesis can be assumed. With that exception, the history and physical examination, serum FSH, leutinizing hormone (LH), testosterone levels, and vasography are of little use in diagnosis.

Diagnostic Testicle Biopsy

The open technique for diagnostic testicle biopsy (which we recommend) is very simple and should be a quick outpatient procedure under local anesthesia *(25)*. The spermatic cord is injected with about 6 mL of 0.5% marcaine (bupivacaine) via a 25-gage needle just distal to the external inguinal ring. Then, an additional 2 mL of 0.5% marcaine is injected over the anterior scrotal skin in the area where a 1-cm incision is made down to the tunica albuginea. With this method, a small "window" is created through which the testis can be visualized. Then an incision is made in the tunica albuginea. A 1.5- to 1-cm long piece of testicular tissue is excised and placed in Zenker's (or Bouins) fixative with an atraumatic "no touch" technique. This clinical proceedure is completely painless (except for the initial injection of local anesthetic). The patient is able to get up and walk away immediately afterward with no greater pain than if he had had a vasectomy.

Needle biopsy is another alternative, but it is no less painful than the open biopsy as described previously, and the open biopsy always yields a sufficient number of seminiferous tubules (>20 cross-sections) to perform an adequate quantitative analysis. Needle biopsy cannot accomplish this unless performed multiple times, which is then ironically more invasive than the open biopsy technique.

The biopsy must be of adequate quality to determine (1) Does the patient have normal spermatogenesis, and therefore obstruction, which might be amenable to microsurgical repair? (2) If he has nonobstructive azoospermia, will the TESE have a good or poor prognosis? Many testis biopsies are fixed incorrectly in formalin or so traumatized as to create artifacts and absurd readings like "sloughing and disorganization" that are not valid diagnoses *(21,26–28)*. Testicle biopsy has been used by most clinicians, including most pathologists, in a nonquantitative manner only. This has severely limited its usefulness and has led to many errors in interpretation *(29–32)*.

A simplified quantitative evaluation of the testicle biopsy is based on the normal histology and kinetics of spermatogenesis in humans *(33)*. The rate or speed of spermatogenesis in humans (or in any species) is constant for any variety of sperm counts, whether high or low. Reduced sperm production is

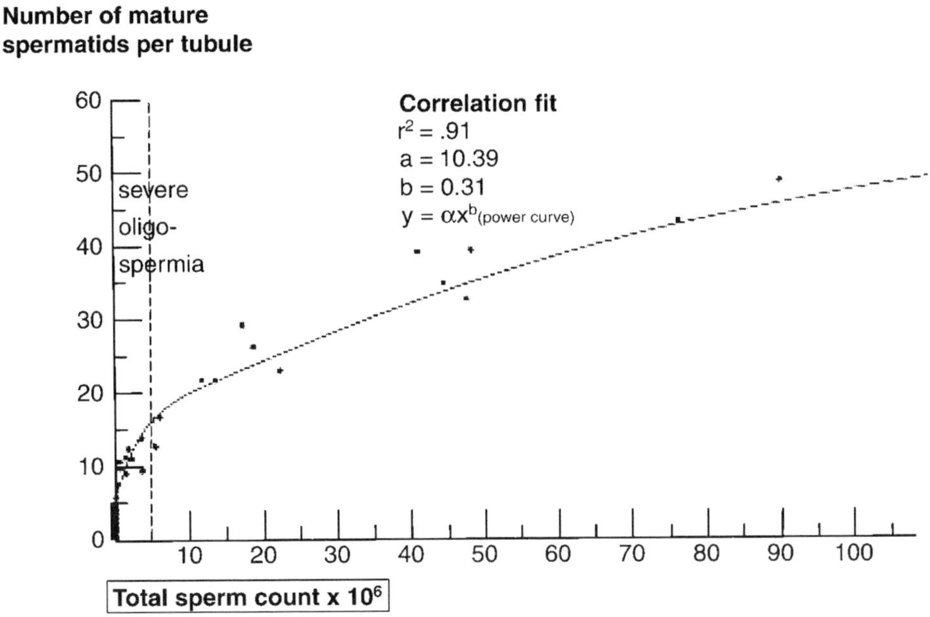

Fig. 1. An exponential curve that relates sperm count in the ejaculate to the average number of mature spermatids seen in each seminiferous tubule. A threshold of three to six mature spermatids per tubule has to be exceeded for sperm to appear in the ejaculate. (From ref. *21*.)

always caused by a lower number of sperm, not by a diminished rate of sperm production. Therefore, the daily sperm quantity being produced in the ejaculate by the testicle is reflected quite accurately by the testicle biopsy. Thus, testicle biopsies of patients with both oligospermia and normal sperm counts have been found to be predictive of mean sperm count in the ejaculate *(21,26–28,33–36)*. For patients who are severely oligospermic after a vasovasostomy, a quantitative testicle biopsy can thus clarify if partial blockage or just poor spermatogenesis is causing the oligospermia (Fig. 1).

The quantitative testicle biopsy is evaluated as follows. At least 25 seminiferous tubules are included in the count from each testis. The mature spermatids (oval-shaped cells with dark, densely stained chromatin) and large pachytene spermatocytes are the easiest to count (Fig. 2A). These cells have the greatest correlation with sperm count and are the easiest to recognize. All steps of spermatogenesis—from spermatogonia to leptotene, zygotene, and pachytene spermatocytes, and to early spermatids—may be observed, but the only clinically important cells are the number of "mature spermatids" (i.e., condensed oval-shaped sperm heads) counted in a minimum of 25 tubules and divided by the number of tubules (Fig. 2A).

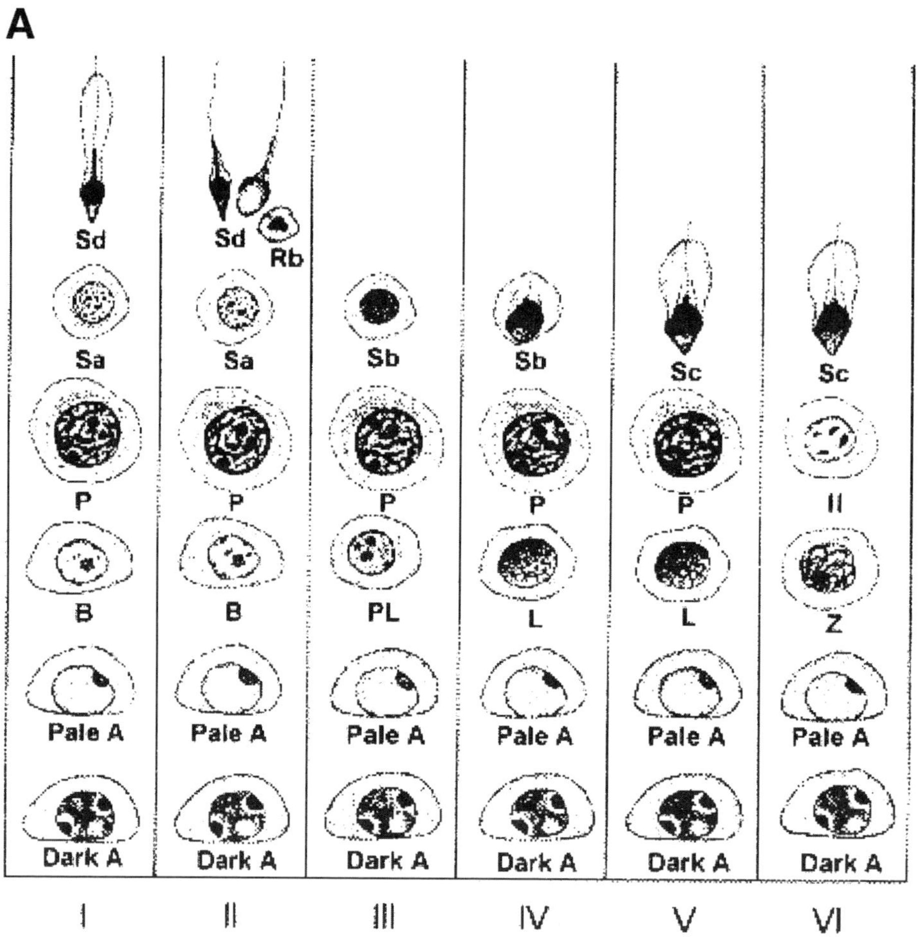

Fig. 2. (A) The six stages of spermatogenesis in the human testicle. (From ref. *7*.)

Pachytene spermatocytes represent the final preparation stage of the chromosomes for the first meiotic division. This is equivalent to the germinal vesicle phase of the oocyte. Nearly all cases of maturation arrest in the testis are at this stage of spermatogenesis, just before the first meiotic division. If spermatogenesis goes beyond this, mature (elongated) spermatids will always develop.

Using an exponential curve (Fig. 1), the number of mature spermatids per tubule can be used to predict the anticipated sperm count. In the absence of obstruction, the correlation is remarkably close. For example, when the patient has 40 mature spermatids per tubule, the sperm count should be just under 60 million per cc; when there are 45 mature spermatids, the sperm count should be just over 85 million. The patient with a sperm count of more than 3 million would

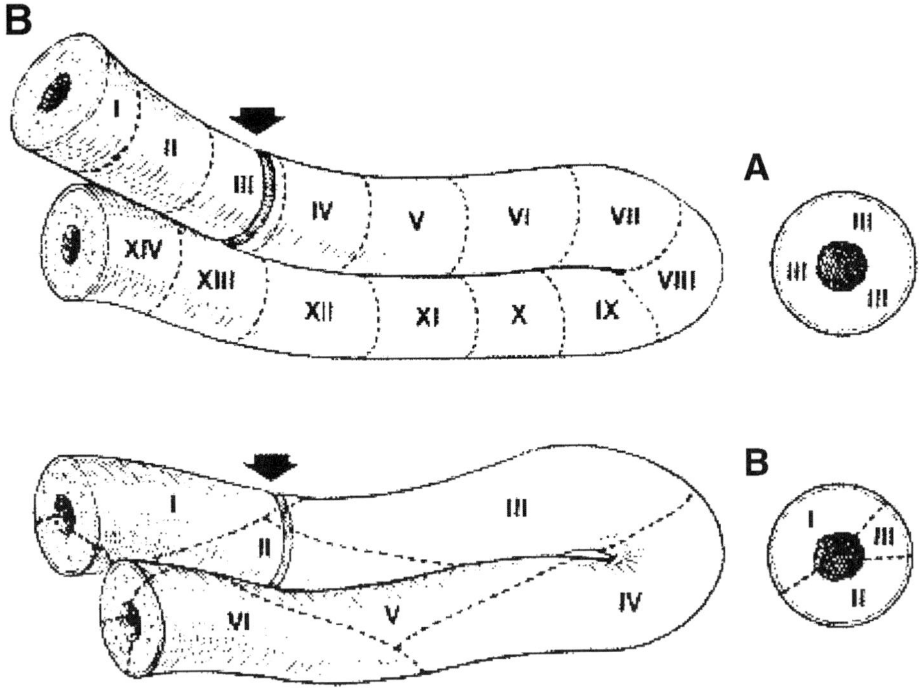

Fig. 2. (B) Drawings of the progression stages of spermatogenesis in the rat seminiferous tubule (a) and human seminiferous tubule (b). In most animals, there is a wave of spermatogenesis in an orderly manner down the seminiferous tubule. Howeverr in the human, there is a mosaic arrangement of the six stages of spermatogenesis. (From ref. *7*.)

be expected to have only 6 to 10 mature spermatids per tubule. When there are less than three mature spermatids per tubule, the patient is virtually always azoospermic.

Frequently, patients undergo vasoepididymostomy inappropriately because the pathology report is incorrectly read as "normal spermatogenesis." Such readings are usually not quantitative, but are instead qualitative impressions that tubules are filled with spermatocytes and have some mature sperm. When the biopsy shows thick tubules with a large amount of spermatocytes but only two or three mature spermatids per tubule, obstruction is not the cause of the patient's azoospermia. Such patients require TESE with ICSI for nonobstructive azoospermia owing to incomplete maturation arrest.

Considerable unnecessary confusion exists about the interpretation and counting of mature spermatids in the testis biopsy. The mature spermatid always has a tail, but it is rarely seen on histological section. This is because the sperm head is 4 μ wide and likely to be in the cut of the microtome's thin section, but the sperm tail is less than 1 μ in thickness and is unlikely to be seen in this cut section. Therefore, when viewing a histologic section, the spermatids will appear to be without tails, despite the fact that with TESE, they will appear just like sperm.

Some clinicians have attempted to use the serum FSH level to monitor the amount of spermatogenesis. They might mistakenly assume that a normal FSH level in an azoospermic patient would indicate obstruction. Unfortunately, this correlation is very poor *(20)*. Patients with azoospermia casued by maturation arrest have a normal FSH level. The FSH level correlates more closely with total number of spermatogonia and testicular volume, not with the number of mature sperm.

Ironically, it is the scattered mosaic arrangement of the various spermatogenesis stages in the human seminiferous tubule (as opposed to the orderly wave moving across the tubule in most other species) that makes quantifying the human testicular biopsy so simple. In rats, a cut through any particular seminiferous tubule shows only one particular stage (Fig. 2B). In humans, a cut through any area of the testicle reveals a scattered array of all the stages. Thus, in humans (unlike most other animals), it requires only 25 seminiferous tubules from any location in the testis for a good statistical sample of the total range of spermatogenesis in the entire testicle.

SPERM RETRIEVAL AND INTRACYTOPLASMIC SPERM INJECTION FOR OBSTRUCTIVE AZOOSPERMIA

CBVAD occurs in about 1% of infertile couples *(37)*. Until the last 12 yr, it was a frustrating and dismal problem with very poor prognosis for treatment. Since the first successful use of epididymal sperm aspiration and in vitro fertilization (IVF) for CBVAD was reported, ICSI has now made it possible for all these men to have children *(18,37–42)*. In fact, with ICSI, the pregnancy rate with microsurgical epididymal sperm retrieval (MESA) is only related to female factors *(18,41,43)*.

A simple "window" scrotal exploration under local anesthesia (just like for diagnostic testis biopsy) is performed on the same day that the female undergoes oocyte aspiration. Alternatively, MESA does not have to be coordinated with ICSI cycles. Frozen epididymal sperm provides results with ICSI no different than fresh. Under ×10 to ×40 magnification with an operating microscope, a 0.5-mm incision is made with microscissors into the epididymal tunic to expose the tubules in the most proximal portion of the congenitally blind-ending epididymis. Sperm are aspirated with a micropipet (0.7 mm/22 mm; Cook Urological, Spencer, IN) on a tuberculin syringe directly from the opening in the epididymal tubule. The specimens are immediately diluted in HEPES-buffered Earle's medium, and a tiny portion is examined for motility and quality of progression.

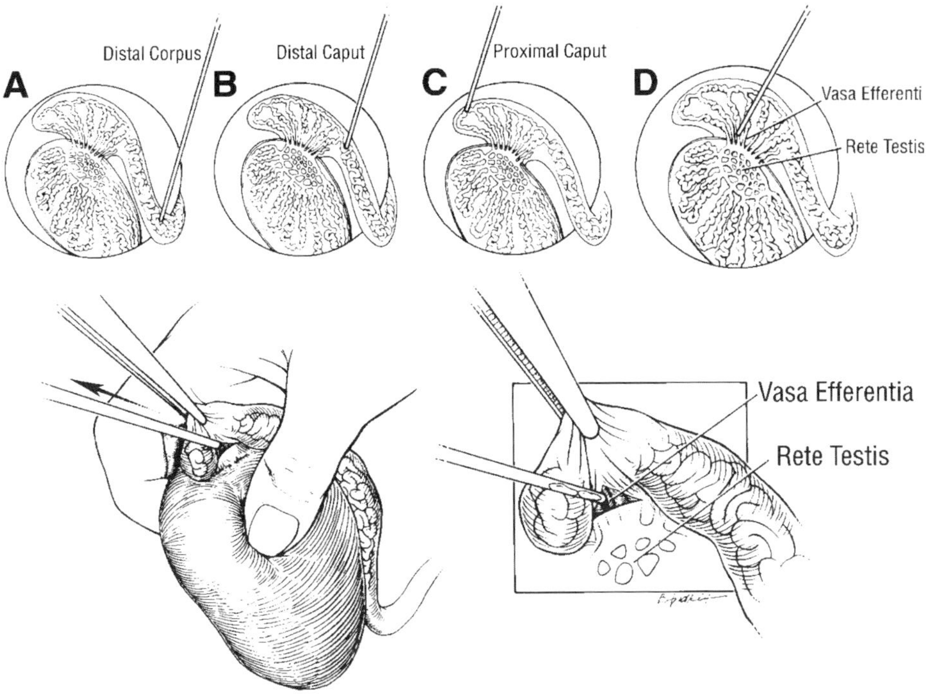

Fig. 3. A depiction of microsurgical epididymal sperm aspiration beginning at the distal corpus (A) and moving proximally to the distal caput, proximal caput, and the vasa efferentia (B–D). With obstructive azoospermia, there is an inversion of the usual physiological location of greatest and least sperm motility. With obstruction, the most motile sperm are always the most proximal. Because of senescence, distal sperm are the least motile. (From ref. *17*.)

If sperm motility is absent or poor, another 0.5-mm incision is made more proximally. Sperm are obtained from successively more proximal regions until progressive motility is found (Fig. 3).

Motile sperm are usually not obtained until the most proximal portion of the caput epididymis or vasa efferentia is reached, which is the opposite of what would be found in a normal nonobstructed epididymis. In the obstructed epididymis, the most recently produced sperm are the most proximal and are therefore the most viable and motile. The distal epididymal sperm are the most senescent and clearly nonviable. Once the area of motile sperm is found, an aliquot of epididymal fluid is used for ICSI, and the remainder is frozen.

There are virtually no cases of obstructive azoospermia that cannot be successfully treated with sperm retrieval methods and ICSI as long as the female does not have insurmountable problems. For obstructive azoospermia, we prefer to use epididymal sperm, although testicular sperm works just as well. The advantage of epididymal sperm as a first choice is that it freezes easily and represents a simple, clean, easy, and indefinite supply of sperm for the laboratory without need for future invasive procedures.

There have been many trivial debates over how best to collect epididymal or testicular sperm from azoospermic patients for ICSI. What works best in the reader's own particular setting can be decided, but our preference is as follows. For obstructive azoospermia, there is typically some epididymis present regardless how severe the congenital defect. In these instances, we prefer MESA. All of our sperm retrievals are done under local anesthesia without sedation. Although the approach is microsurgical and careful, it is an outpatient procedure performed with minimal postoperative discomfort.

The spermatic cord is first grasped between thumb and forefinger by the urologist and, similarly to testis biopsy, the cord is then infiltrated with several cc of 0.5% marcaine. This produces anesthesia of the testicle and epididymis, but not the scrotum. Then, several cc of 0.5% marcaine are used to infiltrate the anterior scrotal skin with a 25-gage needle along a proposed 1- to 2-cm incision line. Once the tunica vaginalis is entered, the epididymis and testicle are exposed and brought into the field of an operating microscope. Indeed, the patient can watch the entire procedure on a video monitor and should be wide awake and comfortable. The advantage of epididymal sperm retrieval performed in this way is the large number of the most motile sperm that can be readily obtained from the most proximal duct and frozen for an unlimited amount of future ICSI cycles.

Often, there is only one specific area of the proximal epididymis where motile sperm can be retrieved, and this can be found more easily through microsurgery than via a blind-needle stick (which, in truth, is a more painful than this microsurgical MESA procedure).

An important warning is that for nonobstructive azoospermia: epididymal sperm can never be retrieved because the walls are collapsed. Nonetheless, for nonobstructive azoospermia, an open testicular biopsy performed under the microscope can still be accomplished in the same manner under the same type of local anesthetic with the patient wide awake and minimal postoperative discomfort.

TESTICULAR SPERM EXTRACTION FOR NONOBSTRUCTIVE AZOOSPERMIA

Shortly after introducing sperm retrieval for obstructive azoospermia, we made the observation that even in men with the most severe spermatogenic defects (causing complete azoospermia), there were frequently a very minute number of sperm sparsely present in an extensive testicular biopsy, and these occasional testicular sperm could be used for ICSI *(19,21,22,42–44)*. We coined this procedure "testicular sperm extraction" or TESE. This approach was based

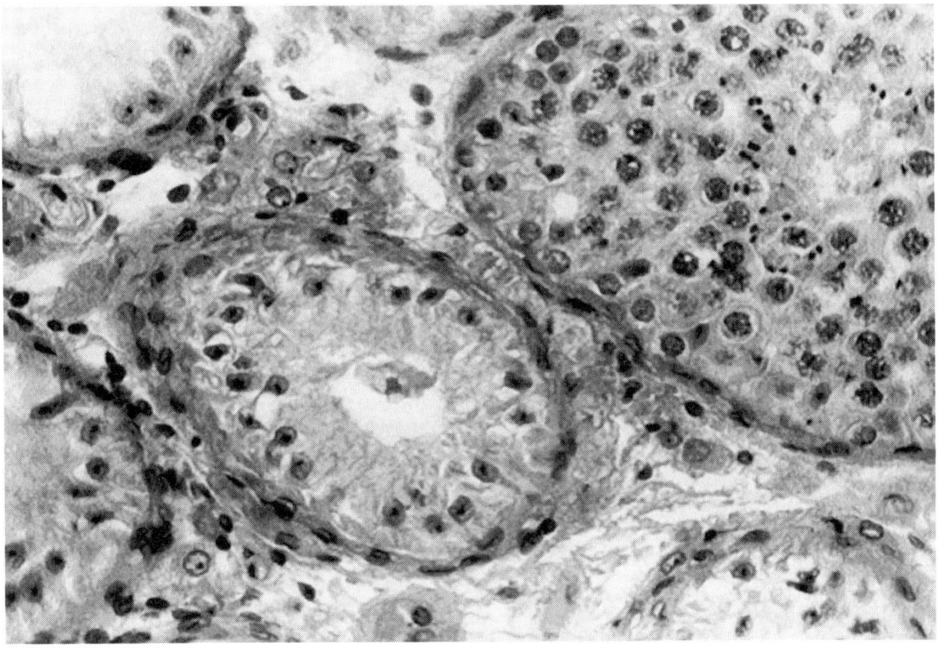

Fig. 4. A histologic section of testicle biopsy in a patient with Sertoli-cell only, elevated follicle-stimulating hormone, and occasional tubules with normal spermatogenesis. Upper right-hand tubule exhibits normal spermatogenesis, but all the other tubules are Sertoli cell-only (From ref. *50*.)

on quantitative studies of spermatogenesis dating back to the late 1970s *(27,28,34–36)*. Examination of the testicular histology of azoospermic, oligospermic, and normospermic men shows that the number of sperm in the ejaculate is directly correlated to the number of mature spermatids found quantitatively in the testis. The average mature spermatid count per tubule in a large amount of tubules is predictive of the sperm count in the ejaculate. Intriguingly, the majority of patients with complete azoospermia have a few mature spermatids in their testis histology (Fig. 4).

These studies of quantitative spermatogenesis in the late 1970s and early 1980s gave the theoretical basis for our efforts to extract sperm, however few, from men with azoospermia caused by Sertoli cell-only or maturation arrest and to use these sperm for ICSI *(45)*. An extremely diminished quantity of sperm production in the testis will result in the absolute absence of sperm in the ejaculate, even though there is some sperm being produced in the testicle. A minimal threshold of sperm production is necessary before any sperm can actually spill over into the ejaculate. Thus, severe oligospermia, which is readily treated with

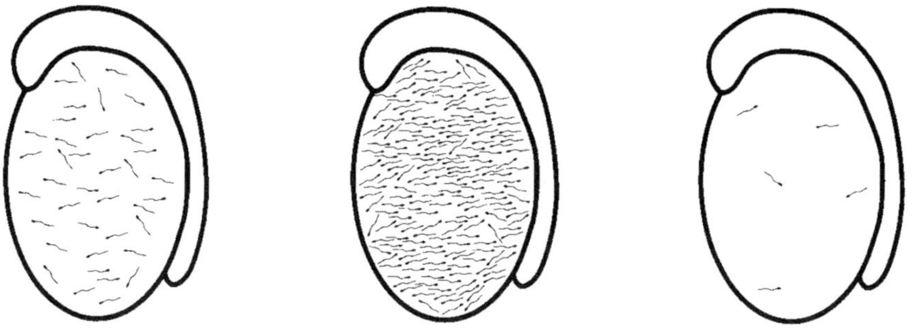

Fig. 5. Various degrees of azoospermia. Normal spermatogenesis (center drawing) is associated with obstructive azoospermia. With nonobstructive azoospermia, the testicular sperm extraction process may be as easy as in the drawing depicted on the left or very difficult as depicted in the drawing on the right.

ICSI, is just a quantitative variant of azoospermia where more than three mature spermatids per tubule are found in the testis. There is some minute presence of spermatogenesis is in 60% of azoospermic men (Fig. 5). However, the amount of spermatogenesis present in these men is below the threshold (three mature spermatids per tubule) necessary for these few sperm to spill over into the ejaculate *(21)*.

The initial approach to TESE for nonobstructive azoospermia was very crude, often involving numerous extensive biopsies from multiple areas of the testis until sperm were located. Legitimate concerns were raised. (1) How is the couple to be counseled for IVF and ICSI (with all that it entails for the female) when there is only a 55 to 60% chance that any sperm will be found? (2) Can the success or failure of sperm retrieval be predicted? (3) In cases of severely compromised testes, should the couple be assured that multiple repeat procedures will result in successful sperm retrievals in future cycles? (4) Is it possible simply to freeze unused sperm derived from a TESE procedure without diminishing the results, thereby avoiding the necessity of timing the female's stimulation cycle to the male's sperm retrieval?

Although it is clear that effective results can often be obtained with thawed testicular sperm for cases of obstructive azoospermia, frozen sperm from the testicle in the most severe nonobstructive azoospermia cases will not give a result equivalent to that of fresh sperm. Therefore, our two major goals were to determine (1) whether a prior diagnostic biopsy or any other test could predict the success or failure of a future TESE, and (2) whether or not a TESE technique could be used that would be harmless and relatively painless, so as not to compromise future attempts at fresh sperm retrieval? In fact, a small prior diagnostic testis biopsy is quite predictive of the likelihood of finding sperm in a TESE procedure in 90% of cases *(21)*. But in 10% of cases, prior diagnostic testis biopsy is not predictive. Our solution to this dilemma is a microsurgical approach to testicular sperm extraction (micro-TESE).

MICROSURGICAL TESTICULAR SPERM EXTRACTION

When extensive multiple biopsies from every area of the testis are performed to find sufficient sperm for TESE, much testicular damage can result and may limit "successful" patients to only one attempt *(23–24)*. An effort to limit damage by using multiple needle sticks rather than open biopsy to obtain sperm for ICSI is just as invasive and quite risky as well *(46)*. Furthermore, controlled studies have shown that for difficult cases of nonobstructive azoospermia where spermatogenesis is very meager, needle biopsy is much less likely to find the rare foci of spermatogenesis than open biopsy *(47,48)*.

We studied the distribution of spermatogenesis in azoospermic men and have outlined a *microsurgical* approach to TESE that minimizes tissue loss and pain and maximizes the chance of finding sperm. Knowledge of the distribution of spermatogenesis and microsurgical technique helps to prevent testicular damage and postoperative pain, making multiple repeat TESE procedures (if needed) safe and reliable *(21,26)*.

Unnecessary confusion exists with testicular sperm, mature spermatids, and round spermatids. Sperm tails are seldom seen on histology, and only the thicker sperm head shows up in thin sections, and usually only an oval-shaped head is observed. Mature spermatids at TESE are no different in appearance than sperm. The solution in cases with no sperm seen on TESE is *not* to look for "round spermatids" *(49,50)*. We never see round spermatids in the absence of mature spermatids, which at TESE are what appear to be sperm (Fig. 6A–C) *(49–51)*. The solution is to search for the few sperm that are sparsely and diffusely present.

Technique

All microsurgical TESE cases are performed under local anesthesia. Just like for MESA or for diagnostic testis biopsy, the procedure is truly painless. The tunica vaginalis is opened and the testicle is exteriorized. The operating microscope is then used under ×16 to ×40 magnification. After microdissection and evaluation of tubular dilation, a tiny microscopic removal of single dilated tubules can often be employed to retrieve large numbers of sperm.

However, large strips of tissue (no greater than the total amount of tissue that would have been removed in the conventional "blind" TESE technique) can be excised if necessary with no damage to blood supply and no pressure atrophy. The tunica albuginea is closed with 9-0 nylon interrupted sutures after meticulous hemo-

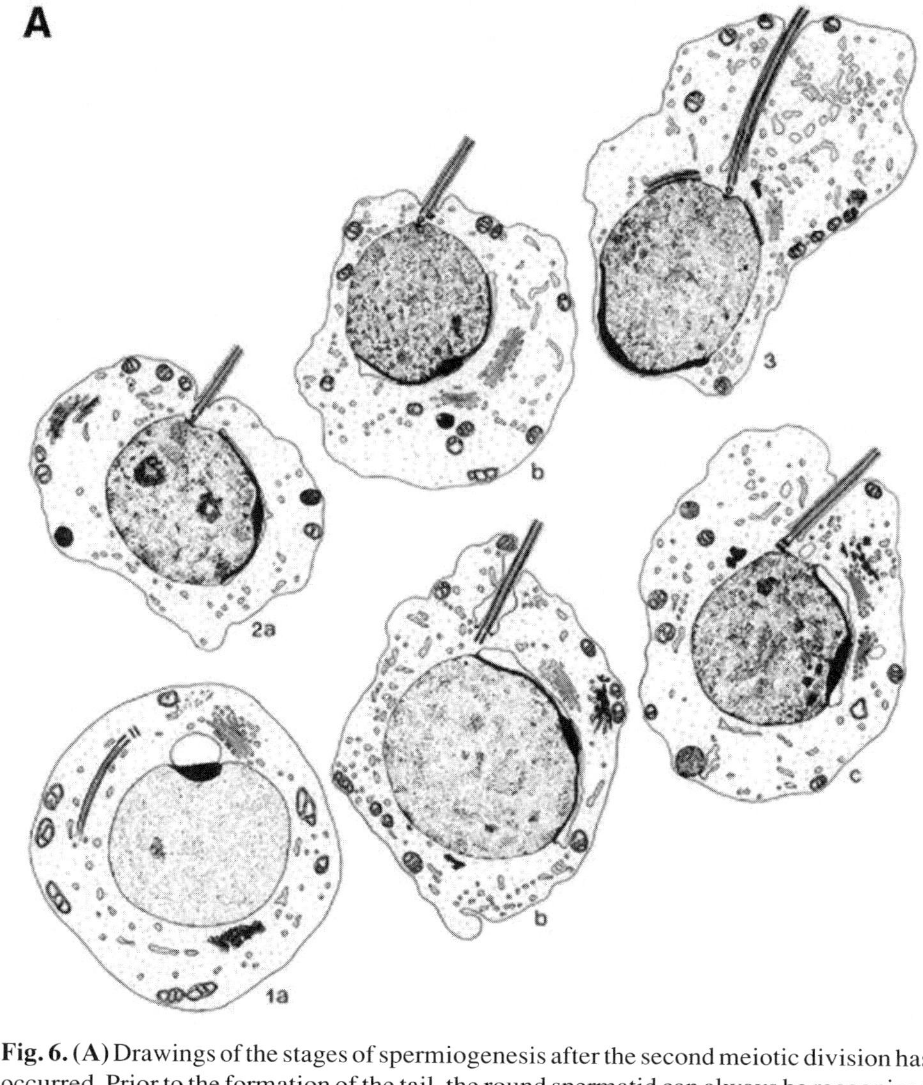

Fig. 6. (A) Drawings of the stages of spermiogenesis after the second meiotic division has occurred. Prior to the formation of the tail, the round spermatid can always be recognized by the prominent acrosomal vesicle (1a). As the acrosomal vesicle recedes, the tail begins to form. (From ref. *51*.)

stasis with microbipolar forceps (Figs. 7 and 8). This prevents any increase in intratesticular pressure, resulting in minimal pain and absence of subsequent atrophy.

Of the total cases subjected to microsurgical TESE for nonobstructive azoospermia, about 60% yield sperm sufficient for ICSI. In Sertoli cell-only, microsurgical dissection often (but not always) allows the removal of only a

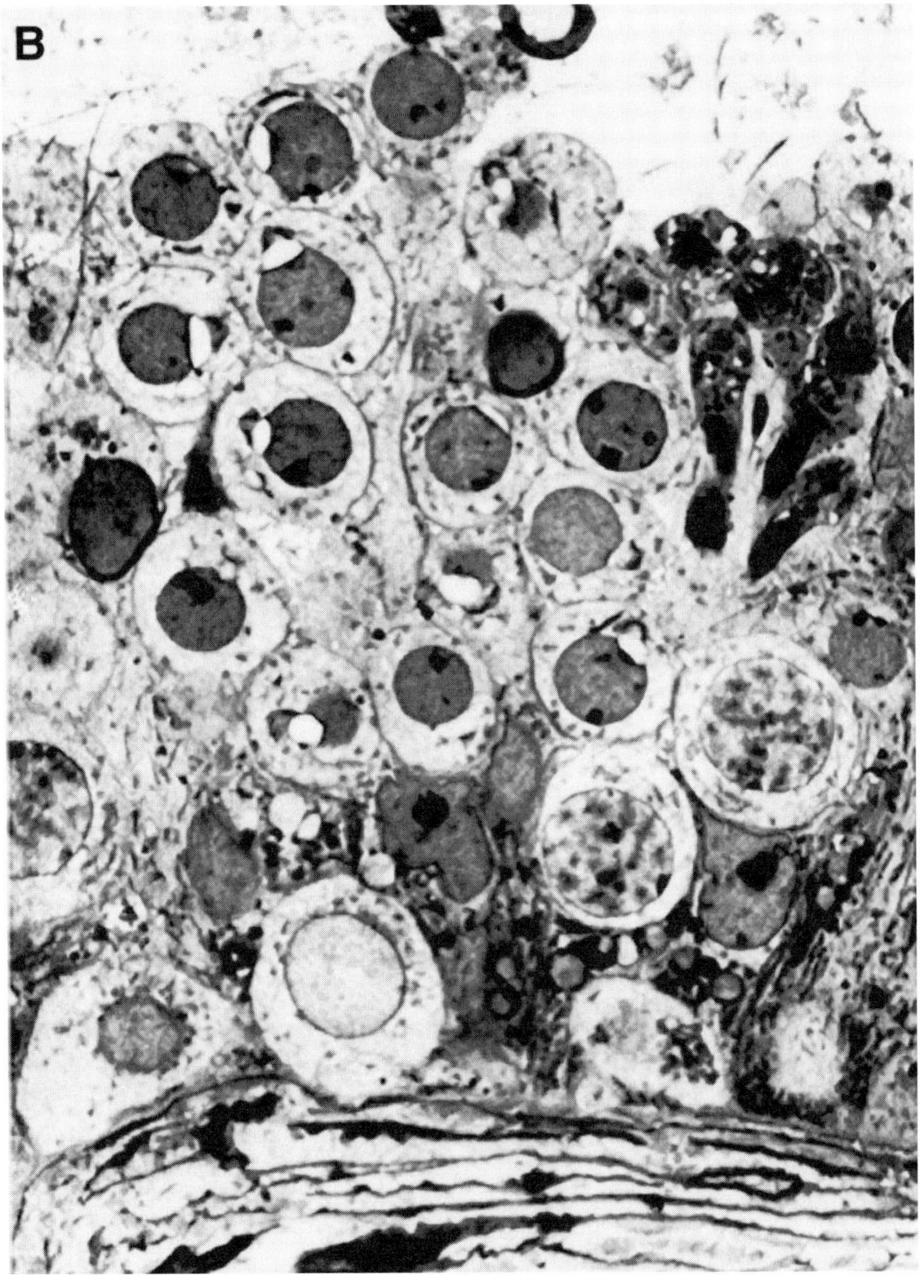

Fig. 6. (B) Electron micrograph of a section of human spermatogenesis demonstrating pale "type A" spermatogonia, Sertoli cell nuclei, pachytene spermatocytes, early round spermatids with acrosomal vesicle, and mature spermatids with an oval dark-staining head. (From ref. *51*.)

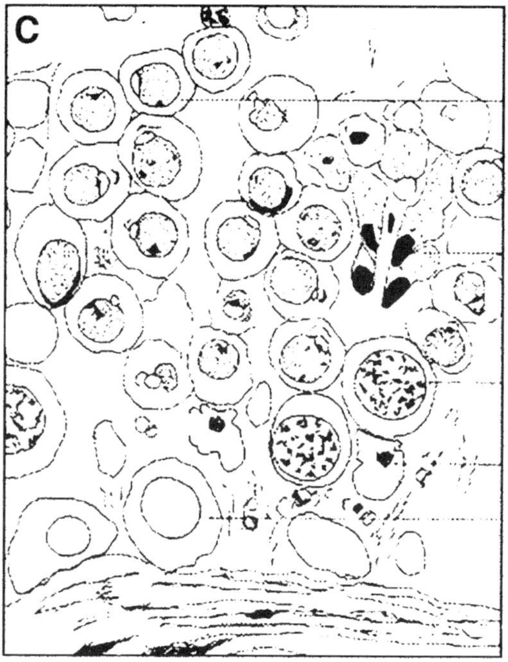

Fig. 6. (C) Diagrammatic depiction of Fig. 6B with labeling of the specific cells involved in spermatogenesis. (From ref. *51*.)

small amount of testicular tissue to find this sperm because normal tubules are full in thickness, and Sertoli cell-only tubules are usually thin and empty. In maturation arrest, a larger amount of testicular tissue usually has to be removed because all tubules are normal size, and the foci of spermatogenesis are not easily discernible. Nonetheless, even in those microsurgical cases where relatively large amounts of tissue have to be removed, minimal damage is incurred with micro-TESE because blood supply is not interrupted; microscopic bleeders are meticulously coagulated; and the tunica albuginea is not encroached because of the closure with 9-0 nylon interrupted stitches. Consequently, there is no increase in intratesticular pressure, no testicular damage, and minimal pain (Figs. 7 and 8).

Our direct mapping provides evidence for a diffuse, rather than regional, distribution of spermatogenesis in nonobstructive azoospermia *(21,26–28)*. Furthermore, the variation in sparseness of spermatogenesis, verified by observation of contiguous strips of testicular tissue, explains why a single random biopsy may or may not yield sperm. Also explained is how, removal of small amounts of tissue blindly with a needle, yeilds sperm in most cases with obstructive azoospermia, but does not work for nonobstructive azoospermia (Fig. 5). Microsurgery under the operating microscope trivializes any testicular damage.

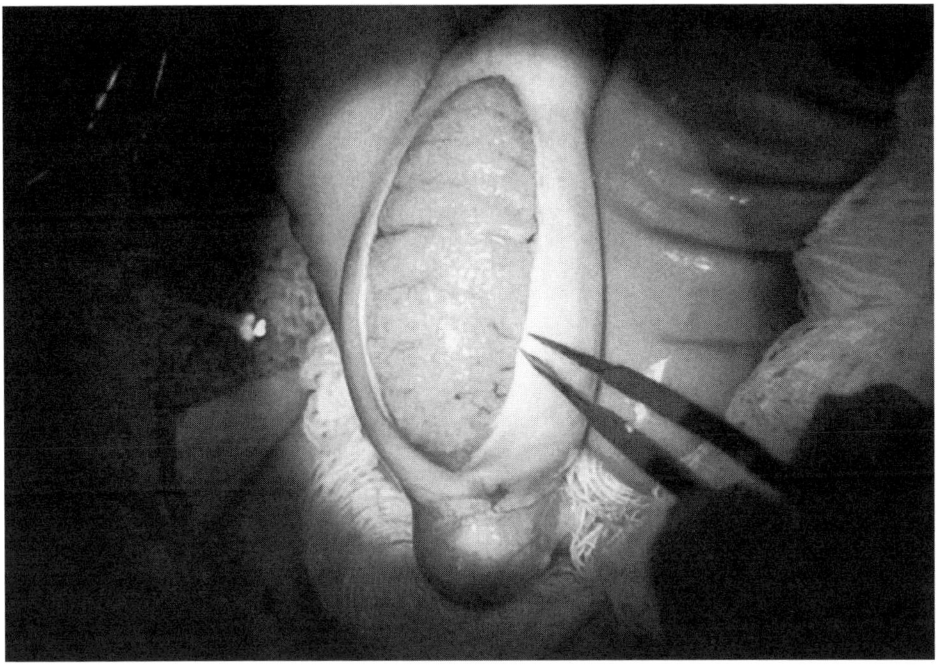

Fig. 7. A single large testicular incision for a testicular sperm extraction procedure under the operating microscope results in minimal to no testicular damage, minimal-to-no postoperative pain, and an ability to analyze each specific seminiferous tubule for the presence of spermatogenesis. (From ref. *26*.)

The formidable testicular deterioration that has been observed with overly aggressive TESE procedures is caused by either direct interference with microvascular supply of the seminiferous tubules or, even more commonly, increased intratesticular pressure because of minor amounts of bleeding within the enclosed tunica albuginea. The tunica albuginea is a very nonflexible enclosure. A small degree of intratesticular bleeding causes a noticeable increase in intratesticular pressure, which can be readily observed by those doing conventional, multiple-testicle biopsy samplings for TESE. Furthermore, the closure of open biopsies with the usual nonmicrosurgical suture, particularly in a running manner with conventional TESE, further compromises the intratesticular volume and thereby adds to the increased pressure (Figs. 7,8).

CHROMOSOMAL ERRORS, EMBRYO QUALITY, AND PREGNANCY RATES FOR INTRACYTOPLASMIC SPERM INJECTION WITH TESTICULAR SPERM

Early studies demonstrated that the major determinant of success with ICSI was not the quality or origin of the sperm, but instead the age and fertility of the

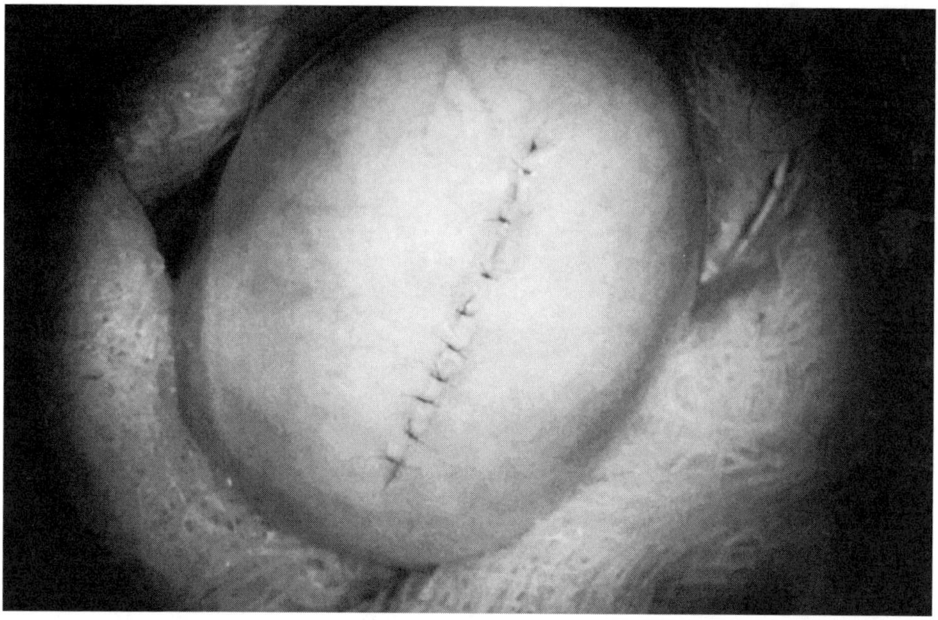

Fig. 8. Microsurgical closure of the tunica albigunea of the testes after a microsurgical testicular sperm extraction procedure results in no increase in intratesticular pressure and subsequently no loss of testicular function. (From ref. *26*.)

wife *(18,19,41–43,52,53)*. However, a detailed review of delivery rates with ICSI in couples with varying degrees of severity of spermatogenic defect, as well as fluoresence *in situ* hybridization (FISH) studies of both sperm and embryos derived from this sperm, indicates that sperm may also have an impact on ICSI results.

FISH analysis of embryos from ICSI cycles for nonobstructive azoospermia (requiring TESE) vs ICSI cycles for oligospermia demonstrates that embryos derived from TESE have a significantly higher rate of chromosome mosaicism *(54)*. In our initial research describing this phenomenon, ICSI cycles with ejaculated sperm produced 830 embryos: 41.8% were normal, 26.2% were aneuploid, and 26.5% were mosaic. In contrast, ICSI cycles with TESE for nonobstructive azoospermia produced 100 embryos: only 22% were normal, 17% were aneuploid, and 53% were mosaic. The difference in mosaicism rates between the two groups was highly significant ($p < 0.001$). Most mosaic embryos were chaotic. We continue to find a higher number of chromosomally abnormal embryos derived from TESE cases with severe spermatogenic deficiency. Sperm derived from TESE for nonobstructive azoospermia probably have a higher rate of comprised or immature centrosome structures, and this may be the cause of increased rates of chaotic chromosome errors in the subsequently derived embryos. Nonetheless, for oligospermia, the rate of chromosome abnormalities found in embryos produced by ICSI is similar to that found with conventional IVF. Thus, ICSI itself does not appear to be a teratogenic *(55,56)*. It is only the severity of spermatogenic defect, not the ICSI procedure itself, that causes this increase in chromosomal errors.

A slightly lower clinical pregnancy rate has been found for testicular sperm derived from men with nonobstructive vs obstructive azoospermia *(57)*. Also, a slightly increased incidence of chromosomal anomalies is found in ICSI offspring when compared to a normal newborn population *(58–63)*. Additionally, there is an increased incidence of abnormalities found in peripheral lymphocytes of males who require ICSI *(64–69)*. Even if the infertile male is chromosomally normal in his peripheral lymphocytes, meiotic disruption still generates higher rates of sperm chromosome abnormalities *(70)*. Thus, these few sperm in TESE cases have a higher rate of chromosomal errors.

In fact, we have observed a higher percentage of aneuploidy in testicular sperm from men with nonobstructive azoospermia (21%) than in ejaculated sperm from men with oligospermia (11%). However, this increased aneuploidy in the testicular sperm of azoospermic men cannot easily explain the dramatic increase in chaotic chromosomal abnormalities of TESE embryos. For this reason, we suspect other sperm abnormalities may be the cause. Most FISH studies on sperm of infertile males have found higher rates of aneuploidy than in fertile males *(71)*. However, with the exception of the most severe defects in spermatogenesis requiring TESE, the increase in sperm sex chromosomal abnormalities was very small and not correlated with an increase in spontaneous abortions of neonatal abnormalities *(72)*. However, it does likely explain the slight, but definite, increase in sex chromosomal anomalies indicated in ICSI offspring *(61)*.

Although most chromosomal studies of the sperm of infertile men had focused on aneuploidy, chromosomal abnormalities in human embryos are not limited to aneuploidy *(73)*. In younger women, the most common abnormality in cleavage-stage embryos is mosaicism, not aneuploidy *(74,75)*. These mosaic embryos can reach blastocyst stage, but still do not result in viable offspring *(73,76,77)*. Different mosaic types have been described in cleavage-stage embryos, and possible mechanisms that produce mosaicism have been proposed *(56,78–80)*. Occasionally, an infertile male in multiple IVF cycles produces mostly chaotic mosaics, but when donor sperm is used, produces normal embryos *(81)*. Significantly, chaotic mosaic embryos are more likely to be of poor quality in appearance than aneuploid embryos, which usually look quite normal. Therefore, the increase in chromosomal abnormalities (chaotic) in TESE embryos results in a higher incidence of poor-quality embryo appearance. This is different from the simple aneuploidy found to be increased in embryos from older women, and which can appear quite deceptively normal. Therefore, the chromosomal abnormalities associated with TESE sperm can be deleted with standard embryo morphology assessment, and do not lead to birth defects or increased miscarriages but do lead to slightly lower pregnancy implantation rates.

Early chromosomal studies of embryos obtained after conventional IVF vs ICSI (in cases of moderate oligospermia) have shown no difference in the incidence of chromosomal abnormalities *(55,56)*. However, there have been growing concerns regarding possible chromosomal anomalies in ICSI offspring of men with the most severe spermatogenic defects. Consistently, there has been a 0.8% to 1% incidence of sex chromosomal anomalies in ICSI offspring in comparison to a population norm of 0.14% to 0.2% *(59,61–66)*. These newborns would appear normal at birth, and the sex chromosomal anomaly (most frequently Klinefelter's) would not be identified without a prenatal karyotype. Autosomal aneuploidies in this population were no different than what would be expected based on maternal age in a non-ICSI population *(61)*. Perhaps a more alarming problem in ICSI-produced neonatal karyotypes was the 0.36% incidence of *de novo*-balanced translocations in comparison to the normal newborn population of 0.07% *(61)*. Additionally, there was a 0.92% incidence of inherited translocations transmitted via ICSI from the father. Of those inherited translocations, 10% were unbalanced. Thus, the total incidence of chromosomal aberrations in the ICSI population was 2.5%.

It is the sperm of infertile men that is the source of this low, but definite increase in chromosomal abnormalities of ICSI offspring, instead of the ICSI procedure itself *(55)*. Since 1994, many studies have been reported on the chromosomal analysis of spermatozoa by FISH *(73,74,85–94)*. A great deal of controversy was generated by these studies about the percentages of aneuploid sperm in infertile men. Although there seems to be a mathematically and statistically significant increase in sperm aneuploidy from infertile men, these differences were so slight to subsequently negate a major biological impact *(95)*. However, there have been several conflicting studies (Levron et al., Martin et al., and Palermo et al.) of the sperm found in the testes of men with nonobstructive azoospermia *(91–94)*. Our data confirm no significant increase in sperm aneuploidy with oligospermia, but about twice the rate of sperm aneuploidy in nonobstructive azoospermia.

It is known that aneuploidy of embryos is not closely associated or correlated with embryo morphology. As women age and the rates of aneuploidy increase, abnormalities in embryo morphology do not increase *(56)*. However, mosaicism, chaotic mosaicism, and polyploidy are associated with an increase in morphologic abnormalities in the embryos and do not increase with age. Aneuploidy appears to rise with maternal age and is related to defects in the egg, but mosaicism and chaotic mosaicism may be linked more to defects in the sperm and can result in a high percentage of chaotic mosaic embryos derived from ICSI with nonobstructive azoospermia.

The high rate of mosaic embryos observed as a result of TESE-ICSI may be more related to defects in the sperm centriole than to a higher incidence of numerical chromosome abnormalities. Our TESE-ICSI-derived embryos had no greater incidence of aneuploidy than ICSI with ejaculated sperm from men with higher sperm-production rates. However, a dramatically increased rate of mosaic errors was found in these embryos because of abnormal mitosis, which could be related to defects in the sperm centriole *(96)*. Similarly, an early report on MESA-ICSI for obstructive azoospermia in which distal (senescent) epididymal sperm were utilized demonstrated an inexplicably high miscarriage rate despite the young age of the female partners *(97)*. This phenomenon might also be explained by defects in embryo cleavage associated with centriole dysfunction *(98,99)*. Thus, the most severe degrees of spermatogenic defect, resulting in nonobstructive azoospermia and requiring TESE, or even senescent nonmotile sperm from distal epididymis, may result in a higher frequency of chromosomal abnormalities. But those abnormalities may be more related to errors in mitosis during early cleavage of the embryo than to sperm aneuploidy.

Present data points to a male origin of chaotic embryos. Because the first mitotic divisions are controlled by the spermatozoon centrosome *(100)*, this may result in abnormal chromosome distribution among sister cells. For instance, dispermic embryos have high rates of first mitotic mosaicism that appear as chaotic mosaics, and they are produced by an abnormal number of male centrioles (no haploids and two polyspermics) or suboptimal centriole function *(101–103)*. Sperm integrity is clearly necessary for normal mitotic division and early embryonic development *(104)*.

Alternatively, another possible explanation is that the higher incidence of autosomal aneuploidy in these TESE-derived sperm might possibly result in initially aneuploid zygotes. Then, the chaotic mosaicism in the subsequent blastomere could be a result of a cellular attempt during early embryo cleavage for mitotic correction of the initial aneuploidy. However, that would not explain the absence of this phenomenon in aging aneuploid eggs.

Severe spermatogenic defects, as in nonobstructive azoospermia, may result in a higher percentage of mosaic and chaotic mosaic embryos, causing less efficient implantation and live birth rates. The live birth rate for TESE with nonobstructive azoospermia is slightly lower than for obstructive azoospermia (normal spermatogenesis). ICSI for nonobstructive azoospermia is also associated with poorer embryo quality (corresponding to the increased incidence of chromosomal mosaicism) and lower live birth rates. Thus, despite the dramatic success of TESE-ICSI for azoospermic men with severe spermatogenic defects, the results are nonetheless adversely affected by sperm factors in these severe cases.

However, the negative impact of sperm factors is only modest (causing mosaicism) when compared to the negative impact of the female's age (causing aneuploidy).

REFERENCES

1. Mosher W. Infertility: why business is booming. Am Demograph 1987;42,43.
2. Mosher WD. Fecundity and infertility in the United States 1965-1982. Adv Data 1985;1:1.
3. Hull MGR, Glazener CMA, Kelly MJ, et al. Population study of causes treatment and outcome of infertility. Brit Med J 1985;291:1693–1697.
4. Silber SJ. Pregnancy after vasovasostomy for vasectomy reversal: a study of factors affecting long-term return of fertility in 282 patients followed for 10 years. Hum Reprod 1989;4:318–322.
5. Silber SJ. Results of microsurgical vasoepididymostomy: role of epididymis in sperm maturation. Hum Reprod 1989;4:298–303.
6. Silber SJ. Microsurgery. The Williams & Wilkins Company, Waverly Press, Baltimore, MD, 1979.
7. Silber SJ. Reproductive Infertility Microsurgery in the Male and Female. Williams & Wilkins, Waverly Press, Baltimore, MD, 1984.
8. Silber SJ. Microscopic vasoepididymostomy: specific microanastomosis to the epididymal tubule. Fertil Steril 1978;30:565–571.
9. Silber SJ. Microscopic technique for reversal of vasectomy. Surg Gynecol Obst 1976;143: 630,631.
10. Silber SJ. Perfect anatomical reconstruction of vas deferens with a new microscopic surgical technique. Fertil Steril 1977;28:72–77.
11. Silber SJ. Microscopic vasectomy reversal. Fertil Steril 1977;28:1191–1202.
12. Silber SJ. Vasectomy and vasectomy reversal. Modern Trends 1978;29:125–140.
13. Silber SJ. Sperm granuloma and reversibility of vasectomy. Lancet 1977;2(8038):588–589.
14. Silber SJ. Vasoepididymostomy to the head of the epididymis: recovery of normal spermatozoal motility. Fertil Steril 1980;34:149–154.
15. Silber SJ. Epididymal extravasation following vasectomy as a cause for failure of vasectomy reversal. Fertil Steril 1979;31:309–316.
16. Silber SJ. Ejaculatory duct obstruction. J Urol 1980;124:294–297.
17. Silber SJ. Congenital absence of the vas deferens. N Engl J Med 1990;323:1788–1792.
18. Silber SJ, Nagy Z, Devroey P, et al. The effect of female age and ovarian reserve on pregnancy rate in male infertility: treatment of azoospermia with sperm retrieval and intracytoplasmic sperm injection. Hum Reprod 1997;12:2693–2700.
19. Silber SJ. Intracytoplasmic sperm injection (ICSI) today: a personal review. Hum Reprod 1998;13:208–218.
20. DeKretser DM, Burger HG, Hudson B. The relationship between germinal cells and serum FSH levels in males with infertility. J Clin Endocrinol Metab 1974;38:787–793.
21. Silber SJ, Nagy Z, Devroey P, et al. Distribution of spermatogenesis in the testicles of azoospermic men: the presence or absence of spermatids in the testes of men with germinal failure. Hum Reprod 1997;12:2422–2428.
22. Silber SJ, Van Steirteghem A, Nagy Z, et al. Normal pregnancies resulting from testicular sperm extraction and intracytoplasmic sperm injection for azoospermia due to maturation arrest. Fertil Steril 1996;66:110–117.
23. Tournaye H, Liu J, Nagy PZ, et al. Correlation between testicular histology and outcome after intracytoplasmic sperm injection using testicular spermatozoa. Hum Reprod 1996; 11:127–132.

24. Tournaye H, Verheyen G, Nagy P, et al. Are there any predictive factors for successful testicular sperm recovery in azoospermic patients? Hum Reprod 1997;12:80–86.
25. Silber SJ. Evaluation and treatment of male infertility. In: Blanco, JD, Keye, RK, eds. Clinical Obstetrics and Gynecology. 2000;43:854–888.
26. Silber SJ. Microsurgical testicular sperm extraction and the distribution of spermatogenesis in non-obstructive azoospermia. Hum Reprod 2000;15:2278–2284.
27. Silber SJ, Rodriguez-Rigau LJ. Quantitative analysis of testicle biopsy: determination of partial obstruction and prediction of sperm count after surgery for obstruction. Fertil Steril 1981;36:480–485.
28. Silber SJ, Patrizio P, Asch RH. Quantitative evaluation of spermatogenesis by testicular histology in men with congenital absence of the vas deferens undergoing epididymal sperm aspiration. Hum Reprod 1990;5:89–93.
29. Charny CW. Testicular biopsy: its value in male sterility. JAMA 1940;115:1429–1432.
30. Nelson WO. Interpretation of testicular biopsy. JAMA 1953;151:1449.
31. Mannion RA, Cottrell TLC. Correlation between testicular biopsy and sperm count. J Urol 1961,85:953.
32. Albert A. The mammalian testis. In: Young WC, ed. Sex and Secretions, 3rd ed. Williams & Wilkins, Baltimore, MD, 1961, pp. 305–365.
33. Heller CG, Clermont Y. Kinetics of the germinal epithelium in man. Recent Prog Horm Res 1964;20:545.
34. Steinberger E, Tjioe DY. A method for quantitative analysis of human seminiferous epithelium. Hum Rreprod 1968;19:960–970.
35. Zukerman Z, Rodriguez-Rigau L, Weiss DB, et al. Quantitative analysis of the seminiferous epithelium in human testicle biopsies and the relation to spermatogenesis to sperm density. Fertil Steril 1978;30:448–455.
36. Clermont Y. Kinetics of spermatogenesis in mammals: seminiferous epithelium cycles in spermatogonial renewal. Physiolog Rev 1978;52:198–236.
37. Silber SJ, Ord T, Balmaceda J, et al. Congenital absence of the vas deferens. The fertilizing capacity of human epididymal sperm. New Eng J Med 1990;323:1788–1792.
38. Silber SJ. New treatment for infertility due to congenital absence of vas deferens. Lancet 1987;850–851.
39. Silber SJ, Balmaceda J, Borero C, et al. Pregnancy with sperm aspiration from the proximal head of the epididymis: a new treatment for congenital absence of the vas deferens. Fertil Steril 1988;50:525–528.
40. Tournaye H, Devroey P, Liu J, et al. Microsurgical epididymal sperm aspiration and intracytoplasmic sperm injection: a new effective approach to infertility as a result of congenital bilateral absence of the vas deferens. Fertil Steril 1994;61:1045–1051.
41. Silber SJ, Nagy ZP, Liu J, et al. Conventional in-vitro fertilization versus intracytoplasmic sperm injection for patients requiring microsurgical sperm aspiration. Hum Reprod 1994;9:1705–1709.
42. Silber SJ, Van Steirteghem AC, Liu J, et al. High fertilization and pregnancy rate after intracytoplasmic sperm injection with spermatozoa obtained from testicle biopsy. Hum Reprod 1995;10:148–152.
43. Silber SJ, Nagy Z, Liu J, et al. The use of epididymal and testicular spermatozoa for intracytoplasmic sperm injection: the genetic implications for male infertility. Hum Reprod 1995;10:2031–2043.
44. Devroey P, Liu J, Nagy Z, et al. Pregnancies after testicular sperm extraction and intracytoplasmic sperm injection in non-obstructive azoospermia. Hum Reprod 1995;10:1457–1460.

45. Silber SJ. Sertoli cell only revisited. Hum Reprod 1995;10:1031,1032.
46. Craft I, Tsirigotis M, Courtauld E, Farrer-Brown G. Testicular needle aspiration as an alternative to biopsy for the assessment of spermatogenesis. Hum Reprod 1997;12:1483–1487.
47. Friedler S, Raziel A, Strassburger D, et al. Testicular sperm retrieval by percutaneous five needle sperm aspiration compared with testicular sperm extraction by open biopsy in men with non-obstructive azoospermia. Hum Reprod 1997;12:1488–1491.
48. Rosenlund B, Kvist U, Ploen L, et al. A comparison between open and percutaneous needle biopsies in men with azoospermia. Hum Reprod 1998;13:1266–1271.
49. Silber SJ, Johnson L. Are spermatid injections of any clinical value? ROSNI and ROSI revisited. Hum Reprod 1998;13:509–523.
50. Silber SJ, Johnson L, Verheyen G, Van Steirteghem A. Round spermatid injection. Fertil Steril 2000;73:897–900.
51. Holstein AF, Roosen-Runge ED, eds. Atlas of human spermatogenesis. Grosse Verlag, Berlin, 1981.
52. Nagy ZP, Liu J, Joris H, et al. The result of intracytoplasmic sperm injection is not related to any of the three basic sperm parameters. Hum Reprod 1995;10:1123–1129.
53. Silber SJ, Devroey P, Tournaye H, et al. Fertilizing capacity of epididymal and testicular sperm using intracytoplasmic injection (ICSI). Reprod Fertil Dev 1995;7:281–293.
54. Silber S, Escudero T, Sadowy S, et al. Chromosomal abnormalities in embryos derived from testicular sperm extraction. Fertil Steril 2003;79:30–38.
55. Munne S, Marquez C, Reing A, et al. Chromosome abnormalities in embryos obtained after conventional in vitro fertilization and intracytoplasmic sperm injection. Fertil Steril 1998a; 69:904–908.
56. Munne S, Cohen J. chromosome abnormalities in human embryos. Hum Reprod Update 1998b;4:842–855.
57. Silber SJ, Colls P, Zheng X, et al. Spermatogenic deficiency and chromosomal abnormalities. ESHRE 2004, Abstract.
58. Bonduelle M, Wilikens J, Buysse A, et al. Prospective study of 877 children born after intracytoplasmic sperm injection with ejaculated, epididymal, and testicular spermatozoa, and after replacement of cryopreserved embryos obtained after ICSI. Hum Reprod 1996;11:131–159.
59. Bonduelle M, Aytoz A, Wilikens A, et al. Prospective follow-up study of 1,987 children born after intracytoplasmic sperm injection (ICSI). In: Filicori, M, Flamigni C, eds. Treatment of Infertility: the New Frontiers. Communications Media for Education, Princeton, NJ, 1998, pp. 445–461.
60. Palermo GD, Schleel PN, Hariprashad JJ, et al. Fertilization and pregnancy outcome with intracytoplasmic sperm injection for azoospermic men. Hum Reprod 1999;14:741–748.
61. Bonduelle M, Aytoz A, Van Assche E, et al. Incidence of chromosomal aberrations in children born after assisted reproduction through intracytoplasmic sperm injection. Hum Reprod 1998b;13:781,782.
62. Bonduelle M, Camus M, De Vos A, et al. Seven years of intracytoplasmic sperm injection and follow-up of 1,987 subsequent children. Hum Reprod 1999;14:243–264.
63. Bonduelle M, Ponjaert I, Van Steirteghem A, et al. Developmental outcome at 2 years of age for children born after ICSI compared with children born after IVF. Hum Reprod 2003;18:342–350.
64. Vernaeve V, Bonduelle M, Tournaye H, et al. Pregnancy outcome and neonatal data of children born after ICSI using testicular sperm in obstructive and non-obstructive azoospermia. Hum Reprod 2003;18:2093–2097.
65. Bonduelle M, Van Assche E, Joris H, et al. Prenatal testing in ICSI pregnancies: incidence of chromosomal anomalies in 1586 karyotypes and relation to sperm parameters. Hum Reprod 2002;17(10):2600–2614.

66. Aboulghar H, Aboulghar M, Mansour R, et al. A prospective controlled study of karyotyping for 430 consecutive babies conceived through intracytoplasmic sperm injection. Fertil Steril 2001;76:249–253.
67. Abyholm T, Stray-Pedersen S. Hypospermiogenesis and chromosomal aberrations. A clinical study of azoospermic and oligospermic with normal and abnormal karyotype. Int J Androl 1981;4:546–558.
68. Egozcue J, Templado C, Vidal F, et al. Meiotic studies in a series of 1100 infertile and sterile males. Hum Genet 1983;65:185–188.
69. Pandiyan N, Jequier AM. Mitotic chromosomal anomalies among 1210 infertile men. Hum Reprod 1996;11:2604–2608.
70. Testart J, Gautier E, Brami C, et al. Intracytoplasmic sperm injection in infertile patients with structural chromosome abnormalities. Hum Reprod 1996;11:2609–2612.
71. Van Assche EV, Bonduelle M, Tournaye H, et al. Cytogenetics of infertile men. Hum Reprod 1996;11:1–26.
72. Yoshida A, Miura K, Shirai M. Chromosome abnormalities and male infertility. Assisted Reprod Rev 1996;6:93–99.
73. Huang WJ, Lamb DJ, Kim ED, et al. Germ-cell nondisjunction in testes biopsies of men with idiopathic infertility. Am J Hum Genet 1999;64:1638–1645.
74. Vegetti W, Van Assche E, Frias A, et al. Correlation between semen parameters and sperm aneuploidy rates investigated by fluorescence in situ hybridization in infertile men. Hum Reprod 2000;15:351–365.
75. Colombero LT, Hariprashad JJ, Tsai MC, et al. Incidence of sperm aneuploidy in relation to semen characteristics and assisted reproductive outcome. Fertil Steril 1999;72:90–96.
76. Verlinsky Y, Cieslak J, Ivakhnenko V, et al. Birth of healthy children after preimplantation diagnosis of common aneuploidies by polar body fluorescent in situ hybridization analysis. Fertil Steril 1996;66:126–129.
77. Munné S, Alikani M, Tomkin G, et al. Embryo morphology developmental rates and maternal age are correlated with chromosome abnormalities. Fertil Steril 1995b;64:382–391.
78. Marquez C, Sandalinas M, Bahce M, et al. Chromosome abnormalities in 1255 cleavage-stage embryos. Reprod Biomed Online 2000;1:17–27.
79. Evsikov S, Verlinsky Y. Mosaicism in the inner cell mass of human blastocysts. Hum Reprod 1998b;11:3151–3155.
80. Liu J, Nagy Z, Joris H, et al. Intracytoplasmic sperm injection does not require a special treatment of the spermatozoa. Hum Reprod 1994;9:1127–1130.
81. Munné S, Weier HUG, Grifo J, Cohen J. Chromosome mosaicism in human embryos. Biol Reprod 1994c;51:373–379.
82. Harper JC, Coonen E, Handyside AH, et al. Mosaicism of autosomes and sex chromosomes in morphologically normal, monospermic preimplantation human embryos. Prenatal Diagn 1995a;15:41–49.
83. Delhanty JDA, Harper JC, Ao A, et al. Multicolour FISH detects frequent chromosomal mosaicism and chaotic division in normal preimplantation embryos from fertile patients. Hum Genetics 1997;99:755–760.
84. Obasaju M, Kadam A, Sultan K, et al. Sperm quality may adversely affect the chromosome constitution of embryos that result form intracytoplasmic sperm injection. Fertil Steril 1999; 72:1113–1115.
85. Miharu N, Best RG, Young SR. Numerical chromosome abnormalities in spermatozoa in fertile and infertile men detected by fluorescence in situ hybridization. Hum Genet 1994; 93:502–506.

86. Moosani N, Pattinson HA, Carter MD, et al. Chromosomal analysis of sperm from men with idiopathic infertility using sperm karyotyping and fluorescence in situ hybridization. Fertil Steril 1995;64:81–817.
87. Bernardini I, Martini E, Geruedts PM, et al. Comparison of gonosomal aneuploidy in spermatozoa of normal fertile men and those with severe male factor detected by in situ hybridization. Mol Hum Reprod 1997;3:431–438.
88. Rives N, Mazurier S, Sibert L, et al. Incidence of aneuploidy in sperm nuclei of infertile men. Hum Reprod 1998;13(Suppl);Abstract O-245, 126,127.
89. Rives N, Mazurier S, Bellet D, et al. Assessment of autosome and gonosome disomy in human sperm nuclei by chromosome painting. Hum Genets 1998;102:616–623.
90. Pang MG, Hoegerman SF, Cuticchin AJ, et al. Detection of aneuploidy for chromosomes 4, 6, 7, 8, 9, 10, 11, 12, 13, 17, 18, 21, X and Y by fluorescence in situ hybridization in spermatozoa from nine patients with oligoasthenoteratospermia undergoing intracytoplasmic sperm injection. Hum Reprod 1999;14:1266–1273.
91. Martin RH, Greene C, Rademaker A, et al. Chromosome analysis of spermatozoa extracted from men with non-obstructive azoospermia. Hum Reprod 2000;15:1121–1124.
92. Palermo GD, Colombero LT, Hariprashad JJ, et al. Chromosome analysis of epididymal and testicular sperm in azoospermic patients undergoing ICSI. Hum Reprod 2002;17:570–575.
93. Yogev L, Paz G, Yavetz H. Chromosome analysis of spermatozoa extracted from testes of men with non-obstructive azoospermia. Hum Reprod 2000;15:2685–2688.
94. Levron J, Aviram-Goldring A, Madjar I, et al. Sperm chromosomal abnormalities in men with severe male factor infertility who are undergoing in vitro fertilization with intracytoplasmic sperm injection. Fertil Steril 2001;63:479–484.
95. McInness B, Rademaker A, Greene CA, et al. Abnormalities for chromosomes 13 and 21 detected in spermatozoa from infertile men. Hum Reprod 1998;13:2787–2790.
96. Sathananthan AH, Ratnam SS, Ng SC, et al. The sperm centriole: Its inheritance, replication and perpetuation in early human embryos. Hum Reprod 1996;11:345–356.
97. Tournaye H, Devrowy P, Liu J, et al. Microsurgical epididymal sperm aspiration and intracytoplasmic sperm injection: a new effective approach to infertility as a result of congenital bilateral absence of the vas deferens. Fertil Steril 1994;61:1045–1051.
98. Schatten G. The centrosome and its mode of inheritance: the reduction of the centrosome during gametogenesis and its restoration during fertilization. Dev Biol 1994;155:299–335.
99. Schatten H, Schatten G, Mazia D, et al. Behavior of centrosomes during fertilization and cell division in mouse oocytes and in sea urchin eggs. Proc Natl Acad Sci USA 1986;83: 105–109.
100. Palermo G, Munné S, Cohen J. The human zygote inherits its mitotic potential from the male gamete. Hum Reprod 1994;9:1220–1225.
101. Zhou H, Kuang J, Zhong L, et al. Tumor amplified kinase STK15/BTAK induces centrosome amplification, aneuploidy and transformation. Nature Genet 1998;20:189–193.
102. Doxsey S. The centrosome - a tiny organelle with big potential. Nature Genet 1998;20:104–106.
103. Sathasivam K, Woodman B, Mahal A, et al. Centrosome disorganization in fibroblast cultures derived from R6/2 Huntington's disease (HD) transgenic mice and HD patients. Human Molec Genet 2001;21:2425–2435.
104. Moomjy M, Colombero LT, Veeck L, et al. Sperm integrity is critical for normal mitotic division and early embryonic development. Molec Hum Reprod 1999;5(9):836–844.

16 Intracytoplasmic Sperm Injection

The Process, the Outcomes, and the Controversies

David E. Battaglia, PhD, HCLD

CONTENTS

INTRODUCTION

As illustrated in this book, many medical and surgical options improve male factor infertility and permit couples to conceive naturally, or with minimal medical intervention. But there are still many conditions where sperm function will remain compromised and thus prevent the fertilization of an egg. Even standard in vitro fertilization (IVF) is ineffective with significant male factor situations. Through the introduction of intracytoplasmic sperm injection (ICSI), Palermo et al. *(1)* made it possible for many male complications to be overcome in the laboratory. Since that time, ICSI has arguably become one of the most important tools in the IVF laboratory. ICSI has provided the successful treatment of many levels of male infertility that were originally untreatable by any available technology.

Using ICSI, more than 100,000 children have been born worldwide, but like the introduction of IVF in 1978, broad interest has been in the follow-up of children born from this technology to assure patients and practitioners that ICSI is safe. Recent reports have presented the birth outcome data from studies comparing the rates of congenital malformations and anomalies between ICSI-derived children and those from IVF and natural conception. These studies have raised the important issue of whether there is, indeed, an increased incidence of

From: *Contemporary Endocrinology: Office Andrology*
Edited by: P. E. Patton and D. E. Battaglia

complications and, if so, whether this is a result of the ICSI procedure itself or a matter of patient selection. This chapter cannot answer the ultimate question of whether ICSI is safe for all patients because more data are needed. Recent studies suggest that certain severe male patients may present somewhat elevated genetic risks to their offspring by pursuing ICSI, indicating that comprehensive patient counseling is prudent in these cases. But it must also be noted that evidence indicates that the ICSI procedure does not appear to be the cause of any particular anomalies per se. By examining the reports on birth outcome data in this chapter situations are illustrated where comprehensive patient counseling would be strongly recommended.

Following the first introduction of ICSI into the clinical arena, the procedure has raised questions about whether it is too artificial or invasive in comparison to natural fertilization or IVF. But the issues surrounding ICSI cannot be discussed without at least a rudimentary knowledge of how fertilization naturally takes place and how the ICSI process is different. Successful fertilization is dependent on the mutual activities of both the sperm and egg. It is an elegant choreography of biochemical and cell biological processes that must be timed appropriately because the fertilizable lifespan of the ovulated egg is relatively short. Disruptions of any of the myriad events attendant to the process of fertilization can prevent its completion, thereby resulting in infertility. ICSI was clearly designed to circumvent potential breakpoints in the process of fertilization. However, there are certain misconceptions about ICSI that may have an influence on the acceptance or rejection of this technology. Many misconceptions can be eliminated by a comparison between natural fertilization and fertilization achieved through microinjection.

NATURAL FERTILIZATION

As described in Chapter 1, many characteristics of sperm physiology are integral to the fertilization process. Vigorous sperm motility and massive numbers of sperm are required for their transport through specific areas of the female reproductive tract. Low-sperm counts and/or poor-sperm motility may prevent conception at the early phases of sperm transport to the egg. There is enormous wastage of the millions of sperm is present in an ejaculate so that once sperm reaches the site of fertilization in the fallopian tube, the sperm-to-egg ratio is extremely low, perhaps as low as 10:1 or even 1:1. Thus, individuals with oligozoospermia or asthenozoospermia may be at risk of not achieving natural conception. In this situation, the fertilizing sperm must be fully primed for the culminating event of its life history. As it passes through the reproductive tract, it undergoes a series of biochemical changes, which are collectively termed "capacitation." These changes alter the sperm's motility pattern and biochemistry to permit it to pass through the egg investments, in addition to exposing specific surface receptor molecules.

When it encounters an ovulated egg on its journey, the capacitated sperm migrates through the cumulus cell matrix that surrounds the recently ovulated egg. Upon completing its transit through the cumulus matrix, the sperm will encounter the egg's "shell"—the zona pellucida. Sperm must recognize and bind to the zona pellucida using receptors exposed on the sperm surface during capacitation. The sperm bind to a specific glycoprotein on the zona pellucida and undergo the acrosome reaction (induced by the zona glycoprotein). Without successful capacitation, the sperm will neither bind to the zona pellucida nor undergo the acrosome reaction, and the fertilization process will end here.

The acrosome reaction is simply the secretion process of the acrosomal vesicle in the sperm head. Enzymes contained in the acrosome soften the zona matrix and aid the sperm making a path through this glycocalyx toward the egg surface. As zona penetration proceeds, the sperm binds to yet another zona protein to keep the sperm in close contact with this matrix. Continued softening of the matrix is accomplished by the presence of surface-bound acrosin on the sperm as it actively pushes its way toward the egg. Although vigorous sperm motility is essential to get the sperm through the zona, sperm cannot "push" their way through the firm gel-like zona matrix without proteolytic digestion. Therefore, sperm without functional acrosomes cannot fertilize an egg. An extreme example of this condition is the globozoospermic patient whose sperm have normal motility but completely lack acrosomes and subsequently cannot penetrate the zona pellucida. Also, sperm with poor postcapacitation motility also cannot cross this barrier because enormous energy output is required to complete this phase of sperm–egg interaction.

Once the zona is penetrated, sperm bind to receptors on the egg surface. This binding facilitates the fusion of the plasma membranes of both gametes. The sperm's plasma membrane is eventually left behind and becomes an integral part of the egg surface. Upon fusion, sperm motility immediately ceases owing to the depolarization of the sperm plasma membrane and mitochondrial membranes. This process alters adenosine triphosphate (ATP) gradients, thereby interrupting the energy supply to the axoneme. Sperm motility will never resume, but sperm function is certainly not finished. The fusion event marks the onset of the incorporation of the entire sperm (without its plasma membrane) into the egg. The first components to enter the egg cytoplasm are soluble activating peptides located in the postacrosomal region of the sperm head. These peptides, along with membrane depolarization, mediate the release of free Ca^{2+} ions from the endoplasmic reticulum and mitochondria of the egg. This process "activates" the egg, permitting it to undergo the cortical reaction and eventually complete its meiotic divisions. Sperm lacking these activating molecules will fail to activate the egg, and the fertilization process will cease at this point. Some globozoospermic patients again represent an example where sperm lack crucial molecules for fertilization—in this case the activating peptides *(2,3)*.

Through a process that takes several hours, from nucleus through axoneme, the entire sperm is incorporated into the egg by cytoskeletal action. During incorporation, egg activation stimulates several elaborate and complex events. The resultant Ca^{2+} flux induces the activation of several enzyme cascades that alter egg metabolism and induce the secretion of thousands of secretory vesicles called "cortical granules." These vesicles contain myriad enzymes that destroy receptors for sperm on the oocyte plasma membrane and zona pellucida. This overall chemical reaction represents the zona reaction that may be important to two phenomena observed during fertilization. First, it is believed by some that the destruction of the sperm receptors on the egg and zona pellucida surfaces is needed to prevent penetration of more than one sperm into the oocyte (polyspermy). However, as mentioned previously, under natural conditions, very few sperm actually reach the ovulated egg. Therefore, the importance of this block to polyspermy may actually be less important than it appears. However, the effectiveness of oocyte mechanisms to prevent multiple sperm penetrations is best exemplified during IVF where 10,000 to 100,000 sperm or more may surround an oocyte in culture. Although polyspermic penetration is extremely rare even under these artificial conditions, it must be stressed that evolution of the zona reaction did not consider IVF. Thus, the theoretical idea regarding the prevention of polyspermy via the zona reaction has little biological basis in humans. More importantly, the cortical reaction modifies the zona pellucida glycoproteins to change its physical characteristics and create a controlled microenvironment in which the cleavage-stage embryo will develop. There is a growing body of evidence that indicates that the confines of this hardened "shell" may allow for the concentration of important growth factors and other molecules that are secreted by specific cell types in the early embryo.

After egg activation, the second meiotic division is completed, resulting in a haploid pronucleus. During this time, the sperm nucleus loses its nuclear membrane, and enzymes in the egg cytoplasm alter protamine bonds, causing the sperm nucleus to decondense. The sperm's nucleus, which became haploid in the testis, will also transform into a pronucleus.

At this point, another key component of the sperm is utilized. Fertilizing sperm contain a functional centrosome that carries the necessary biochemistry to assemble microtubule-based structures. Nearly all cells possess a centrosome that is used to form mitotic spindles for cell division. However, the human egg loses much of its original centrosomal molecules and cannot easily generate microtubule-based structures after it becomes arrested in the second meiotic metaphase of meiosis near the time of ovulation. During fertilization, the specialized sperm centrosome is still competent and is used by the egg to create a microtubule matrix to capture both the female and male pronuclei, moving them centrally into the egg, and affecting nuclear fusion. Thus, the fertilization process is completed by the syngamy of both gametes' pronuclei. The sperm-derived centrosome will eventually organize the first embryonic cleavage divisions by orchestrating the assembly of the mitotic spindle for each division. Sperm that lack centrosomal components, or an egg cytoplasm that is unable to affect the decondensation of the sperm nucleus will clearly interrupt the fertilization process.

INTRACYTOPLASMIC SPERM INJECTION

The dozens of cell processes involved to produce a fertilized egg are all critical to success. Lesions in any of the biochemical pathways attendant to these processes will likely result in fertilization failure. Fertilization dysfunction can occur at any of the steps described previously, and probably in many subtle steps that have yet to be identified. But many of these potential dysfunction sites can be overcome with ICSI. The driving force behind the successful development of ICSI in 1992 stems from years of observations of IVF cases where male conditions caused dramatically reduced fertilization efficiency or prevented fertilization altogether. These included conditions of low-sperm counts, poor motility, abnormal sperm morphology, inability of sperm to undergo capacitation and the acrosome reaction, or combinations of these situations. Additionally, unexplained fertilization failures occurred after IVF where no overt male conditions could be identified by the semen analysis or any available tests of sperm function.

ICSI overcomes many male problems in that it bypasses the initial steps in the fertilization process. The direct injection of sperm into the egg cytoplasm with ICSI eliminates the need for sperm to undergo capacitation, convert to hyperactivated motility, bind to zona receptors, undergo an acrosomal reaction, and bind to the egg plasma membrane. It can be used with nearly any male factor situations, but is particularly effective in treating severely low-sperm counts and even azoospermia (if sperm can be retrieved from the testis).

The ICSI process begins with the selection of a motile (i.e., living) and morphologically normal sperm. Even in cases of teratozoospermia, every attempt is made to find morphologically normal sperm to be used for microinjection because it is evident that sperm with abnormal morphology may possess a higher risk of chromosome abnormalities than morphologically normal sperm *(4)*. After the appropriate sperm is selected, it is immobilized by slight crushing of its midpiece with the ICSI needle. Although this seems brutal, this action performs two functions. By creating a tear in the sperm plasma membrane, the ATP gradient created by the mitochondria is lost, and sperm motility is abolished. Also, this permits the soluble peptides in the sperm to eventually be released into the egg cytoplasm after injection. The overall effect of this membrane tear is akin to natural fertilization at the time of fusion of the sperm and egg plasma membranes as already described. Similar to natural fertilization, the "activating factors" create oscillations in free Ca^{2+} release from egg stores. Without this membrane disruption, an injected sperm is ineffective in fertilizing an egg because the soluble-activating peptides cannot be released at the appropriate time. The activation response in the presence of the activating peptides and sperm, including Ca^{2+} oscillations, is similar to that seen with IVF *(5,6)*.

The now immobilized sperm is maneuvered tail-first into the ICSI needle. The egg is secured by a holding pipet and oriented so the first polar body is away from the injection site (usually at the 6 or 12 o'clock position). This action assumes that the polar body is a presumptive marker of where the meiotic spindle may be located. But it has been shown that the polar body is unreliable as a marker for spindle position *(7,51)*. Although the meiotic spindle is located within 45° of the polar body in the majority of eggs, this position can range up to 180 degrees. Nonetheless, the chance of spindle disruption by the ICSI needle has proven to be extremely low as indicated by the fact that the normal fertilization rate with ICSI is actually slightly higher than with IVF. Moreover, if disruption of chromosomes on the meiotic spindle by the ICSI needle were a common event, then chromosome-related anomalies would be prevalent in all types of ICSI cases. Dumoulin et al. *(8)* demonstrated that very few embryos display the potential aneuploid conditions that would be created by spindle disruption. Furthermore, genetic information from birth data also reflects that physical damage of the spindle during injection is apparently very rare.

Injection is performed by needle passage through the zona pellucida, then through the egg plasma membrane. The human egg's plasma membrane is an extremely elastic structure, and the skill of the embryologist is needed to ensure that the needle actually pierces it. The entire sperm is then injected into the cytoplasm with minimal volume. Human eggs tolerate ICSI remarkably well. For experienced programs, egg survival should be more than 95%, and average fertilization rates more than 70 to 80% should be expected.

Studies have shown that the fertilization sequelae after ICSI are relatively equivalent to events seen with natural fertilization. The largest difference between ICSI and natural fertilization stems from the fact that the sperm plasma membrane is brought into the egg along with an intact acrosome during injection. Because of this, concerns have been raised that the formation of the male pronucleus may be altered or inhibited because of the presence of the acrosome overlying the sperm nucleus of the injected sperm. Studies in the monkey have suggested that pronucleus formation may be slower than normal after ICSI, and a particular layer between the nucleus and acrosome—the perinuclear theca—is unusually persistent during this process *(9)*. Slow pronucleus formation after ICSI has also been suggested in experiments where human sperm are injected into hamster eggs *(10)*. It has also been suggested that the chromosomes may be packed into the sperm nucleus in an ordered manner with sex chromatin being at the apex in 60% of the sperm *(12)*. But this study failed to correlate the DNA positioning with sperm morphology, and this finding has not been replicated. Nonetheless, it has been postulated that orderly DNA packaging and delayed decondensation and pronucleus formation (seen in the monkey) may be the cause of a higher incidence of gonosomal anomalies during development after ICSI. However, it has actually been shown with human ICSI that the process of pronucleus formation is slightly accelerated from that seen with natural fertilization *(11)*. Thus, in this instance, the animal studies do not appear to be reflective of the human situation. Moreover, the rate of gonosomal anomalies with ICSI is more likely a result of intrinsic genetic conditions of the sperm in selected patients and not because of the ICSI process itself or irregularities in the unpacking of DNA in the sperm during ICSI fertilization.

It has been argued by some practitioners that ICSI removes all natural sperm selection processes and is therefore far more artificial than IVF. But it must be noted that the vast majority of so-called sperm "selective" processes have already been removed even with standard IVF procedures. Under natural conditions, the female reproductive tract effectively reduces the prodigious sperm quantities viewed at ejaculation to the very small number that eventually arrive in the fallopian tubes. It does so primarily on the basis of sperm motility characteristics before and during capacitation. Perhaps sperm receptivity to the zona pellucida may be considered another part of the selection process. Although these processes certainly select for physiologically vigorous sperm capable of getting through the egg's barriers, none of them has been demonstrated to "select" for genetically normal or vital sperm. In IVF, egg cultures are surrounded by 10,000 to 100,000 sperm or even more depending on the laboratory. Under these conditions, fertilization is achieved in a statistical process where a biochemically competent sperm binds to zona receptors and passes through to the egg surface before its neighbor. There is no evidence that only more "genetically normal" sperm succeed other than those with superior motility and the ability to undergo capacitation at the right time. But, importantly, this situation with IVF is in contrast to natural fertilization where the egg encounters very few sperm after their transit through the reproductive tract. These few sperm tend to be morphologically normal and vigorous in motility, but the egg is not exposed to significant amounts of sperm metabolic byproducts. "Competition" among sperm for fertilization is very low or possible nonexistent. Thus, in one sense, ICSI is closer to natural conditions because the egg is not exposed to an enormous concentration of sperm and their metabolic byproducts. Morphologically normal sperm are selected for microinjection by the embryologist. There is actually no objective evidence that ICSI is significantly more artificial than IVF in terms of sperm selection.

BIRTH OUTCOME DATA

In early 2002, a study was published that showed an increased risk of congenital malformations in ICSI births when compared to IVF *(13)*. This report received considerable amount of attention, but its conclusions were based on only 301 ICSI infants from a localized geographical area vs 4000 naturally conceived births. Questions exist regarding reporting bias between the groups in this retrospective analysis, in addition to failure to account for maternal age effects, medical history, and separation of severe male factor patients in the analysis. This study could not address the issue of whether ICSI itself may be a cause of congenital problems. Moreover, the issue that patient selection, particularly those with severe conditions, may have significant impact on birth outcomes could not be discerned. This study is a good example of the need for consistent and unbiased evaluation of study groups before conclusions are made. Nonetheless, such reports have raised important awareness about whether ICSI possesses a potential risk to the infants born from this procedure.

Numerous recent studies have analyzed the birth outcomes of thousands of ICSI births. A comprehensive series of reports on birth outcomes from ICSI have been published over nearly a decade using data from multiple locations, ethnic groups, and concerted attempts to standardize comparisons between treatment groups *(14–17)*. These extensive analyses have found no increase in the incidence of major congenital malformations with ICSI when compared with IVF or the general population. In the most extensive analysis of this series *(17)*, pregnancy loss rates, follow-up rates, and maternal age were shown to be equivalent between ICSI and IVF cases. Thus, the data showing similar congenital malformation rates between the procedures was apparently not influenced by data omissions. Malformation of specific organ systems after IVF has been suggested. In two reports, it was determined that the incidence of hypospadias was elevated with IVF children in comparison to the general population *(18,19)*. However, in a larger study, no rise in the incidence of this anomaly was seen with ICSI cases *(17)*.

The source of sperm used for ICSI (ejaculated, epididymal, and testicular) has been compared with the prevalence of significant congenital malformations *(17,18)*. Although no differences in congenital birth anomalies have been seen between these sperm sources, it must be acknowledged that there were relatively few cases ($n = 311$) of testicular sperm included in the study. Follow-up of more cases is needed to determine whether testicular sperm used in ICSI pose a significant risk for congenital anomalies.

Unfortunate controversy has also been generated regarding the developmental outcomes of ICSI children. An early report by Bowen et al. *(20)* suggested that the mental development of ICSI children lagged significantly behind children born from IVF or natural conception. However, this study methodologically suffered by unequal inclusion of socioeconomic groups, language background, and possible evaluation bias between the ICSI and non-ICSI groups. Other studies have corrected the methodology and have reported no differences in the mental development between ICSI and non-ICSI children *(21–23)*.

It is encouraging that the majority of these studies do not reveal particular congenital or developmental problems associated with ICSI *(23,24)*. But it must also be noted that follow-up data from birth outcomes is still relatively limited. The mechanisms for comprehensive postnatal follow-up are often neglected, and multicenter studies would certainly aid in answering this important question with complete accuracy.

GENETIC ISSUES

Some of the earliest chromosomal studies comparing pregnancy outcomes between ICSI and IVF indicated that there was no increased rate of chromosomal abnormalities with ICSI *(25,26)*. These studies provided evidence that the ICSI procedure itself is not a cause of genetic anomalies. However, these earlier studies focused on moderate male factor conditions (generally, moderate oligozoospermia) as the source of sperm for ICSI. It is evident that as more severe patients are treated with ICSI, particularly with the wider use of testicular sperm biopsy to obtain sperm from azoospermic patients, the incidence of chromosome irregularities has increased. While congenital malformation rates have been shown to be similar between ICSI and IVF in the majority of reports, several studies have found a low, but statistically significant, increased risk of chromosomal anomalies in some ICSI groups. Of particular note is the observation that the incidence of sex chromosomal abnormalities with ICSI babies appears to be higher than the general population *(15,17)*. Significantly, the actual incidence of this situation is low (up to 1% in ICSI vs 0.2% in the general population), but the finding has been confirmed in several studies *(14–17,27)*. Additionally, there is an apparent increase in translocations of paternal origin and *de novo*-balanced translocations (0.36% with ICSI vs 0.07% in the general population) *(15)*. Again, to keep an accurate perspective, it must be noted that the actual incidence of chromosomal problems in ICSI offspring is relatively low, but the elevation over IVF or the general population is statistically significant and of concern to all practitioners.

Growing research shows that the origin of these chromosomal anomalies stems from the sperm source, not the ICSI procedure itself *(25,26,28,52)*. Analysis of sperm chromosomes in many studies has revealed that patients with significant male factor conditions (i.e., oligozoospermia, asthenozoospermia, or teratozoospermia) often exhibit elevated levels of aneuploidy in their sperm *(29–34)*. In cases of severe oligozoospermia, the rate of aneuploidy may reach 70% *(35)*. Of particular interest, specific chromosomes (X, Y, and 21) have been shown to exhibit extremely high rates of aneuploidy in sperm from men with abnormal semen analyses, thus providing the basis for the findings of elevated sex chromosome anomalies in ICSI cases. Interestingly, patients have also been shown to exhibit higher levels of genetic anomalies in their peripheral lymphocytes *(36–39)*, providing further evidence of paternal origin for the ICSI findings.

There has been some disagreement about the actual level of aneuploidy in male factor patients. For example, in a small study of 45 infertile patients exhibiting abnormal semen analyses, Guttenbach et al. *(40)* found no increased prevalence of aneuploidy. A few other studies have had varying results *(41–43)*, but nearly all studies would agree that there is a rise in aneuploidy's incidence in the more severe male factor categories, particularly severe oligozoospermia and azoospermia.

The concept that sperm may be the source of genetic anomalies in patients with certain diagnoses is further supported by a recent study by Silber et al. *(28)*, who compared ICSI outcomes between nonobstructive azoospermic and oligozoospermic patients. This study found that embryos derived from nonobstructive azoospermic patients using testicular sperm extraction procedure (TESE) exhibited a significantly higher rate of mosaicism than those obtained using ejaculated sperm from oligozoospermic patients. With the use of preimplantation genetic diagnosis, it was revealed that for the embryos derived from the oligozoospermic patients, 26.2% exhibited aneuploidy, and 26.5% were mosaic. By comparison, the embryos derived from nonobstructive azoospermic patients (TESE cases) exhibited 17% aneuploidy and 53% mosaicism. Indeed, many of the affected embryos from the TESE cases exhibited "chaotic mosaicism" in which there were different chromosomal complements in every cell. The difference in mosaicism between these two groups was highly significant, giving support to the concept that the sperm source, not the ICSI procedure, has a very significant impact on the chromosomal conditions of embryos derived from ICSI. These results were not related to maternal age. But, in fact, mosaicism is the most common chromosomal abnormality in embryos derived from either IVF or ICSI *(44,45)*. These reports suggest that the sperm is the likely source. This concept is further supported by the finding that male-factor patients who produce embryos with chaotic mosaicism can avoid this through the use of donor sperm *(46)*.

Importantly, such studies also demonstrate that irregularities in embryos from nonobstructive azoospermic patients may not be derived entirely from the sperm genetic makeup. As described earlier in this chapter, the mature human egg at fertilization does not possess fully functional centrosomal domains at the time of fertilization and therefore cannot assemble the mitotic machinery needed for embryonic cleavage. It is the sperm that provides the majority of the functional centrosome that is responsible for orchestrating early embryonic cleavage *(47,48)*. Along with a higher incidence of chromosomal anomalies, there is compelling evidence that sperm from some severe male factor patients possess dysfunctional centrosomes *(49,50)*. Although not yet proved, this situation may contribute to the embryonic aneuploidy or even chaotic mosaicism seen in some ICSI cases.

In light of the broad variety of reports on the ICSI procedure and birth outcome data, it appears that the procedure itself is relatively safe. While there are some slight differences in the process of natural fertilization vs ICSI, these differences do not appear to alter the outcomes in these cases. But it is clear from the data that patient selection may have a very significant impact on birth outcomes. The rates of genetic anomalies seen with severe male factor cases, while low, are indeed elevated above those seen with IVF or natural conception. Considering that severe male factor patients have been shown to present a variety of genetic irregularities in their sperm, the anomalies seen after ICSI can be likely attributed to the sperm source. It is evident that patient counseling and appropriate genetic testing should be offered to patients seeking ICSI treatment—this is particularly important for the severely infertile male. Although these patients may have no other options to be a genetic contributor to pregnancy than to use ICSI, they need to be aware of the risks that this approach may pose to their offspring.

REFERENCES

1. Palermo GD, Joris H, Devroey P, Van Steirteghem AC. Pregnancies after intracytoplasmic injection of a single spermatozoon into an oocyte. Lancet 1992;340:17,18.
2. Battaglia DE, Koehler JA, Klein NA, Tucker MJ. Failure of oocyte activation after intracytoplasmic sperm injection using round-headed sperm. Fert Steril 1997;68:118–122.
3. Rybouchikin AV, Van der Straeten F, Quatacker J. Fertilization and pregnancy after assisted oocyte activation and intracytoplasmic sperm injection in a case of round-headed sperm associated with deficient oocyte activation capacity. Fert Steril 1997;68:1144–1147.
4. Yanagimachi R. Intracytoplasmic sperm injection experiments using the mouse as a model. Hum Reprod 1998;13(suppl. 1):87–98.
5. Tesarik J, Sousa M, Testart J. Human oocyte activation after intracytoplasmic sperm injection. Human Reprod 1994;9:511–518.
6. Ludwig M, Scroder AK, Diedrich K. Impact of intracytoplasmic sperm injection on the activation and fertilization process of oocytes. Reprod Biomed Online 2001;3:230–240.
7. Hewitson L, Dominko T, Takahashi D, et al. Unique checkpoints during the first cell cycle of fertilization after intracytoplasmic sperm injection in rhesus monkeys. Nat Med 1999;5:431–433.
8. Dumoulin JCM, Coonen E, Bras M, et al. Embryo development and chromosomal anomalies after ICSI:effect of the injection procedure. Human Reprod 2001;16:306–312.

9. Sutovsky P, Hewitson L, Simerly CR, et al. Intracytoplasmic sperm injection for Rhesus monkey fertilization results in unusual chromatin, cytoskeletal, and membrane events, but eventually leads to pronuclear development and sperm aster assembly. Human Reprod 1996;11:1703–1712.
10. Terada Y, Leutjens CM, Sutovsky P, Schatten G. Atypical decondensation of the sperm nucleus, delayed replication of the male genome, and sex chromosome positioning following intracytoplasmic human sperm injection ICSI into the golden hamster egg. Does ICSI itself introduce chromosome anomalies? Fertil Steril 2000;74:454–460.
11. Nagy ZP, Janssenswillen C, Janssens R, et al. Timing of oocyte activation, pronucleus formation and cleavage in humans after intracytoplasmic sperm injection (ICSI) with testicular sperm and after ICSI or in vitro fertilization on sibling oocytes with ejaculated spermatozoa. Human Reprod 1998;13:1606–1612.
12. Leutjens CM, Payne C, Schatten G. Non-random chromosome positioning in human sperm and sex chromosome anomalies following intracytoplasmic sperm injection. Lancet 1999;353:1240–1241.
13. Hansen M, Kurinczuk JJ, Bower C, Webb S. The risk of major birth defects after intracytoplasmic sperm injection and in vitro fertilization. N Engl J Med 2002;346:725–730.
14. Bonduelle M, Wilikens J, Buysse A, et al. Prospective study of 877 children born after intracytoplasmic sperm injection with ejaculated, epididymal, and testicular spermatozoa, and after replacement of cryopreserved embryos obtained after ICSI. Hum Reprod 1996;11 (suppl. 4):131–159.
15. Bonduelle M, Aytoz A, Van Assche E, et al. Incidence of chromosomal aberrations in children born after assisted reproduction through intracytoplasmic sperm injection. Hum Reprod 1998;13:781,782.
16. Bonduelle M, Camus M, De Vos A, et al. Seven years of intracytoplasmic sperm injection and follow-up of 1,987 subsequent children. Hum Reprod 1999;14(suppl. 1):243–264.
17. Bonduelle M, Van Assche E, Joris H, et al. Prenatal testing in ICSI pregnancies: incidence of chromosomal anomalies in 1586 karyotypes and relation to sperm parameters. Hum Reprod 2002;17:2600–2614.
18. Wennerholm UB, Bergh C, Hamberger L, et al. Incidence of congenital malformations in children born after ICSI. Hum Reprod 2000;15:944–948.
19. Ericson A, Kallen B. Congenital malformations in infants born after IVF: a population-based study. Hum Reprod 2001;16:504–509.
20. Bowen JR, Gibson FL, Leslie GI, Saunders DM. Medical and developmental outcome at 1 year for children conceived by intracytoplasmic sperm injection. Lancet 1998;351:1529–1534.
21. Suttcliffe AG, Taylor B, Li J, et al. Children born after intracytoplasmic sperm injection: population control study. Br Med J 1999;318:704,705.
22. Suttcliffe AG, Saunders K, Thornton S, et al. Outcome in the second year of life after in vitro fertilization by intracytoplasmic sperm injection: a UK case-control study. Lancet 2001;357:2080–2084.
23. Bonduelle M, Ponjaert I, Van Steirteghem A, et al. Developmental outcome at 2 years of age for children born after ICSI compared with children born after IVF. Hum Reprod 2003;18: 342–350.
24. Van Steirteghem A, Bonduelle M, Devroey P, Liebaers I. Follow-up of children born after ICSI. Hum Reprod Update 2002;8:111–116.
25. Munne S, Cohen J. Chromosome abnormalities in human embryos. Hum Reprod Update 1998;4:842–855.

26. Munne S, Marquez C, Reing A, et al. Chromosome abnormalities in embryos obtained after conventional in vitro fertilization and intracytoplasmic sperm injection. Fertil Steril 1998; 69:904–908.
27. Aboulghar H, Aboulghar M, Mansour R, et al. A prospective controlled study of karyotyping for 430 consecutive babies conceived through intracytoplasmic sperm injection. Fertil Steril 2001;76:249–253.
28. Silber S, Escudero T, Sadowy S, et al. Chromosomal abnormalities in embryos derived from testicular sperm extraction. Fertil Steril 2003;79:30–38.
29. Bernardini L, Martini E, Geraedts JP, et al. Comparison of gonosomal aneuploidy in spermatozoa of normal fertile men and those with severe male factor detected by in situ hybridisation. Mol Hum Reprod 1997;3:431–438.
30. Martin RH, Greene C, Rademaker A, et al. Chromosome analysis of spermatozoa extracted from men with non-obstructive azoospermia. Hum Reprod 2000;15:1121–1124.
31. McInness B, Rademaker A, Greene CA., et al. Abnormalities for chromosomes 13 and 21 detected in spermatozoa from infertile men. Hum Reprod 1998;13:2787–2790.
32. Colombero LT, Hariprashad JJ, Tsai MC, et al. Incidence of sperm aneuploidy in relation to semen characteristics and assisted reproductive outcome. Fertil Steril 1999;72:90–96.
33. Vendrell JM, Garcia F, Veiga A, et al. Meiotic abnormalities and spermatogenic parameters in severe oligoasthenozoospermia. Hum Reprod 1999;14:357–378.
34. Vegetti W, Van Assche E, Frias A, et al. Correlation between semen parameters and sperm aneuploidy rates investigated by fluorescence in situ hybridization in infertile men. Hum Reprod 2000;15:351–365.
35. Pang MG, Hoegerman SF, Cuticchin AJ, et al. Detection of aneuploidy for chromosomes 4, 6, 7, 8, 9, 10, 11, 12, 13, 17, 18, 21, X and Y by fluorescence in situ hybridization in spermatozoa from nine patients with oligoasthenoteratospermia undergoing intracytoplasmic sperm injection. Hum Reprod 1999;14:1266–1273.
36. Egozcue J, Templado C, Vidal F, et al. Meiotic studies in a series of 1100 infertile and sterile males. Hum Genet 1983;65:185–188.
37. Pandiyan N, Jequier AM. Mitotic chromosomal anomalies among 1210 infertile men. Hum Reprod 1996;11:2604–2608.
38. Testart J, Gautier E, Brami C, et al. Intracytoplasmic sperm injection in infertile patients with structural chromosome abnormalities. Hum Reprod 1996;11:2609–2612.
39. Van Assche EV, Bonduelle M, Tournaye H, et al. Cytogenetics of infertile men. Hum Reprod 1996;11(suppl. 4):1–26.
40. Guttenbach M, Martinez-Exposito MJ, Michelmann HW, et al. Incidence of diploid and disomic sperm nuclei in 45 infertile men. Hum Reprod 1997;12:468–473.
41. Palermo GD, Colombero LT, Hariprashad JJ, et al. Chromosome analysis of epididymal and testicular sperm in azoospermic patients undergoing ICSI. Hum Reprod 2002;17:570–575.
42. Yogev L, Paz G, Yavetz H. Chromosome analysis of spermatozoa extracted from testes of men with non-obstructive azoospermia. Hum Reprod 2000;15:2685–2688.
43. Levron J, Aviram-Goldring A, Madjar I, et al. Sperm chromosomal abnormalities in men with severe male factor infertility who are undergoing in vitro fertilization with intracytoplasmic sperm injection. Fertil Steril 2001;63:479–484.
44. Munné S, Alikani M, Tomkin G, et al. Embryo morphology developmental rates and maternal age are correlated with chromosome abnormalities. Fertil Steril 1995;64:382–391.
45. Marquez C, Sandalinas M, Bahce M, et al. Chromosome abnormalities in 1255 cleavage-stage embryos. Reprod Biomed Online 2000;1:17–27.

46. Obasaju M, Kadam A, Sultan K, et al. Sperm quality may adversely affect the chromosome constitution of embryos that result form intracytoplasmic sperm injection. Fertil Steril 1999;72:1113–1115.
47. Sathananthan AH, Ratnam SS, Ng SC, et al. The sperm centriole: its inheritance, replication and perpetuation in early human embryos. Hum Reprod 1996;11:345–356.
48. Palermo G, Munné S, Cohen J. The human zygote inherits its mitotic potential from the male gamete. Hum Reprod 1994;9:1220–1225.
49. Hewitson L, Simerly CR, Schatten G. Fate of sperm components during assisted reproduction: implications for infertility. Hum Fertil 2002;5:110–116.
50. Simerly C, Zoran SS, Payne C, et al. Biparental inheritance of gamma-tubulin during human fertilization: molecular reconstitution of functional zygotic centrosomes in inseminated human oocytes and in cell-free extracts nucleated by human sperm. Mol Biol Cell 1999;10: 2955–2969.
51. Silva CP, Kommineni K, Oldenbourge R, Keefe DL. The first polar body does not predict accurately the location of the metaphase II meiotic spindle in mammalian oocytes. Fertil Steril 1999;71:719–721.
52. Wennerholm UB, Bergh C, Hamberger L, et al. Obstetric outcome of pregnancies following ICSI, classified according to sperm origin and quality. Hum Reprod 2000;15:1189–1194.

17 Treatment of Human Immunodeficiency Virus-Discordant Couples

Joseph E. Peña, MD *and Mark V. Sauer,* MD

CONTENTS

INTRODUCTION

HIV infection is a global epidemic, with more than 47 million infected individuals, many of whom are of reproductive age. More than 730,000 AIDS cases have been reported to the Centers for Disease Control and Prevention (CDC) in the United States. The great majority of infections (70%) result from unprotected intercourse, emphasizing heterosexual contact as a major risk factor for women *(1)*. Although the length of time from initial infection to the development of clinical disease varies, the median time for untreated patients is approx 10 yr. In addition, the use of highly active antiretroviral therapy in the last several years has brought significant improvements in survival expectations *(2–5)*, and HIV infection is now considered to be a chronic ailment. The improvement in the quality of life and increase in survival rates of infected individuals have given

From: *Contemporary Endocrinology: Office Andrology*
Edited by: P. E. Patton and D. E. Battaglia

many the hope of living a normal life. Accordingly, many individuals naturally desire to have children.

Regarding family planning, most HIV-serodiscordant couples in which the male is seropositive face the risk of viral transmission to the female partner and possibly the unborn child through unprotected intercourse. The rate of male-to-female transmission of HIV in stable heterosexual relationships is estimated to be approximately 1 in 500 to 1 in 1000 acts of unprotected intercourse *(6–10)* or perhaps greater with advanced stages of the disease, presence of ulcerative genital infection, history of previous sexually transmitted disease in the female partner, and presence of postcoital bleeding *(6,9,10)*.

TREATMENT OPTIONS AND ALTERNATIVES

HIV-seropositive males with seronegative partners have traditionally been counseled on the use of HIV-negative donor sperm, consideration of adoption, or refraining from having children to prevent HIV transmission *(11)*.

Recent advances in sperm processing have given these HIV-serodiscordant couples the chance to have a biological and genetic child of their own while decreasing the risk of viral transmission. The pioneering work of Semprini in the preparation and washing of semen from HIV-positive men *(12)* has led to its adjunctive use with intrauterine insemination (IUI) *(12–16)*. The use of in vitro fertilization (IVF) with intracytoplasmic sperm injection (ICSI) has been investigated *(16–20)* with a potential reduction of virus exposure to a few gametes. Using IVF alone (without ICSI) has also been reported *(15,16,21)*.

HIV AND SEMEN

Poor correlation between plasma and semen viral loads has been noted by several investigators *(22–24)*, as well as discordance in infected cell frequencies in blood and semen *(25)*. The distinct compartmentalization of blood and semen infection suggests that HIV-1 in semen arises from a unique reservoir of HIV-1 infections when compared to that of blood. This is supported by the genetic analysis of HIV strains of peripheral blood cells and semen cells *(25–27)*. In addition, the disease stage of HIV/AIDS, CD4+ T-cell count in blood, or antiretroviral therapy does not correlate with semen viral load *(22,27)*. Therefore, timed intercourse for the purpose of conception is discouraged in HIV-serodiscordant couples who hope to minimize viral transmission despite favorable CD4+ T-cell counts and serum viral loads. Although preliminary, we believe offering to intervene using the husband's processed sperm in assisted reproduction technology (ART) is a more viable alternative.

HIV DNA has been localized to T cells and macrophages of the cellular fraction of semen, and these cells are the likely targets of HIV infection. The association between HIV and spermatozoa is not as clear and remains a topic of controversy. The presence of proviral DNA has been reported in human spermatozoa *(28,29)*, even after processing the semen *(30)*. Alternatively, others have reported that viral nucleic acids have not been detected in spermatozoa, which lack the CD4 receptor, especially after careful sperm washing and separation techniques were used to incorporate swim-up techniques. These techniques isolate mature motile spermatozoa and remove nonmotile cell fractions *(24,31,32)*.

Assisted reproduction (IUI, IVF, and IVF-ICSI) using processed semen to minimize viral transmission appears to be a safe and reasonable alternative for HIV-serodiscordant couples, but larger multicenter studies are needed to confirm preliminary results *(12–21)*. Despite the presumed safety of the different methods of assisted reproduction, IVF-ICSI may potentially offer advantages over IUI. Whereas the IUI of processed sperm involves millions of sperm placed into the uterine cavity, IVF-ICSI only exposes individual oocytes to single sperm cells, thus decreasing viral exposure by a magnitude of 10^6. Additionally, as only mature motile sperm cells are microscopically selected for ICSI, the risk of the sperm cell harboring the virus is greatly minimized, as the virus is not thought to be present in mature motile spermatozoa *(24,31,32)*. At this time, the routine laboratory testing of semen is too preliminary and experimental to ensure the safety of individual samples. In consultation with our infectious disease department, HIV testing of semen for the purposes of triage for IVF-ICSI treatment is not advised because there is no current test available to detect the virus from the individual sperm selected for injection. We do not perform IUI of processed sperm from HIV-seropositive men. However, in centers that do provide IUI services, semen is generally frozen, HIV-tested, and released for later use if found to be virus-free.

SPERM PROCESSING

Various methods of sperm preparation of semen from HIV-seropositive men is described in the literature for use for IUI or ART *(12,14,18,33)*. Processing semen samples basically involves "washing," which utilizes centrifugation through a discontinuous gradient or separation medium, resuspension and incubation of the sperm pellet, followed by collection of supernatant-containing motile spermatozoa allowed to swim up over a 45 to 60 min interval. If specific testing of the washed specimen is performed, then it is usually at the end of the sperm-processing technique. Virus is commonly detected in unwashed whole ejaculates from HIV-seropositive men.

The sperm-processing technique utilized in our laboratory for semen samples from HIV-seropositive men is described as follows *(19,20)*. The handling of semen samples is performed in a separate class II biologic safety cabinet located outside the embryology laboratory with strict universal precautions. Semen used for ICSI is processed by centrifugation through a discontinuous density gradient (PureCeption, cat. no. PAP U12 human tubal fluid [HTF] and cat. no. PAP CL12; Sage BioPharma, Bedminster, NJ) as follows: 1.5 mL of the lower (90%) layer is pipetted into one or more (depending on semen volume) Falcon 35 2095 tubes; 1.5 mL of the upper (47%) layer is carefully pipetted on top of this; and 1 to 2 mL of semen is pipetted directly on top of the upper layer. The gradient tubes are centrifuged for 10 to 20 min at 300*g*. After centrifugation, the pellets are transferred to a clean Falcon 35 2095 tube and diluted with 5 mL of modified HTF (cat. no. 9963; Irvine Scientific, Santa Ana, CA) supplemented with 5% (v/v) human serum albumin (HSA; Sage BioPharma, cat. no. ART-3001). Sperm are centrifuged for a maximum of 10 min at 300*g*, and the supernatant (wash no. 1) is removed. The pellet is resuspended in 3 mL of fresh modified HTF-HSA and spun again for a maximum of 5 min. The supernatant (wash no. 2) is removed, and the pellet resuspended in a small volume of modified HTF-HSA for swim-up. The purified sperm is counted, and the concentration lowered, if necessary, to approx 5 to 10×10^6 motile sperm/mL (final sperm preparation). The tube is tightly capped and incubated until it used for ICSI.

PROTOCOL FOR IN VITRO FERTILIZATION-INTRACYTOPLASMIC SPERM INJECTION

The protocol for providing ART to HIV-serodiscordant couples using IVF-ICSI at our institution was reviewed and approved by the Institutional Review Board and Ethics Committee of Columbia-Presbyterian Medical Center in New York.

The treatment protocol for providing ART to eligible HIV-serodiscordant couples has been previously described *(19,20)* and is as follows. Briefly, entry requires men to be under current medical care for their infection and, when appropriate, treated with antiviral medications. A letter from the physician providing HIV care must be received, stating the patient's present and past medical status, including recent plasma viral load (HIV-RNA-polymerase chain reaction, highly sensitive detecting as low as 50 copies of HIV-1 RNA per milliliter of plasma) and CD4+ T-cell counts. The male patient must be in general good health, with a viral load less than 30,000 copies per milliliter and a stable CD4+ T-cell count for the past 6 mo. Men with azoospermia or leukospermia as assessed by formal semen analysis with hematoxylin and eosin stain are excluded.

Female partners are HIV tested using an HIV-enzyme-linked immuno-absorbent assay (ELISA) antibody screen and are required to be seronegative.

The long-term practice of safe sex with condoms is ascertained at interview. A general reproductive screen is performed on couples prior to attempting assisted reproduction. Counseling by specialists in maternal fetal medicine and psychiatry is encouraged and readily available. Treatment is rendered in a manner similar to the care provided for conventional patients undergoing IVF-ICSI. Informed consent is obtained from patients before each IVF cycle, including a statement that warns patients of the chance for infection.

Female partners undergo ovarian downregulation using leuprolide acetate (estradiol < 30 pg/mL), which is decreased once human menopausal gonadotropin or follicle-stimulating hormone is initiated. The gonadotropin dose is individualized on the basis of the patient's age and previous responses. Ovarian response is assessed by serial ultrasound and serum estradiol levels, and human chorionic gonadotropin (hCG) is administered when lead follicles reach 18 to 20 mm in diameter. Ultrasound-guided transvaginal oocyte retrieval is performed 34 to 36 h later with intravenous conscious sedation. At the time of retrieval, all recovered oocytes are graded for maturity. Mature oocytes are injected via ICSI using the processed sperm as already described *(34)*.

Approximately 18 h after ICSI, embryos with two visualized pronuclei are considered normally fertilized. Embryos are cultured in separate incubators from those of HIV-seronegative infertile couples. Progesterone (200 mg vaginal suppository once daily) is prescribed to women the day after retrieval and maintained until instructed to discontinue use. All embryo transfers are performed 72 h postretrieval.

Before embryo transfer, embryos are morphologically graded according to a 1 to 5 scale *(35)*. A grade 5 embryo would be optimal, whereas grade 1 embryo would be very poor quality. The program's policy on the number of embryos recommended for embryo transfer is in accordance with guidelines set forth by the American Society for Reproductive Medicine *(36)*. Excess embryos of high quality (grades 4–5) are cryopreserved using a programmable freezer with a similar protocol as described by Lassalle *(37)*. Cryopreserved embryos are stored in separate freezers from those of HIV-seronegative infertile couples.

Following embryo transfer, supplemental progesterone therapy is continued until a negative pregnancy test is demonstrated, or if pregnant, until an embryonic heartbeat is evident on ultrasonography. Clinical pregnancy is defined as the visualization of a gestational sac on ultrasound, and an ongoing pregnancy is defined as a viable pregnancy past the first trimester.

Ongoing pregnancies are followed by physician specialists in maternal fetal medicine, and HIV-RNA tests are performed on pregnant women every 3 mo during pregnancy. Infants and mothers are tested by either HIV-RNA or HIV-DNA-PCR (highly sensitive detecting of 10 or less copies of HIV-1 DNA per milliliter of whole blood of DNA) at birth and 3 mo later. In nonpregnant patients, HIV-ELISA antibody screens are performed 3 mo following embryo transfer.

RESULTS OF IN VITRO FERTILIZATION-INTRACYTOPLASMIC SPERM INJECTION FOR HIV-SERODISCORDANT COUPLES

We have reported our experience using IVF-ICSI in the treatment of HIV-1-serodiscordant couples in which the male was infected and the female was seronegative *(20)*. Since first offering treatment in 1997, we have performed 113 IVF-ICSI cycles in 61 eligible couples (73.5% of interested couples satisfied enrollment criteria and proceeded with IVF). Table 1 illustrates the characteristic profile of the HIV-serodiscordant couples who underwent IVF-ICSI during that time. The overall clinical pregnancy rate was 44.8% per embryo transfer; ongoing/delivered PR was 36.5% per embryo transfer, including 12 twins, 7 triplets, 1 quadruplet (57.1% multiple gestation rate). Cumulatively, 50.8% of couples achieved a pregnancy through IVF-ICSI; 54.1% by IVF-ICSI or frozen embryo transfer (FET) cycle (Table 2). Four couples had two successful pregnancies from IVF-ICSI. Pregnancy data for HIV-1-serodiscordant couples who underwent IVF-ICSI are shown in Table 2. All female recipients tested negative for HIV 3 mo postembryo transfer and, if pregnant, tested negative for HIV at delivery and 3 mo postpartum as well. All delivered babies tested negative for HIV at birth and 3 mo postpartum. Five women (8.2%) required treatment for moderate-to-severe ovarian hyperstimulation syndrome (OHSS)—a known risk when using fertility drugs.

In a review of the literature of HIV-1-serodiscordant couples undergoing ART *(38)*, there have been several studies reporting IUI, IVF, or IVF-ICSI using specifically processed semen to decrease the risk of viral transmission. Briefly, in 2884 reported IUI cycles in 1058 patients, 470 pregnancies are reported. There have been 93 reported IVF cycles in 75 patients that resulted in 28 pregnancies and 108 pregnancies in 191 patients following 302 IVF-ICSIs. Most importantly, no reported HIV seroconversions are noted in the treated women or their offspring.

With the baseline male-to-female transmission rate approx 0.1 to 0.2%, results regarding seroconversion following ART are far from conclusive. Much greater numbers, possibly gained through a multicenter study or a meta-analysis, are needed to assess seroconversion rate. However, to date, the results (although preliminary) are encouraging.

RISKS AND COMPLICATIONS

HIV-serodiscordant couples undergoing ART should understand the risks and complications involved, both those unique to them (viral transmission) as well as those similar to that faced by other infertile couples uninfected with HIV (i.e., OHSS in ovarian stimulation cycles and multiple pregnancy).

The CDC currently recommends against the use of semen from HIV-infected men for insemination of HIV-seronegative women *(39)*. In 1990, the CDC

Table 1
Characteristic Profile of 61 HIV-1-Serodiscordant Couples Deemed Suitable for IVF-ICSI

	N (%)	*Mean ± SD (range)*
Couples		
Deemed suitable for enrollment and proceeded to IVF	61 (73.5%)	
Total number of IVF cycles	113	
Number of IVF attempts per couple		1.8 ± 1.1 (1–6)
Male partner		
Age (years)		38.1 ± 5.6 (22–48)
Known HIV diagnosis (years)		8.8 ± 5.1 (1–19)
On antiretroviral therapy	51 (83.6%)	
Viral load (copies/mL)		946 ± 2909 (50–19300)
CD4+ T-cell count (mm^3)		574 ± 301 (50–1558)
Route of viral transmission		
Transfusion of blood products	15 (24.6%)	
Sexual contact (male or female)	19 (31.1%)	
Intravenous drug use	7 (11.5%)	
Unknown	20 (32.8%)	
Female partner		
Age (years)		34.1 ± 4.8 (24–43)
Day 3 estradiol (pg/mL)		36.2 ± 17.0 (14–72)
Day 3 FSH (mIU/mL)		5.5 ± 2.5 (2.4–14.4)

IVF-ICSI, in vitro fertilization-intracytoplasmic sperm injection; SD, standard deviation; FSH, follicle-stimulating hormone.

reported a woman infected with HIV-1 from insemination with washed semen from her HIV-1 seropositive husband *(40)*. However, in this case, the semen was simply centrifuged with the resulting pellet, potentially containing infected T lymphocytes and macrophages, inserted into the uterus. No attempt was made at extracting the other cells from the pellet prior to insemination; thus, this may account for the HIV-1 transmission. Using recent sperm preparation methods that minimize contamination, the risk of this complication should be significantly reduced. Nevertheless, it must be stressed to the couple that despite the careful sperm processing techniques, the risk of viral transmission to the female partner and/or infant cannot be totally eliminated, and complete safety cannot be guaranteed.

In our experience of offering IVF-ICSI to HIV-serodiscordant couples, we reported an incidence of moderate and severe OHSS in initiated IVF cycles of 4.5% *(41)*. This is similar to the 2 to 4% incidence reported in the literature for

Table 2
IVF Performance and Pregnancy Data From 113 IVF-ICSI Cycles in 61 HIV-1-Serodiscordant Couples

	N (%)	*Mean ± SD (range)*
Oocyte retrievals (*N* = 100)		
Cycle cancellation rate	13 (11.5%)	
Number of oocytes retrieved per retrieval		17.1 ± 9.5 (2–47)
Number of mature oocytes for ICSI per retrieval		14.0 ± 8.1 (1–42)
Number of normally fertilized oocytes per retrieval		9.3 ± 5.5 (0–24)
Embryo transfers		
Retrievals with enough embryos for fresh transfer	96 (96.0%)	
Number of embryos transferred per embryo transfer		3.5 ± 1.1 (1–6)
Cycles with embryo transfer and cryopreservation		
Retrievals with enough embryos for fresh transfer and cryopreservation	31 (31.0%)	
Number of embryos cryopreserved per cryopreservation		5.1 ± 3.5 (1–19)
Clinical pregnancy rate		
Per IVF cycle	38.1%	
Per oocyte retrieval	43.0%	
Per embryo transfer	44.8%	
Ongoing/delivered pregnancy rate		
Per IVF cycle	31.0%	
Per oocyte retrieval	35.0%	
Per embryo transfer	36.5%	
Per couple—IVF cycles only[a]	50.8%	
Per couple—IVF and FET cycles[a,b]	54.1%	
Pregnancies resulting from IVF-ICSI (*N* = 35)		
Singletons	15 (42.9%)	
Twins	12 (34.3%)	
Triplets	7 (20.0%)	
Quadruplets	1 (2.9%)	
Multiple gestation rate	57.1%	
Delivery data (26 deliveries, 39 infants)[c]		
Vaginal birth	9 (34.6%)	
Cesarean section	17 (65.4%)	
Term delivery (37-wk gestation)	17 (65.4%)	
Number of infants	22	
Estimated gestational age (wk)		39.3 ± 1.2 (37.1–41.3)
Birth weight (g)		3183 ± 714 (1984–4396)
Preterm delivery (< 37-wk gestation)	9 (34.6%)	
Number of infants	17	
Estimated gestational age (wk)		33.1 ± 3.8 (26.0–36.9)
Birth weight (g)		1806 ± 630 (678–2940)

[a] Four couples with two pregnancies.
[b] Two pregnancies in 11 frozen embryo transfer cycles.
[c] Eleven ongoing pregnancies.
IVF-ICSI, in vitro fertilization-intracytoplasmic sperm injection; SD, standard deviation.

conventional infertility patients using IVF *(42)*. Only one of the six women with moderate and severe OHSS had ovaries that were polycystic in appearance. Three of six were younger than 35 yr old, with only one younger than 30 yr of age. All the women utilized protocols with gonadotropin-releasing hormone agonists, which is thought to abolish the body's protective mechanism of early luteinization, prolonging the stimulatory phase and resulting in greater estradiol levels and number of follicles selected *(43)*. However, only a single patient attained an estradiol level greater than 3800 pg/mL on the day of hCG administration, and only one had an excessive number of oocytes recovered. Not surprisingly, the majority of cases were associated with conception cycles (five of six patients), and the one woman who did not conceive had her embryo transfer postponed and her embryos cryopreserved owing to the development of symptoms before the scheduled transfer.

Although elimination of OHSS cannot be guaranteed, there are several prevention strategies that can significantly decrease its occurrence *(42,43)*. Vigilant monitoring of serum estradiol levels and follicular characteristics during the COH-IVF cycle is of principal importance.

Another common IVF complication is the occurrence of higher order multiple gestations (i.e., triplets or greater). In our experience with IVF-ICSI to HIV-serodiscordant couples *(41)*, the complication occurred in 16.3% of pregnancies. This incidence is greater than that of triplets or more (7.7%) reported by the CDC from ART technology *(44)*, which may be attributed to the three to four embryos transferred in this relatively young and "fertile" population. One patient had five embryos transferred after failing to become pregnant after five IVF attempts.

Higher order multiple gestations (triplets or greater) carry a significant risk to both the mother and fetus. Triplet pregnancy is associated with a high rate of perinatal complications primarily attributed to prematurity (i.e., retinopathy of prematurity and intraventricular hemorrhage), with median gestational age at delivery of 33 wk and 14% of pregnancies delivered prior to 28-wk gestation *(45)*. Triplet pregnancy is also associated with significant maternal morbidity.

For HIV-serodiscordant couples who have decided to pursue pregnancy through IVF-ICSI, strategies to reduce complications from ART may not be well-accepted. Decreasing the number of embryos transferred may adversely affect the pregnancy rate. Aggressive embryo freezing in patients at risk for OHSS may not be as readily accepted because the transfer of frozen thawed embryos is associated with lowered success; but with increasing success rates of FET cycles, this is becoming a more viable option. Financial concerns and travel restrictions (with limited infertility services available to this unique cohort of patients) make multiple attempts at treatment difficult for most couples. Typically, great pressure is on the physician to transfer more embryos, rather than less, with the hope to increase the chance for pregnancy. Infertility patients generally appear willing to accept the increased risk for the opportunity to conceive. This is undoubtedly true for HIV-serodiscordant couples—most believe they would not be given the chance to reproduce.

CONCLUSIONS

The development of sperm processing techniques of semen from HIV-seropositive men has given many HIV-serodiscordant couples involving an HIV-infected man the opportunity to have a biological and genetic child of their own through various means of ART. Using carefully processed sperm for IUI, IVF, and IVF-ICSI can be reasonable alternatives for HIV-1-serodiscordant couples who hope for a child of their own while also minimizing the risk of viral transmission. This has led to the recent ethical and political endorsements supporting assisted reproduction without regard to HIV status *(11,38,46–50)*. Thus, we advocate extensive counseling, thorough informed consent, and specific advanced directives in this cohort of patients, who must deal with the nature of their HIV disease (risk of infection and death) and the complications related to assisted reproduction (multiple pregnancy and OHSS) as it relates to themselves, their partner, and their unborn child.

REFERENCES

1. Gayle H. An overview of the global HIV/AIDS epidemic, with a focus on the United States. AIDS 2000;14(Suppl 2):S8–S17.
2. Survival after introduction of HAART in people with known duration of HIV-1 infection. The CASCADE Collaboration. Concerted action on seroconversion to AIDS and death in Europe. Lancet 2000;355:1158,1159.
3. Tam HK, Zhang ZF, Jacobson LP, et al. Effect of highly active antiretroviral therapy on survival among HIV- infected men with Kaposi sarcoma or non-Hodgkin lymphoma. Int J Cancer 2002;98:916–922.
4. Morris A, Wachter RM, Luce J, et al. Improved survival with highly active antiretroviral therapy in HIV- infected patients with severe Pneumocystis carinii pneumonia. AIDS 2003;17:73–80.
5. Diagnosis and reporting of HIV and AIDS in states with HIV/AIDS surveillance—United States, 1994-2000. MMWR Morb Mortal Wkly Rep 2002;51:595–598.
6. de Vincenzi I. A longitudinal study of human immunodeficiency virus transmission by heterosexual partners. European Study Group on Heterosexual Transmission of HIV. N Engl J Med 1994;331:341–346.
7. Downs AM, De Vincenzi I. Probability of heterosexual transmission of HIV: relationship to the number of unprotected sexual contacts. European Study Group in Heterosexual Transmission of HIV. J Acquir Immune Defic Syndr Hum Retrovirol 1996;11:388–395.
8. Mandelbrot L, Heard I, Henrion-Geant E, Henrion R. Natural conception in HIV-negative women with HIV-infected partners. Lancet 1997;349:850,851.
9. Padian NS, Shiboski SC, Glass SO, Vittinghoff E. Heterosexual transmission of human immunodeficiency virus (HIV) in northern California: results from a ten-year study. Am J Epidemiol 1997;146:350–357.

10. Gray RH, Wawer MJ, Brookmeyer R, et al. Probability of HIV-1 transmission per coital act in monogamous, heterosexual, HIV-1-discordant couples in Rakai, Uganda. Lancet 2001;357: 1149–1153.
11. Human immunodeficiency virus and infertility treatment. Fertil Steril 2002;77:218–222.
12. Semprini AE, Levi-Setti P, Bozzo M, et al. Insemination of HIV-negative women with processed semen of HIV-positive partners. Lancet 1992;340:1317–1319.
13. Semprini AE, Fiore S, Pardi G. Reproductive counselling for HIV-discordant couples. Lancet 1997;349:1401,1402.
14. Marina S, Marina F, Alcolea R, et al. Human immunodeficiency virus type 1—serodiscordant couples can bear healthy children after undergoing intrauterine insemination. Fertil Steril 1998;70:35–39.
15. Gilling-Smith C. HIV prevention. Assisted reproduction in HIV-discordant couples. AIDS Read 2000;10:581–587.
16. Weigel MM, Gentili M, Beichert M, et al. Reproductive assistance to HIV-discordant couples—the German approach. Eur J Med Res 2001;6:259–262.
17. Marina S, Marina F, Alcolea R, et al. Pregnancy following intracytoplasmic sperm injection from an HIV-1- seropositive man. Hum Reprod 1998;13:3247–3249.
18. Loutradis D, Drakakis P, Kallianidis K, et al. Birth of two infants who were seronegative for human immunodeficiency virus type 1 (HIV-1) after intracytoplasmic injection of sperm from HIV-1-seropositive men. Fertil Steril 2001;75:210–212.
19. Sauer MV, Chang PL. Establishing a clinical program for human immunodeficiency virus 1-seropositive men to father seronegative children by means of in vitro fertilization with intracytoplasmic sperm injection. Am J Obstet Gynecol 2002;186:627–633.
20. Peña JE, Thornton MH, Sauer MV. Assessing the clinical utility of in vitro fertilization with intracytoplasmic sperm injection in human immunodeficiency virus-1 serodiscordant couples: report of 113 consecutive cycles. Fertil Steril 2003;80:356–362.
21. Semprini AE, Vucetich A, Oneta M, et al. IVF-ET with processed semen of HIV-positive males in infertile HIV-discordant couples. Fertil Steril 1999;72:S40.
22. Liuzzi G, Chirianni A, Clementi M, et al. Analysis of HIV-1 load in blood, semen and saliva: evidence for different viral compartments in a cross-sectional and longitudinal study. AIDS 1996;10:F51–56.
23. Hamed KA, Winters MA, Holodniy M, et al. Detection of human immunodeficiency virus type 1 in semen: effects of disease stage and nucleoside therapy. J Infect Dis 1993;167:798–802.
24. Kim LU, Johnson MR, Barton S, et al. Evaluation of sperm washing as a potential method of reducing HIV transmission in HIV-discordant couples wishing to have children. AIDS 1999;13:645–651.
25. Byrn RA, Kiessling AA. Analysis of human immunodeficiency virus in semen: indications of a genetically distinct virus reservoir. J Reprod Immunol 1998;41:161–176.
26. Byrn RA, Zhang D, Eyre R, et al. HIV-1 in semen: an isolated virus reservoir. Lancet 1997;350:1141.
27. Kiessling AA, Fitzgerald LM, Zhang D, et al. Human immunodeficiency virus in semen arises from a genetically distinct virus reservoir. AIDS Res Hum Retroviruses 1998;14(Suppl 1):S33–41.
28. Bagasra O, Farzadegan H, Seshamma T, et al. Detection of HIV-1 proviral DNA in sperm from HIV-1-infected men. AIDS 1994;8:1669–1674.
29. Baccetti B, Benedetto A, Collodel G, et al. The debate on the presence of HIV-1 in human gametes. J Reprod Immunol 1998;41:41–67.
30. Leruez-Ville M, de Almeida M, Tachet A, et al. Assisted reproduction in HIV-1-serodifferent couples: the need for viral validation of processed semen. AIDS 2002;16:2267–2273.

31. Quayle AJ, Xu C, Mayer KH, Anderson DJ. T lymphocytes and macrophages, but not motile spermatozoa, are a significant source of human immunodeficiency virus in semen. J Infect Dis 1997;176:960–968.
32. Hanabusa H, Kuji N, Kato S, et al. An evaluation of semen processing methods for eliminating HIV-1. AIDS 2000;14:1611–1616.
33. Weigel M. HIV-infected people who wish to have children—chances and limits of assisted reproductive techniques. Andrologia 2003;35:186–188.
34. Palermo GD, Cohen J, Alikani M, et al. Development and implementation of intracytoplasmic sperm injection (ICSI). Reprod Fertil Dev 1995;7:211–217.
35. Veeck L. Atlas of Human Oocyte and Early Conceptus. Williams & Wilkins, Baltimore, MD, 1991, pp. 121–150.
36. American Society of Reproductive Medicine. Guidelines on number of embryos transferred. American Society of Reproductive Medicine, Birmingham, AL, 1999.
37. Lassalle B, Testart J, Renard JP. Human embryo features that influence the success of cryopreservation with the use of 1,2 propanediol. Fertil Steril 1985;44:645–651.
38. Sauer MV. Providing fertility care to those with HIV: time to re-examine healthcare policy. Am J Bioeth 2003;3:33–40.
39. Jamieson DJ, Schieve L, Duerr A. Semen processing for HIV-discordant couples. Am J Obstet Gynecol 2001;185:1433,1434.
40. HIV-1 infection and artificial insemination with processed semen. MMWR Morb Mortal Wkly Rep 1990;39:249,255–246.
41. Peña JE, Thornton MH, II, Sauer MV. Complications of in vitro fertilization with intracytoplasmic sperm injection in human immunodeficiency virus serodiscordant couples. Arch Gynecol Obstet 2003;268:198–201.
42. Schenker JG. Clinical aspects of ovarian hyperstimulation syndrome. Eur J Obstet Gynecol Reprod Biol 1999;85:13–20.
43. Navot D, Bergh PA, Laufer N. Ovarian hyperstimulation syndrome in novel reproductive technologies: prevention and treatment. Fertil Steril 1992;58:249–261.
44. Centers for Disease Control and Prevention. 2000 Assisted reproductive technology success rates: National summary and fertility clinic reports. Centers for Disease Control and Prevention, Atlanta, GA, 2002.
45. Devine PC, Malone FD, Athanassiou A, et al. Maternal and neonatal outcome of 100 consecutive triplet pregnancies. Am J Perinatol 2001;18:225–235.
46. ACOG Committee Opinion. Committee on Ethics. Human immunodeficiency virus: ethical guidelines for obstetricians and gynecologists. Obstet Gynecol 2001;97(Suppl):1-6.
47. Sharma S, Gilling-Smith C, Semprini AE, et al. View 1: assisted conception in couples with HIV infection. Sex Transm Infect 2003;79:185–188.
48. Gilling-Smith C, Smith JR, Semprini AE. HIV and infertility: time to treat. There's no justification for denying treatment to parents who are HIV positive. BMJ 2001;322:566,567.
49. Nahvi S, Flanigan T, Cu-Uvin S. Processing of semen from human immunodeficiency virus-seropositive men for use in insemination of seronegative women. Am J Obstet Gynecol 2001; 184:1048,1049.
50. Englert Y, Van Vooren JP, Place I, et al. ART in HIV-infected couples: has the time come for a change of attitude? Hum Reprod 2001;16:1309–1315.

18 Sperm and Egg Retrieval for Posthumous Reproduction

Practical, Ethical, and Legal Considerations

Lisa V. Brock, JD, MA
and Anna C. Mastroianni, JD, MPH

Contents

INTRODUCTION

Posthumous reproduction refers to a deliberate decision to produce a child after one or both potential biological parents die *(1)*. For purposes of this chapter, we are also using this term to refer to reproduction when one or both of the biological parents is in a permanent unconscious condition *(2)*. Posthumous reproduction may involve several distinct levels of physician involvement: (1) in the procurement ("harvesting") of the biological specimens; (2) in the preparation and/or storage of those specimens; and (3) in the use of the specimens for reproduction. Posthumous reproduction may include the use of "banked" specimens that were knowingly procured and stored by explicit consent of the individual. However, this chapter focuses on a more recent phenomenon of harvesting and use of specimens collected *after death or a diagnosis of a permanent unconscious condition* of the "donating" individual *(3)*. The medical and legal communities have debated what physicians should or should not do in response to requests for posthumous reproduction for a number of years without achieving a complete consensus. In the United States, there are currently no uniform laws

From: *Contemporary Endocrinology: Office Andrology*
Edited by: P. E. Patton and D. E. Battaglia © Humana Press Inc., Totowa, NJ

or regulations for governing assisted reproduction *(4)*. Through a series of questions listed below, this chapter poses the common questions and examines the trends in posthumous reproduction.

This chapter gives health care providers a guide to understand the fundamental concerns raised by posthumous reproduction. It also strongly encourages them to consider developing a personal, clinic, and/or institutional policy to guide decision making on this issue. The authors believe that ad hoc decision making may result in actions that are not grounded in solid principled reasoning, whereas decisions made consistent with developed policy allow for reflective choices based on the facts of each individual situation. This chapter does not focus on fact patterns involving anonymous donors, nor does it provide a review of all applicable state laws. The information in this chapter is not definitive guidance because readers need to also consider their own institutional policies (if any), applicable state laws and regulations; and, if the procedure falls within the realm of human experimentation, applicable federal law and institutional review board (human subjects review committee) policies and procedures.

COMMON QUESTIONS

What Medical Procedures and Practical Limitations Are Involved in Posthumous Reproduction?

Posthumous reproduction takes place in two distinct phases separated by time, involving multiple medical procedures: (1) the harvesting, preparation, and storage of gametes; and (2) the use of the gametes in assisted reproduction efforts. In the first phase, current medical technology permits the harvesting and cryopreservation of sperm *(5)* and current experimental technology allows harvesting of ovarian tissue and cryopreservation of eggs *(6)*. The second phase involves the application of assisted reproductive technologies (ART) in embryo creation and implantation. For a male specimen, it may involve intrauterine insemination (IUI) or in vitro fertilization (IVF) techniques; for a female specimen, it would also require the involvement of another woman to serve as a gestational carrier. Note, however, that the technology needed for conception from cryopreserved eggs is still experimental. If and when it becomes medically available, it is anticipated to require a complex and expensive application of ART *(7)*.

Gametes remain viable for a limited time postmortem, which constrains the time in which harvesting decisions must be made. It is generally understood that sperm must be collected within 24 to 36 h after death, and eggs must be collected within a few hours after death *(8)*. Because perfusion continues to testes and ovaries while the patient is in a permanent unconscious state, the same time constraints on harvesting may not apply. However, other medical and social considerations should be noted, such as decisions on when to withdraw ventilatory support, treatment, or hydration and nutrition, along with the availability of beds. These elements may place considerable time pressures on decision making related to gamete harvesting in those who are in a permanent unconscious condition.

What Are the Circumstances in Which Posthumous Reproduction Requests Arise?

Retrieval or harvesting requests are usually made to physicians by grieving family members who wish to preserve potential biological reproduction of a loved one. Such requests may arise in an emotionally charged situation following the loved one's sudden death or a diagnosis of coma or persistent vegetative state *(9)*. The following reports illustrate some actual fact patterns for these requests.

- After a young man's sudden death in a California hospital, his wife's family asks a urologist to harvest his sperm at the morgue. His sperm is harvested 30 h after his death for future reproductive use by his wife *(10)*.
- A 25-yr-old married man was in a car accident, resulting in being comatose. His prognosis for recovery is poor. Purportedly, he and his wife had been trying to conceive a child, and his wife asks his treating physician to have his sperm extracted *(11)*.
- A 21-yr-old woman calls a physician (the director of reproductive endocrinology at an academic medical center) to request harvesting assistance when her 19-yr-old sister was declared braindead following a car accident. The requesting family member wishes to have her sister's ovaries harvested and her eggs preserved for future reproduction *(12)*. (This will require use of a gestational carrier—a surrogate to carry the resulting embryo.)

One survey reported that most requests occurred after the male's accidental death (males ages ranged from 15–60 yr) and were made by wives, girlfriends, and parents *(13)*. The survey also showed that a single physician was frequently the only decision maker about whether to honor these requests *(14)*. Another study found that 22% of these requests were made by wives of deceased men *(15)*. The wives were usually the intended recipients (28%), but there were also other proposed recipients, such as fiancées (1.2%), girlfriends (4.9%), and even anonymous donations (1.2%) *(16)*.

In sudden death situations, there is little time for reflection by all participants in the process before the window of time for harvesting viable gametes closes. A harvesting request is made during an emotionally stressful time. Harvesting requests may place physicians in a difficult position because of: (1) time constraints for viability of specimens; (2) the potential for disagreement among immediate family members; (3) the frequent lack of clinic/institutional policies; and (4) the lack of resources, including professional guidelines, to give clear direction to providers. It is common for a physician to decide whether to grant a particular request in isolation on an ad hoc basis as the sole decision maker. This ad hoc approach is stressful and may result in unnecessary liability exposure for the physician and organization.

Are Physicians Required to Perform Harvesting for Posthumous Reproduction?

Commentators generally agree that a physician does not have a professional duty to carry out a request for posthumous reproduction procedures, and such a position is supported by the ethical principle of provider autonomy *(17)*. At least one hospital's guidelines state that physicians can refuse to perform postmortem sperm harvesting if they believe the procedure "...may result in significant adverse effects to involved individuals" *(18)*. A physician would not be ethically required to enter into a provider–patient relationship unless the procedure is medically necessary, the patient has no other access to such care, and the physician is competent to perform it. A physician may also decline to perform the procedure under the principle of conscientious objection because it is a controversial area of medicine *(19)*.

Before a physician either grants or refuses posthumous reproduction requests, the facts of the situation should be gathered, the clinic or institutional policy reviewed, and if needed, a legal consult obtained. If no clinic or institutional policy is in place at the time of a harvesting request, at minimum, the physician receiving the request should consult with legal counsel to ensure consideration of potentially applicable laws and regulations. This may vary depending on the state where the harvesting will be conducted. The legal approach will differ based on the specific facts present in the request (e.g., male or female donor, dead or alive donor). (*See also* discussion in the following two sections.)

Generally, the medical provider will rely on the deceased or permanent unconscious donor's legally authorized surrogate decision maker to provide consent for any procedure. However, there may be some exceptions in which a physician may refuse to follow a surrogate's choice. These exceptions are: if the physician reasonably believes that the surrogate person(s) cannot give consent owing to mental incapacity; the choice made is not in the patient's best interests; or the choice is inconsistent with what the patient would want. In addition, a physician *may* be justified in declining to perform posthumous harvesting procedures on the basis that specimen retrieval is an elective procedure, not a medically necessary treatment. To decline a harvesting request may or may not create a potential liability concern, especially if there is no other physician readily accessible that the requesting family member could seek assistance from.

It is important to note that there are frequent significant pressures facing a physician confronted with a harvesting request. First, the request arises in an emotionally charged situation of a grieving family member who has lost a loved one to sudden death or a permanent unconscious condition. Second, the timeframe for harvesting viable specimens is very small in sudden death situations. Third, because the deceased or permanent unconscious person is usually treated at the same facility as where the physician practices, there can be a burden to mitigate the loss for the family by allowing them what they want. Fourth, when the patient is dead or permanently unconscious, the remaining family may begin to feel more like the patient than the individual whose specimen is sought. With this shift of patient perception comes less ability to appreciate the risk of harvesting without the deceased or permanently unconscious person's consent. These pressures underscore the profound implications that physicians have in making these decisions on an ad hoc basis and in isolation.

Does the Analysis Differ if the Specimen Donor is Male or Female?

The sex of the specimen donor impacts the type of medical specialist involved, nature and invasiveness of the medical procedures, type of consent required, applicable laws and regulations, and time constraints in responding to a harvesting request. The procedures necessary for posthumous reproduction are harvesting, preparation of specimens, storage, and later use for any future reproductive technologies. For a male specimen donor, the involved medical specialist for harvesting would likely be a urologist, whereas for a female donor it would likely be an obstetrician/gynecologist. Harvesting procedures would always involve surgery for a female donor, but with a male donor's specimen, they may be obtainable using the nonsurgical electroejaculation method. The viability of gametes affects the time needed to respond to a postmortem harvesting request, with sperm estimated to remain viable 24 to 36 h after death, and ovarian tissue remaining viable only for a few hours after death *(20)*. The nature of ART needed to achieve a pregnancy would differ significantly depending on the sex of the donor as well. This phase of posthumous reproduction requires another specialist in reproductive medicine. In a female donor situation, there needs to be a gestational carrier (surrogate for the pregnancy). In a male donor case, the sperm could be used with or without a gestational carrier, depending on the availability and fertility of a female partner. Currently, harvesting ovarian tissue is considered to be experimental so the nature of consent and procedures are significantly different when compared to a male donor situation as well.

Does the Analysis Differ if the Specimen Donor is Dead or in a Permanent Unconscious State?

Whether the specimen donor is alive, but permanently unconscious, or dead impacts the type of medical specialist involved, nature and invasiveness of the medical procedures, type of required consent, and the applicable laws and regulations. If the specimen donor is dead, the body may be in storage at a morgue, and a pathologist may be involved in harvesting procedures, along with a urologist (male donor) or obstetrician/gynecologist (female donor). Medical procedures differ because with a dead donor, there is no need to worry about the impact of the harvesting procedure on the patient's health. For male donors, the invasiveness of sperm harvesting varies because if the donor is dead, it is usually a surgical procedure, but for a permanently unconscious donor, it is nonsurgical electroejaculation. Time is also a crucial difference. With dead donors, there is a finite window of opportunity to harvest viable specimens, whereas a permanently unconscious donor situation would not have these time constraints. Time is also a factor for family members and may affect the consent process because the family of a permanently unconscious donor likely has had more time to reflect on its loss than a family who loses a loved one to a sudden death. The applicable laws and regulations also vary significantly. With dead donors, state laws governing dead bodies and organ donation would apply by analogy, whereas for a permanently unconscious donor, the analogous governing laws would be informed consent for medical treatment. In addition, if a permanently unconscious donor has a "living will" or other health care directive under another state law (e.g., natural death act), then that document should be considered on the consent issue as well.

What Physicians Are Usually Involved in Posthumous Reproduction?

Frequently, posthumous harvesting requires the coordination between medical specialties, such as urology, pathology, and reproductive medicine. Posthumous reproduction crosses over into different medical specialties and may require cooperation among them to preserve the viability of the specimens. Involving medical specialists varies depending on the sex of the deceased donor. Sperm harvesting requires urology expertise, whereas ovary harvesting requires obstetrical and gynecological expertise. Cryopreservation and subsequent use of the gametes requires ART professionals and/or sperm banks. Practically, these professionals should be available on short notice, and the lines of authority for decision-making should be well-established to enable quick responses to requests.

Coordination is critical because the harvesting physicians need to understand the timeframes for obtaining viable specimens *(21)*. Other medical coordination includes offering family members cryropreservation storage and the potential future use of the specimens in ART procedures. Although a harvesting physician may never be in contact with the surviving persons again, he or she needs to be aware of the ramifications that flow from harvesting, as the consent process for the specimen covers distinct procedures and is usually multiphased with ART occurring later.

How Often Are Posthumous Reproduction Harvesting Requests Made?

Electroejaculation was first used in 1996 to obtain sperm from a brain dead man *(22)*. In 1999, the United States had its first known birth of a child conceived when her mother used sperm retrieved from her dead husband *(23)*. A 1997 survey reported that from 1980 through 1995, 82 requests for postmortem sperm harvesting were made at 40 facilities in 22 states *(24)*. More than half of the requests were made between 1994 and 1995. Of the 82 requests, 25 were granted at 14 facilities in 11 states. Because the study did not survey hospitals, the study's authors concluded that the total numbers reported were likely to be low. Harvesting requests have likely increased since this survey was conducted, especially because public awareness of medical technology and harvesting options has grown through cases reported in the news media. Requests are likely to continue to grow as the public becomes better educated about possible options *(25)*. Additionally, with technological advances, it is also anticipated that future requests related to posthumous reproduction will include requests for ovarian and egg harvesting *(26)*. Not much current literature exists on this issue, but there is at least one report of such harvesting being requested *(27)*.

What Should a Physician Do if a Harvesting Request is Made?

If there is no applicable clinic or institutional posthumous reproduction policy, the physician or medical director should contact the organization's attorney for assistance in considering the potentially applicable state and federal laws and regulations.

If there is a clinic or institutional policy, it should be based on and reflect the applicable legal standards, medical practice guidelines, including any applicable medical specialties, and medical (ethics) literature from peer-reviewed journals. It should also identify conditions under which requests are to be granted or refused. In that instance, the physician should follow the policy. As discussed throughout, the authors strongly encourage policy development to eliminate ad hoc decision making under difficult and isolated circumstances.

Does the Law Permit Physicians to Perform Posthumous Reproduction Procedures?

In the United States, there is little settled law to guide physicians in the field of reproductive medicine, including posthumous reproduction *(28)*. The law as established by legislative policymakers has not kept pace with the technology that medically permits posthumous reproduction *(29)*. However, there are other laws that are frequently referred to by analogy as setting some parameters. For example, consent laws used for medical treatment authority may be used as guidance for harvesting from a permanently unconscious patient. This application may be problematic because sperm retrieval likely cannot be characterized as a medically necessary procedure for the benefit of the patient, as generally required under such laws. For harvesting from a deceased individual, the Uniform Anatomical Gift Act (organ donor laws) may be used as guidance, which specifies the persons who can consent to the donation of a deceased's organ or tissue *(30)*. This application may also be problematic because sperm may be characterized as legally distinguishable from organs owing to its genetic reproduction capacity. The existing laws do no explicitly apply to either of these harvesting situations because the underlying facts are significantly different. Any decision making in this context implicates liberty and privacy rights under law. The right to procreate and corresponding right not to procreate are well-established as fundamental and personal decisions deserving constitutional protections *(31)*. But how does one balance a surviving next of kin's right to procreate against traditional notions of respect for the deceased and decedent's right while alive not to reproduce? Courts have evaluated this conflict and found that the decedent's intentions regarding procreation should be used as a guide *(32)*. However, the decedent's intentions frequently fall short of the specific situation presented by posthumous reproduction because even if it is known that the individual wished to become a parent, it usually is not known if that includes a wish for parenthood after death.

If the Law Does Not Provide Explicit Guidance About Posthumous Reproduction, Where Should the Physician Turn?

When there is no directly applicable law, medical organizations and ethics literature may provide the only source of guidance for physicians. When biotechnology jumps ahead of the law, ethical evaluation is paramount, and statements of professional organizations have great weight. Medical ethics can fill in the regulatory gaps and inform lawmakers about what laws should be. Some medical specialties involved may have policy statements about posthumous reproduction. The American Society of Reproductive Medicine (ASRM) has a guidance statement for its members, but it refers only to posthumous use of banked specimens and does not directly address harvesting of specimens from dead or permanently unconscious donors *(33)*. Urologists are being asked more frequently to retrieve sperm from deceased and permanently unconscious patients *(34)*. Interestingly, the American Urological Association (AUA) does not have a published statement that explicitly addresses posthumous reproduction. The AUA's Code of Ethics does direct its members to "obey the law" and regarding "emerging issues," to consider "the best interests of the individual, of society, and of the yet-unforeseen consequences of the various alternative actions" *(35)*. There is no clear consensus, but numerous articles in the medical literature support allowing posthumous harvesting as long as the donor's immediate family is in agreement, and there is evidence that this is what the donor would have wanted.

If There Is No Clinic and/or Institutional Policy Addressing Posthumous Reproduction, What Are the General Parameters to Help Guide a Physician's Decision-Making Process?

Even in the absence of a clinic or institutional policy addressing posthumous reproduction, a physician has parameters to guide consideration and actions on these types of requests. First, a physician is obligated to follow the law. Therefore, the physician should consult the clinic or institution's attorney to review the request. Even in the absence of explicit laws that govern consent for posthumous reproduction procedures, the physician's legal advisor may assist the physician in reviewing applicable state laws and regulations that by analogy provide guidance, or if research, applicable federal laws, regulations, and institutional review board (IRB) procedures. Second, the physician should consider any medical practice guidelines issued by professional organizations. (*See* discussion under the previous section.) Such guidelines may be helpful as indicating any consensus among providers about how to consider these types of requests. Third, the physician should also consider medical literature published in peer-reviewed journals because it may likewise indicate a consensus among providers or be a useful framework for decision-making. Fourth, if the physician practices in an environment with an institutional ethics committee, then exploring the posthumous reproduction request with the committee for guidance may be a helpful decision-making method.

How Is the Informed Consent Process Implemented?

There is legal, medical and ethical consensus that posthumous reproduction requires informed consent *(36)*. But the implementation of consent is debated—should evidence of explicit consent of the deceased or permanently unconscious person be required, or is consent of the next of kin sufficient? Does the evidence of the deceased or permanently unconscious person's wishes for reproduction need to be in writing, or are reported oral statements adequate evidence? What information should be included in a written informed consent, and when should it be obtained?

It is important to note that consent is actually a state of mind, but it is frequently treated as a signed document. Informed consent ensures that information has been provided and a choice made; the written documentation of that choice is evidence that the state of mind was achieved.

It is rare that a posthumous reproduction request is made in reliance on an explicit and written consent or provision previously prepared and signed by the deceased person (e.g., a will), or permanently unconscious person (e.g., a "living will" also known as a "health care directive"). Requests to harvest gametes for later use in reproduction are typically made by the next of kin, or rather, persons acting as surrogate decision makers for the newly deceased or permanently unconscious person. Surrogate decision makers are generally required to make decisions consistent with the best interests and wishes of the patient or deceased person. Even when written evidence of intent to reproduce posthumously exists, family members may disagree among themselves and challenge such a request, which places physicians, clinics, and institutions in a difficult position of mediating family squabbles in a time-pressured and emotional environment *(37)*.

Institutional policies available to the authors show significant variation. At the University of Washington, an ethics committee concluded that explicit written consent from the deceased must indicate both a desire to have gametes harvested and a child conceived after death *(38)*. The Lahey Clinic's policy on sperm retrieval from dead or irretrievably comatose patients indicates that its facility's participation in the gamete retrieval process is not an acknowledgment of responsibility for the subsequent process of procreation. Indeed, that policy places the burden on the gamete recipient to contact and contract with the cryopreservation and storage facility before gamete harvesting *(39)*. The New York Hospital's guidelines include detailed exclusionary criteria to be used in granting a harvesting request *(40)*.

Informed Consent for Harvesting, Preparation, and Storage

Obtaining appropriate informed consent to harvest gametes for posthumous reproduction requires attention to informed consent and organ donation laws particular to the state where the physician practices. When the patient is alive (i.e., in a permanent unconscious state) the informed consent law for medical treatment are most applicable for specimen harvesting. When the patient is dead, the organ donation laws are most applicable for specimen harvesting. Both sets of laws for treatment of incapacitated persons and organ donation for deceased persons contain lists of authorized surrogate decision makers to give informed consent. Importantly, the priority of listing and categories of these surrogate decision makers is likely to be different depending on which law applies, even within the same state. Health care providers should consult an attorney for the requirements of a particular state's laws in both these areas.

The discussion of harvesting options and the content of a written document with consent for the harvesting procedure should also include information about the preparation of the specimen, storage, and its intended future use for reproduction by a specific person or indicate otherwise, e.g., a gestational carrier/surrogate for pregnancy. The rationale for including all this information in the harvesting discussion and written consent is that such information is important to make the decision to harvest the specimen. For example, whoever is consenting to the harvesting should also be aware of the risks of harvesting and storage, known costs, and limits on potential use of the specimen, such as a mandatory waiting period for use or who may use the specimen.

Informed Consent for Use in Reproduction

The physician should obtain the informed consent of all living parties participating in the procedure that involve ART. For the use of sperm posthumously, informed consent for ART typically should include all of the elements required for any medical procedure, including a description of the procedure, risks, benefits, success rates of the procedure, and alternatives. The American Medical Association's ethical guidelines for artificial insemination by a known donor, for example also specifically recommend including information about screening for infectious and genetic disease, costs, confidentiality procedures, and laws regarding the rights of children and rights and obligations of the rearing parent(s) *(41)*. The ASRM statement on posthumous reproduction concludes that it is the "…responsibility of a specialist in assisted reproduction to insist on full disclosure to all participants to ascertain that all appropriate informed consents are obtained and to ensure adequate screening and counseling of all concerned parties" *(42)*. Regarding the rights of subsequently born children, informed consent can include a reference to the uncertainty surrounding inheritance rights and other benefits emanating from the deceased person, such as social security benefits. (*See* the following section.) Indeed, some commentators recommend going further, advising a potential parent to consult with pre-existing siblings before proceeding with posthumous reproduction to avoid property inheritance problems *(43)*.

Because ovarian cryopreservation is still in the experimental phase, the use of eggs obtained from previously frozen ovaries should provoke the additional consideration of consent requirements detailed in human subjects' regulations and related requirements for institutional review and oversight *(44)*. In addition, the use of a gestational carrier will implicate a host of requirements under state laws related to surrogate motherhood *(45)*.

Who Should be Permitted to Use Posthumously Harvested Gametes?

Some commentators suggest that in the absence of evidence a man would approve of anyone besides his wife being inseminated, it would be ethically unjustifiable to permit anyone else to be inseminated *(46)*. One implication is that storage agreements should stipulate that the harvested gametes are to be used only by a specific individual. Others would allow posthumous reproduction only in the context of marriage and when a prior consent exists.

What Additional Social Considerations Might Arise in the Development or Implementation of a Posthumous Reproduction Policy?

A review of the literature reveals several ethics opinions, policies, and commentaries that address additional social and practical concerns with posthumous reproduction. These include questions about who at the institution or clinic is responsible for applying the policy and rendering the final judgment on a particular case, who pays for the medical procedures, whether a waiting period should be required before reproductive use of harvested gametes, exclusionary criteria and screening for disease, whether the subsequently born child will be considered the legitimate child of the deceased biological donor, with inheritance rights and eligibility for other benefits, and what the potential harms are to the subsequently born child and other family members.

Who at the Institution or Clinic Should be Responsible for Applying the Policy and Rendering Judgment on a Particular Case?

From the research, it appears that decisions concerning posthumous reproduction are typically made on a case-by-case basis, e.g., by an institutional ethics committee *(47)* or a specially constituted multidisciplinary committee that may include physicians, clergy, psychiatrists, psychologists, sociologists, medical ethicists, reproductive technology expert, and a male infertility, and legal counsel *(48)*. Where female gametes are intended to be harvested, the clinic or institution should develop mechanisms to seek IRB review should such a medical research situation arise.

Who Pays for the Medical Procedures?

It is highly unlikely that the health insurer for the donor will cover the cost of harvesting, specimen preparation, and storage. Insurance policies typically exclude coverage procedures that are not medically necessary or are experimental, and it would be difficult to claim that the harvesting and storage of gametes is medically necessary in the case of a male or female and not experimental in the case of a female. Also, very few insurers cover the cost of assisted reproduction. Clinics and institutions must be prepared to accurately estimate the costs of the procedures and discuss them with the requestor and should also have the requestor directly arrange and pay for the preparation and storage of gametes in a sperm bank or reproductive clinic before gametes are harvested to ensure the best conditions for viability *(49)*.

Should a Waiting Period be Required Before Reproductive Use of Harvested Gametes?

Professional organizations and institutions with policies in place typically recommend or institute a waiting period before the gametes can be used for reproduction *(50)*. There is a general sense that the circumstances surrounding the harvesting procedure are so emotional that some commentators have recommended it is advisable to harvest on the condition that the gametes will not be used in ART for a particular period of time to allow appropriate bereavement and counseling. One policy specifically does not permit sperm harvesting without a wife's prior agreement not to use the specimen for 1 yr. It is unknown how many women actually attempt pregnancy using sperm collected posthumously. However, this same policy opines without reference, "[e]ven when retrieval has been performed, appropriately counseled women will rarely proceed with an attempt at pregnancy" *(51)*. If the harvesting, storage, and use of gametes are done at separate facilities, it would be difficult (perhaps impossible) to enforce such a waiting period.

Screening of Gametes

Some policies include a requirement that the donor's death not be owing to an infectious disease or a disease known to adversely affect spermatogenesis *(52)*. Others instead disavow any warranty regarding the quality of the sperm *(53)*.

Rights of the Child

The availability of posthumous reproduction also raises new questions about inheritance rights of the subsequently born child. Historically, state law has recognized the inheritance rights of a child born within 9 mo of a biological father's death. Thus, the law accounts for circumstances when a husband or male partner dies after conception but before the resulting birth of a child. Can children born more than 9 mo after a biological parent's death inherit from that parent? There is no consensus among the states on this issue. Some state statutes explicitly prohibit posthumously conceived children from inheriting. States that have adopted the Uniform Parentage Act will allow these children to inherit in limited circumstances (i.e., if a formal record exists of the deceased spouse's prior consent to be a parent if assisted reproduction occurred after death) *(54)*. The highest state court in Massachusetts took the evidentiary requirement one step further, requiring evidence of both the intent to reproduce after death and the intent to support any resulting children *(55)*. Because eligibility of a widow and dependents for federal social security survivor benefits is determined according to state inheritance laws, a particular state's approach toward posthumous inheritance may have far-reaching consequences.

CONCLUSIONS

Institutions and clinics should develop policies on posthumous reproduction to help ensure consistent and principled decision making. Such a policy can relieve individual physicians of the burden of ad hoc decision making in emotionally charged circumstances. These decisions will have practical, legal, and ethical implications for the provider, institutions, clinics, patients, and their families. Any policy created should reflect applicable legal standards and medical practice guidelines. In the absence of such a policy, the provider should obtain a legal consultation and refer to professional guidelines and ethics. Where due consideration has been given to this issue, most commentators and medical policies appear to advocate a conservative approach that requires explicit evidence of permission to harvest and the intent to reproduce even after death.

RECOMMENDED RESOURCES

Articles

Soules MR. Commentary: posthumous harvesting of gametes—a physician's perspective. J Law Med Ethics 1999;27:362–365.

White GB. Commentary: legal and ethical aspects of sperm retrieval. J Law Med Ethics 1999;27:359–361.

Kerr SM, Caplan A, Polin G, Smugar S, et al. Postmortem sperm procurement. J Urol 1997;157:2154–2158.

Strong C. Ethical and legal aspects of sperm retrieval after death or persistent vegetative state. J Law Med Ethics 1999;27:347–358.

Land S, Ross L. Posthumous reproduction: current and future status. Urol Clin N Am 2002;29: 863–871.

Strong C, Gingrich JR, Kutteh WH. Ethics of postmortem sperm retrieval: ethics of sperm retrieval after death or persistent vegetative state. Human Reprod 2000;15:739–745.

Policy Examples

The Lahey Clinic, Sperm Retrieval from Dead or Comatose Patients: Clinical and Administrative Policy and Procedure Manual, Available at: www.lahey.org/pdf/ethics/pdf_policy/5166.pdf. Accessed March 16, 2004.

American Society for Reproductive Medicine, Posthumous Reproduction, Jan. 10, 1997. Available at: www.asrm.org/Media/Ethics/posthum.html. Accessed March 16, 2004. The website for the ASRM indicates that this policy is under review as of January 2004.

New York Hospital Guidelines for Consideration of Requests for Post-mortem Sperm Retrieval. Available at: www.cornellurology.com/uro/cornell/guidelines.shtml. Accessed March 16, 2004.

National Ethics Committee on Assisted Human Reproduction (NECAHR), New Zealand Ministry of Health, Appendix 6: Guidelines for the storage, use and disposal of sperm from a deceased man, February 2000. Available at: www.newhealth.govt.nz/necahr/files/annualreport2001.pdf. Accessed March 16, 2004.

Legal Cases of Interest

R. v. Human Fertilisation and Embryology Authority, ex parte Blood, 2 All ER 687 (1997) per Lord Woolf.

Hecht v. Superior Court, 16 Cal. App. 4th 836, 20 Cal. Rptr. 2d 275 (1993).

Woodward v. Commissioner of Social Security, 760 NE2d 257 (Mass. 2002).

REFERENCES

1. Shuster E. The posthumous gift of life: the world according to Kane. J Cont Health Law Policy 1998;15(2):401–403.
2. As used in this chapter, a diagnosis of permanent unconscious condition includes a diagnosis of coma or persistent vegetative state.
3. It wasn't until May 1998 that a woman used sperm harvested from her dead husband to become pregnant. Andrews LB. The Clone Age: Adventures in the New World of Reproductive Technology, Henry Holt, New York, 1999, p. 226. This is distinct from using sperm that a man chose to donate and bank at a sperm bank where he also would likely sign paperwork indicating his wishes for disposition upon his death. Soules MR. Commentary: posthumous harvesting of gametes-a physician's perspective. J Law Med Ethics 1999;27:362–365.
4. Annas GJ. The shadowlands-secrets, life and assisted reproduction. N Engl J Med 1998;339: 935–939.
5. Kerr SM, Caplan A, Polin G, et al. Postmortem sperm procurement. J Urol 1997;157:2154–2158; Soules MR. Commentary: posthumous harvesting of gametes-a physician's perspective. J Law Med Ethics 1999;27:362–365.
6. Soules MR. Commentary: posthumous harvesting of gametes-a physician's perspective. J Law Med Ethics 1999;27:362–365; Hardy K, et al. Future developments in assisted reproduction in humans. Reproduction 2003;123:171–183.
7. Soules MR. Commentary: posthumous harvesting of gametes-a physician's perspective. J Law Med Ethics 1999;27:362–3658.
8. Ibid.
9. Andrews LB. The Clone Age: Adventures in the New World of Reproductive Technology. Henry Holt, New York, 1999, p. 226.
10. Andrews LB. The Sperminator. New York Times, March 28, 1999, p. 62.
11. *See* ref. *9*.
12. *See* ref. *7*.
13. Kerr SM, Caplan A, Polin G, et al. Postmortem sperm procurement 1997;157:2154–2158.
14. Ibid.
15. Kahan SE, Seftel AD, Resnich MI. Postmortem sperm procurement: a legal perspective. J Urol 1999;161.
16. Ibid.
17. Strong C, Gingrich JR, Kutteh WH. Ethics of postmortem sperm retrieval: Ethics of sperm retrieval after death or persistent vegetative state. Human Reprod 2000;15:739–745; Loughlin KR, ed. Point and Counterpoint, Postmortem Sperm Retrieval: New Technologies, New Dilemmas, Contemporary Urology Archive, July 2001. Available at: www.conturo.com/be_core/content/journals/u/data/2001/0701/ptsperm1.html. Accessed March 16, 2004.
18. New York Hospital Guidelines for Consideration of Requests for Post-mortem Sperm Retrieval. Available at: www.cornellurology.com/uro/cornell/guidelines.shtml. Accessed March 16, 2004.

19. Strong C, Gingrich JR, Kutteh WH. Ethics of postmortem sperm retrieval: Ethics of sperm retrieval after death or persistent vegetative state. Human Reprod 2000;15:739–745.
20. Ibid.
21. Ibid.
22. Land S, Ross L. Posthumous Reproduction: current and future status. Urologic Clin North Am 2002;29:863–871.
23. *See* ref. *9*.
24. *See* ref. *13*.
25. The New York Times, Late Edition (East Coast); New York, March 27, 1999.
26. *See* ref. *7*.
27. Ibid.
28. *See* ref. *4*.
29. Update Conception Inheritance Law. Seattle Post-Intelligencer; Seattle, Washington, DC, Jan. 11, 2002. In the United States, the American Bar Association (ABA), a national legal organization, recognized the void in regulating reproductive technologies, including posthumous reproduction. An ABA committee drafted a model act to provide comprehensive guidance for state legislation on reproductive technologies. American Bar Association, Assisted Reproduction and Genetic Technologies Committee, Family Law Section, Assisted Reproductive Technologies Model Act, December, 1999. The model act recommended adopting a standard of explicit prior consent in a formal written document for harvesting of sperm or egg specimens for posthumous reproduction. The ABA committee developed this proposed standard in recognition of the privacy and liberty rights of individuals to control their destiny about whether to become parents, even after death. As of the date of this writing, the law has not been approved by the ABA.
30. *See* ref. 22.
31. "If the right of privacy means anything it is the right of the individual...to be free from unwarranted governmental intrusion into matters so fundamentally affecting a person as the decision whether to bear or beget a child," holding that a state may not prohibit unmarried individuals from using contraceptives) *Eisenstadt v. Baird*, 405 US at 453; *Skinner v. Oklahoma*, 316 US 535, 541 (1942) (...marriage and procreation are fundamental to the very existence and survival of the race"); *Griswold v. Connecticut*, 381 US 479, 485,486 (1965) (a state may not prohibit a married couple from using contraception).
32. *R. v. Human Fertilisation and Embryology Authority*, ex parte Blood, 2 All ER 687 (1997) per Lord Woolf; *Hecht v. Superior Court*, 16 Cal App. 4th 836, 20 Cal. Rptr. 2d 275 (1993); *Woodward v. Commissioner of Social Security*, 760 NE2d 257 (Mass. 2002).
33. American Society for Reproductive Medicine, Posthumous Reproduction, Jan. 10, 1997. Available at: www.asrm.org/Media/Ethics/posthum.html. Accessed March 16, 2004. The website for the ASRM indicates that this policy is under review as of January 2004.
34. *See* ref. *15*.
35. Code of Ethics. American Urological Association, December 12, 2004, Available at: www.ama-assn.org/ama/pub/category/13355.html. Accessed January 5, 2005.
36. *See* ref. *33*.
37. *See*, e.g., *Hecht v. Superior Court*, 16 Cal App. 4th 836, 20 Cal Rptr. 2d 275 (1993), where a man who committed suicide previously banked his sperm, designated his girlfriend as the beneficiary under the storage contract and in his will, and his living children contested the awarding of the sperm to his girlfriend for posthumous use.
38. *See* ref. *7*.
39. Sperm Retrieval from Dead or Comatose Patients: Clinical & Administrative Policy & Procedure Manual. Available at: www.lahey.org/pdf/ethics/pdf_policy/5166.pdf. Accessed

March 16, 2004. The policy requires execution of a consent form prior to sperm retrieval that acknowledges the "limits of the clinic's responsibility in the process of posthumous procreation and procreation by the irreversibly comatose patient."
40. *See* ref. *18*.
41. American Medical Association, Principles of Medical Ethics, Section E-204, Artificial Insemination by Donor. Available at: www.amaassn.org/ama/pub/category/8391.html. Accessed March 23, 2004.
42. *See* ref. *33*.
43. Benshushan A, Schenker JG. The right to an heir in the era of assisted reproduction. Hum Reprod 1998;13:1407–1410.
44. *See*, e.g., 45 Code of Federal Regulations 46.
45. Andrews LB. Beyond Doctrinal Boundaries: A Legal Framework For Surrogate Motherhood, 81 Va. L. Rev. 2343 (1995).
46. *See* ref. *19*.
47. *See* ref. *7*.
48. *See* refs. *18* and *43*.
49. *See* ref. *7*.
50. *See* refs. *7* and *18*.
51. *See* ref. *18*.
52. Ibid.
53. The Lahey Clinic policy states that it will "make no guarantee as to the quantity, quality, genetic content, safety, viability, or effectiveness of any sperm it collects." The Lahey Clinic, Sperm Retrieval from Dead or Comatose Patients: Clinical & Administrative Policy & Procedure Manual. Available at: www.lahey.org/pdf/ethics/pdf_policy/5166.pdf. Accessed March 16, 2004.
54. Uniform Parentage Act, sec. 707 9B U.L.A. 358 (2001).
55. *Woodward v. Commissioner of Social Security*, 760 NE2d 257 (Mass. 2002).

19 Gender Selection

Separating Fact From Fiction

David S. Karabinus, PhD, HCLD
and Keith L. Blauer, MD

Contents

INTRODUCTION

The mechanisms and possibilities of controlling or predetermining the sex of offspring are likely to have been pondered by humans throughout history. Different cultures, social classes, and races may exhibit different preferences for a child of a given sex. Chromosomal sex is determined at fertilization by the heterogametic parent. For humans, the male is the heterogametic parent, producing both X and Y chromosome-bearing sperm. The mechanisms of meiosis in the production of gametes by the heterogametic parent should, in theory, yield an equal number of male and female offspring. Because the human sex ratio is almost 50:50, it appears that the sex ratio of babies born primarily reflects the ratio of X- and Y-bearing sperm in semen and is probably not significantly impacted by other factors, such as the female reproductive tract environment or differential fetal survival to birth.

Impact of Chance on the Sex Ratio

Although *sex* is defined as the anatomical and physiological differences that distinguish males from females, and *gender* is a grammatical classification/

From: *Contemporary Endocrinology: Office Andrology*
Edited by: P. E. Patton and D. E. Battaglia

distinction that refers to words, the two terms have become synonymous in recent usage. Genetic or chromosomal sex is determined at fertilization when the maternal and paternal gametic haploid genomes combine at syngamy to form the embryo. In humans and most other mammals, the male determines the sex of the offspring: during spermatocytogenesis, one diploid XY spermatogonium undergoes a series of mitotic and meiotic divisions to yield 256 haploid spermatids (assuming 100% spermatogenic efficiency), half of which contain an X chromosome, and half contain a Y chromosome. Spermatids then undergo maturation steps during spermiogenesis to become spermatozoa. Because the sex chromosome complement for the male is XY, and assuming that there is no differential or preferential survival of X- vs Y-bearing gametes during mitosis and meiosis, the proportion of X- vs Y-bearing sperm produced by the testes should be equal. If equal numbers of each type of sperm are produced and subsequently presented to the female, then the X- and Y-bearing sperm have an equal chance of fertilizing an oocyte (containing an X chromosome) to form an XX (female) or an XY (male) embryo. Thus, the chances of a male or female are 50:50 for each conception and the sex of previous babies has no effect on that likelihood. Preimplantation genetic diagnosis (PGD) data generated at the Genetics & IVF Institute on embryos resulting from fertilization by unsorted (random) sperm showed similar proportions of male and female embryos. Similarly, birth data show essentially a 50:50 sex ratio at birth.

Despite biological facts, parents with numerous children of only one sex may find it difficult to believe that chance alone was responsible for the disparity in sex ratio among their children. To address that question, we used fluorescence *in situ* hybridization (FISH) analysis to determine the distribution of X- and Y-bearing sperm in raw (unsorted) semen from 678 participants in the MicroSort® clinical trial. Of the participants, 44 had more than three male children and no female children, and 21 had more than three female children and no male children. The FISH results showed that the X:Y ratio in raw semen was essentially 50:50 overall. The distribution of X- and Y-bearing sperm in raw semen was 50.7 ± 3.2% and 49.3 ± 4.3%, respectively. For couples with more than three boys it was 50.6 ± 3.2% X and 49.4 ± 3.2% Y, and for those with more than three girls it was 50.9 ± 2.2 X and 49.1 ± 2.2% Y.

Choosing the child's sex before birth can be effected before conception (fertilization), after conception but before implantation in the uterus, and after implantation but before delivery. Preconception sex selection involves manipulating the proportion of X- or Y-bearing sperm to the point of considerably increasing the probability that a sperm carrying the desired sex chromosome will fertilize the egg. Postconception but preimplantation sex selection involves acting after identifying the sex of the embryo. Postimplantation sex selection deals with acting after identifying the sex of the fetus or baby. Historically, the choices available to those wishing to have a child of a specific sex have been limited to adoption or continuing to bear children until a child of the desired sex was born. The advent of amniocentesis and chorionic villus sampling, although invasive, permitted accurate fetal sex determination prior to delivery. When the resolving ability of ultrasonography sufficiently improved to allow accurate imaging of fetal genitalia, this noninvasive method of fetal sex determination led to widespread use. Thus informed, the prospective parents could then decide whether to continue with the pregnancy.

PRECONCEPTION SEX SELECTION

Preconception sex selection methods are based on manipulations whose aim is to increase the likelihood that an X- or a Y-bearing sperm will fertilize the oocyte. These methods aim to enhance or interfere with the in vivo access of X- or Y-bearing sperm to the oocyte or may involve the in vitro separation of X- from Y-bearing sperm prior to insemination. The three categories of preconception sex selection methods are so-called "natural" methods, density gradient separation methods, and flow cytometric methods. Natural methods are usually simple and unlikely to harm the sperm. The perceived degree of control the couple can exert on the application of these methods, coupled with their relative low-cost and pseudoscientific underpinnings, likely enhance their appeal. The natural methods fall, more or less, into one of the following categories: the timing of intercourse relative to ovulation, the length of abstinence before intercourse, dietary modifications specific for the desired sex, vaginal pH modifications, egg membrane polarity, and combinations of methods. An Internet search using the key words "sex selection" or "gender selection" reveals the extent of methods currently being promoted.

Natural Methods

The timing method is based on the unsubstantiated claim that Y chromosome-bearing sperm are smaller, less robust, and have a swimming advantage over their larger, slower-swimming X-bearing counterparts. Couples wishing to have a male child are advised to have intercourse as close as possible to ovulation, whereas those wishing for a female should have intercourse at least 2 to 3 d before ovulation. Shettles and Rorvik *(1)*, advocates of this method, claim high success rates that are not universally accepted *(2)*.

The length of abstinence method—a modification of the timing method—was proposed by Chesterman-Phillips *(3)*. Abstinence from ejaculation for at least 1 wk before ovulation is advised for those who desire to conceive a male child. For a female child, frequent ejaculations are advised until several days before ovulation, followed by intercourse 2 to 5 d before ovulation. Of note, the length of abstinence has been shown to not impact the X:Y ratio in ejaculated semen *(4)* or on the sex ratio at birth *(2)*.

Modifications of the female's diet to increase the odds of conceiving a child of the desired sex were proposed by Papa *(5)*. For a boy, food rich in sodium and potassium were recommended, whereas foods rich in calcium and magnesium were recommended for a girl. Proponents claim a high success rate for the baby of the desired sex when the diet is strictly followed for 3 mo prior to conception. Although diet can presumably affect the female reproductive tract environment, it is not clear that such changes (if they occur) truly have differential effects on X- or Y-bearing sperm access to the oocyte.

Sex selection based on changing the vaginal pH with acidic or alkaline douches has been indicated to affect the likelihood of a male or female conception. Some believe alkaline conditions are conducive to Y-bearing sperm success, whereas acidic environments enhance X-bearing sperm success *(6)*. Based on this theory, douching with either a sodium bicarbonate solution (for a boy) or lemon juice or diluted vinegar (for a girl) is recommended 15 to 30 min before intercourse. It is unclear the degree to which these treatments actually impact the pH of the vagina (normally 3.8–4.5), semen (normally 7.2–8.0 with some buffering capacity), or cervical mucus (range 6.4–8.0; preovulatory mucus is most alkaline).

Changes in the charge or polarity of the egg membrane are thought to impact receptivity of the oocyte to X- or Y-bearing sperm. These changes are claimed to occur on certain days of a woman's cycle and are based on details of the most recent menstrual cycle, blood group, and female age. A specific calendar is then constructed that identifies the individual's "polarity cycle" (the most receptive days of each month) for the desired sex over the period of 1 yr. Based on the unpublished work of Patrick Schoun, this method is currently being promoted as the Selnas/Right Baby Method. It is not certain whether this method refers to the polarity of the vitelline membrane (oolemma) or zona pellucida or whether it recognizes the role of the proteins involved in sperm–zona pellucida binding. A blunt comment, referring to this method as "...nonsense," was published in the *British Medical Journal (7)*.

Several natural methods of sex selection are available that combine elements of the individual methods cited earlier. The *Yinyang Solutions*, developed by Dashi Tan and offered through the Yinyang Institute, is a timing method that combines elements of birth information, Chinese astrology, the Chinese lunar calendar, and Feng-shui to construct a personalized calendar for optimizing the likelihood of conceiving a baby of the desired sex. They suggest its use in conjunction with other gender selection methods, such as the Shettles Method. GenSelect is another combined method that promotes nutraceuticals in the form of proprietary formulations, timing of intercourse through ovulation predictor kits, and basal body temperature monitoring, changing the vaginal environment through douching, and dietary guidelines.

Physical Separation of X- and Y-Bearing Sperm Using Density Gradients

Ericsson et al. *(8)* reported that an enriched population of Y-bearing sperm could be recovered using a bovine albumin density gradient. Ericsson *(9)* later described Y-spermatozoa as containing 4% less DNA, 7% less surface area, being faster swimmers, and to be specifically stained by florescent dye when compared to the X-bearing spermatozoa. Quinlivan et al. *(10)* reported verification of the Ericsson method based on the ability of quinacrine chloride, believed to fluorescently label the distal long arm of the Y chromosome, to differentiate Y- from X-bearing sperm. Bovine albumin was later replaced by human serum albumin, and combined clinical results were published for four different protocols *(11)*, reporting over 72% of births being male when desired and more than 68% female births when desired. Others *(12–14)* reported similar results. Success claims were based on birth sex results alone; the actual percentages of X- and Y-bearing spermatozoa isolated from these methods were never quantified in these studies. The results reported by Ericsson et al. *(8)* proved difficult to reproduce, and as molecular biology techniques improved, quinacrine chloride was found to not to be a Y chromosome-specific stain *(15)*. The application of FISH analysis, which allows the simultaneous differential staining of both X- and Y-bearing spermatozoa, has shown that the ratio of X- and Y-bearing sperm before and after application of the Ericsson methods is essentially 50:50 *(16–19)*.

Other density gradient separation methods have employed media, such as Percoll *(16,20,21)*, Ficoll *(22)*, or Sephadex *(23,24)*, based presumably on the differences in density or mass between X- and Y-bearing sperm. Centrifugation of sperm through discontinuous density gradients would theoretically result in an enriched population of X-bearing sperm because of their greater DNA content. Early reports of significant enrichment of this sperm after such treatments were based on results of quinacrine staining. Later studies that employed probes specific to the chromosomes were unable to show enrichment *(16,20,25)*. Although combining density gradient separation with swim-up has been reported to yield shifts in the X:Y ratio of recovered sperm *(26,27)*, others have shown that biologically insignificant changes resulted from the use of those methods when appraised using molecular techniques *(18,28)*.

Efficacy of Natural Methods and Density Gradient Separation

Sex selection through the use of natural methods or sperm processing via swim-up or gradients has not been shown as effective *(29,30)*. Despite claims to the contrary, these methods do not withstand scientific scrutiny, and reported results have proved difficult to reproduce or verify. However, they are unlikely to result in harm, and the patient does have a 50% chance of successful outcome. The American College of Obstetricians and Gynecologists *(31)* does not recommend the use of these methods owing to the lack of demonstrable reliability. Similarly, the American Society of Reproductive Medicine Ethics Committee *(32)* commented that, even with the lack of consistency and validation, such methods continued to be offered by some with claims of success based on "...highly questionable data that could mislead patients." Similarly, the Human Fertilisation and Embryology Authority (HFEA) *(33)*—the governmental agency that regulates assisted reproduction in Great Britain—concluded that gradient methods were of questionable suitability for sex selection resulting from contradictory reports of effectiveness. The HFEA *(34)* also noted that the use of gradient methods would be unreasonable to allow in situations like avoidance of X-linked disease, where efficacy was of great importance.

Flow Cytometric Separation of X- and Y-Bearing Sperm

History

Sorting sperm into their separate X and Y chromosome-bearing populations by flow cytometry is the only preconception method of gender selection with a solid scientific basis and where results can be validated by modern molecular techniques, e.g., FISH or by birth results (phenotypic sex). Flow cytometric sperm sorting is the only sperm selection method that consistently and reliably results in offspring of the desired sex. With this method, sperm are stained with a DNA-specific fluorescent dye and processed through a flow cytometer. The flow cytometer utilizes a laser to cause stained sperm to fluoresce, then detects differences in the amount of fluorescence emitted by stained sperm. The difference in fluorescence intensity enables discrimination between the X- and Y-bearing sperm such that the desired sperm may be recovered in a highly enriched population of X- or Y-bearing sperm. Because the X chromosome is larger and contains more DNA than the Y chromosome in mammals *(35,36)*, and the autosomes in X- and Y-bearing sperm have identical DNA content, X-bearing sperm have more total DNA than its counterpart. Thus, when stained with a DNA-specific fluorochrome, the fluorescent signal emitted by an X-bearing sperm is greater than that emitted by a Y-bearing sperm.

Using the DNA-specific supravital stain Hoechst 33342, Johnson and colleagues *(37)* at the United States Department of Agriculture (USDA) Agriculture Research Station at Beltsville, MD were able to sort mammalian sperm into two enriched populations based varying DNA content. Reports of normal births in different animal species soon followed in rapid succession *(38–41)*. Humans have been shown to have a 2.8% difference in DNA content between X- and Y-bearing sperm *(42,43)*. Johnson et al. *(42)* reported the first successful flow cytometric separation of X- and Y-bearing human sperm into highly enriched populations. The first human pregnancy resulting from the use of flow cytometrically sorted sperm resulted from work done at GIVF *(44)*. In 1998, Fugger and colleagues *(45)* reported the births resulting from the use of flow cytometrically separated human sperm for intrauterine insemination (IUI), in vitro fertilization (IVF), and intracytoplasmic sperm injection (ICSI).

In 1992, the USDA granted GIVF an exclusive license to apply the patented flow cytometric sperm separation technology for development and use in humans. Institutional review board (IRB) approval was received in 1993 to initiate clinical studies to use the process for couples at risk for conception with X-linked disease. The clinical study indications were expanded in 1995 to offer family balancing. The US Food and Drug Administration (FDA) approved an Investigational Device Exemption in 2000 for GIVF to continue to conduct a clinical trial of safety and efficacy of the MicroSort Sperm Separation Technology. To date, more than 400 babies have been born after using MicroSort® for sorting fresh or frozen sperm into enriched X- and Y-bearing sperm populations for use in IUI, IVF, and ICSI. Flow cytometric sperm sorting in the livestock species, most notably by Cogent in Great Britain, Goyaike SA in Argentina, and XY, Inc in the United States, has resulted in the birth of tens of thousands of offspring (Johnson LA, personal communication).

Either freshly collected or cryopreserved semen can be used for sorting. After evaluating semen quality, conventional semen processing methods are employed to recover motile sperm and to remove undesirable seminal components *(46)*. After processing, semen is re-evaluated for quality and then stained for 1 h at 35ºC with Hoechst 33342 at a final concentration of 9 μM, as previously described *(42)*.

Description of the Flow Cytometric Separation Method

Successful flow cytometric sorting of X- and Y-bearing sperm depends on the accurate detection of differences in fluorescent signal intensity (a function of sperm DNA content) between the X- and Y-bearing sperm. Major factors affecting the fluorescent signals that result from the sperm-laser interaction are species-specific. In the human, sperm head shape, degree of sperm head polymorphism, and the difference in DNA content between X- and Y-bearing sperm (2.8%) are primary factors. Human sperm heads are not symmetric in their axes; they have an oval appearance when lying flat but exhibit a narrow, angular, spear-tip profile in longitudinal section. Because of sperm head morphology and the nature of chromatin packaging in the nucleus, the fluorescent signal emitted by the edge of the sperm head is brighter than that emitted by the flat aspect, making sperm head orientation relative to the excitation light a critical factor in analyzing and sorting the sperm *(47)*.

Sperm move through the flow cytometer in a narrow stream of media (sample stream) which, when subsequently surrounded by sheath fluid, is squeezed so that the sperm in the sample stream are aligned (more or less) one behind the other. In the sample stream, the sperm may be positioned head first or tail first. However, the orientation of sperm heads relative to the excitation light source, which is situated perpendicular to the sample stream, is random (at any position in the 360° rotation along the long axis of the sperm). This random orientation results in only a small percentage of sperm, perhaps 10%, being appropriately oriented for accurate analysis of DNA content and sorting. The effects of sperm orientation, coupled with other factors (e.g., sperm-to-sperm variation within a specimen, the impact of sorting time on sperm survival, and the fact that only 50% of those sperm carry the desired sex chromosome) result in a very small proportion of available sperm actually recovered by sorting. As an illustration after processing, a raw specimen containing 130 million sperm may yield 40 million sperm for sorting, which in turn may yield 200,000 to 400,000 sorted sperm or 0.2 to 0.5% of the original, after 4 h of sorting.

Currently, stained sperm are sorted using commercially available flow cytometer cell sorters that have been modified specifically for sorting sperm through the addition of a forward fluorescence detector *(47)* and equipped with argon ion lasers. Fluorescence emitted by each stained sperm after excitation with laser light (100 mW ultraviolet) is detected by forward- (0º) and right-angle (90º) fluorescence sensors. The fluorescent signals from sperm collected at the 90º detector are analyzed, and those exhibiting the greatest intensity (proper orientation) are gated so that their fluorescent signals (to the exclusion of signals from nonproperly oriented sperm) can then be simultaneously analyzed after collection by the forward fluorescence detector. Thus, the fluorescent signals emitted by properly oriented sperm are collected by the forward fluorescence detector, then gated based on lower (YSORT) or higher (XSORT) intensity.

At this time, currently available technology allows human sperm analysis at a rate of 3000 to 3500 cells per second, and sorted sperm may be collected at a rate of 20 to 25 cells per second. The rate of analysis, and the subsequent rate at which sorted sperm are collected, depends on instrumentation limitations and the specimen quality. Specimens containing sperm with a high degree of homogeneity may be sorted at a greater rate than those exhibiting, e.g., a high level of grossly abnormal sperm or cellular debris. By comparison, it is common when sorting bovine sperm, notable for their high degree of sperm-to-sperm morphologic uniformity and greater difference in DNA content between the X- vs Y-bearing sperm, to collect 3000 to 6000 sorted sperm per second *(48–50)*. At the conclusion of sorting, a sample of sorted sperm is evaluated for motility, progression, and the extent of enrichment in X- or Y-bearing sperm (postsort purity) using FISH. Sorted sperm are then utilized fresh for IUI or IVF-ICSI or are cryopreserved for future IVF-ICSI use.

Clinical Trial Participation and Follow-Up

The recipients of MicroSort-sorted sperm include clinical trial participants: married couples meeting inclusion criteria who have sought reduced genetic disease risk or balanced sex distribution among their children (family balancing). Qualified couples with infertility undergoing IVF that desired participation have also been included. Clinical trial participants agree, as part of the informed consent process, to provide birth and pediatric records (through the first year of life) for babies born using MicroSort® sperm. Birth and pediatric records are reviewed by two board-certified medical geneticists who record any major or minor malformations evident in the babies.

Efficacy of Flow Cytometric Separation of X- and Y-Bearing Sperm

Ongoing Clinical Trial Results. As of December 31, 2002, 1530 couples had enrolled in the MicroSort clinical trial; 90% of participants desired to balance the gender distribution among their children, and 10% wished to avoid a sex-linked genetic disease. Most participants desired a girl (97% for genetic disease avoidance and 71% for family balancing). Of the 2570 total sorts performed, 73.3% were used for IUI and 26.6% were used for IVF-ICSI.

Results of sex outcome are summarized in Table 1, which shows that the frequency of X- and Y-bearing sperm after sorting (postsort purity), as determined by FISH, was nearly 90 and 70%, respectively, for XSort® and YSort® and unmistakably skewed away from the 50:50 ratio expected in raw semen. Our experience has shown that postsort purity is unaffected by abstinence up to 175 h, age of the male, or whether fresh- or frozen-thawed sperm are sorted. The postsort purity results are closely matched by the percentage of male and female embryos that result from the use of MicroSort® sperm as determined using PGD (blastomere biopsy). Similarly, the sex of babies born from using MicroSort sperm is consistent with postsort purity and PGD results. These data show that MicroSort® leads to a meaningful, verifiable shift in the X:Y ratio in the sorted sperm population used for insemination ($n = 2570$ sorts), which persists in the sex of resultant embryos ($n = 908$ embryos biopsied) but also in the sex of the babies ($n = 387$) either born or whose sex was determined *in utero*.

Table 2 contains a summary of MicroSort® IUI results. At the current time, IUIs are only performed at MicroSort® sites in Fairfax, VA and Laguna Hills, CA. The 14.9% overall per-cycle pregnancy rate ($n = 1824$ IUI cycles with follow-up) is reasonable when considering that clinical trial participants were generally a normally fertile population, and an average of 169,000 motile sperm were inseminated. With MicroSort® sperm, the per-cycle IUI pregnancy rate

Table 1
MicroSort® Efficacy Results: XSort® and YSort® Outcomes

	*XSort**	*YSort**
Postsort purity	87.6% **X** *n* = 2015	69.3% **Y** *n* = 555
Embryo sex (PGD)	89.1% ♀ *n* = 385	63.7% ♂ *n* = 523
Baby sex	90.8% ♀ *n* = 336	76.5% ♂ *n* = 51

*XSort, YSort: Enriches specimen with X-bearing or Y-bearing sperm to increase chances of having a female or a male baby, respectively. PGD, preimplantation genetic diagnosis.

Table 2
MicroSort® Efficacy Results:
IUI Clinical Pregnancy and Spontaneous
Loss Rates by Female Age

Age	*Pregnancy rate*	*SAB rate*
<30	18.5% (35/189)	5.7% (2/35)
30–34	15.4% (105/681)	12.4% (13/105
35–39	14.6% (119/816)	18.5% (22/119)
40	8.7% (12/138)	33.3% (4/12)
Overall	14.9% (271/1824)	15.1% (41/271)

IUI, intraunterine insemination; SAB, spontaneous loss.

increased from 7.2% (*n* = 152) with approx 65,000 motile sperm inseminated to a consistent 18 to 20% (*n* = 788) with the insemination of 200,000 to 400,000 motile sperm. Because of current limitations, the effect of inseminating more than 450,000 motile sperm has not been tested. In an evaluation of 1678 MicroSort® IUI cycles, the likelihood of pregnancy remained consistent across consecutive and multiple (four or more) IUI cycles when the cycle stimulation regimen was characterized by decreased incidence of natural cycles, increased frequency of follicle-stimulating hormone, and a relatively constant incidence of clomiphene stimulation in subsequent cycles. The spontaneous abortion rate for IUI cycles increases with rising patient age, but overall, it is well within the 20 to 25% loss rate exhibited by the general population *(51)*.

A total of 683 IVF-ICSI cycles have been performed both at the Virginia site and by collaborating physicians in the United States, Europe, and Africa. The cycles for which gamete data is available (*n* = 556) resulted in 3716 fertilized oocytes of the 5639 oocytes inseminated (65.9%); of those fertilized oocytes, 3231 of 3418 two pronuclei embryos underwent cleavage (94.5%). Pregnancy results for the IVF-ICSI cycles for which such data is available (*n* = 502) is

Table 3
**MicroSort® Efficacy Results:
IVF-ICSI Clinical Pregnancy Rate
and Spontaneous Loss Rates by Female Age**

Age	*Pregnancy rate*	*SAB rate**
<30	47.0% (47/100)	20.0% (11/55)
30-34	36.0% (54/150)	12.1% (7/58)
35-39	29.5% (54/183)	16.9% (10/59)
40	16.1% (9/56)	33.3% (3/9)
Egg age unknown	38.5% (5/13)	20.0% (1/5)
Overall	33.7% (169/502)	17.2% (32/186)

*Combined fresh and frozen transfer data.
IVF-ISCI, in vitro fertilization-intracytoplasmic sperm injection; SAB, spontaneous loss.

summarized in Table 3. The IVF-ICSI results are comparable with the most recent Center for Disease Control and Prevention *(52)* results for assisted reproductive technology procedures, showing that pregnancy rates were greatest for patients in the youngest age group and decreased with increased patient age. The pregnancy rate for frozen embryo transfers was 34% per cycle ($n = 50$). The IVF-ICSI spontaneous abortion rate, similar to that for the MicroSort® IUI cycles, increases with patient age and is consistent with that for the general population *(51)*.

The safety of the MicroSort® process can be evaluated by examining the effects on sperm functional competence, fertilization and cleavage rates, IUI and IVF-ICSI pregnancy rates, spontaneous abortion rates, and rates of congenital malformation. An average of 192×10^6 total motile sperm with an average 2.4 (0–4 scale; 0, no sperm movement; 4, hyperactivated movement) motility grade yielded an average of 167.9×10^3 motile sperm with grade 2.5 motility postsort. Sperm sorting is an inefficient process (its effects on numbers of sorted sperm recovered is previously presented), which accounts for the reduction in number of motile sperm numbers in the postsort vs unsorted specimens. Sperm motility grade appears at least to be unaffected, if not slightly improved, after sorting. For IUIs, the per-cycle pregnancy rate (14.9%) is comparable to that reported in the literature and is accomplished after inseminating less than 1% of the 20×10^6 (or more) sperm normally deposited when therapeutic IUI is performed. The functional competence of MicroSort® sperm is further demonstrated through the IVF-ICSI results presented previously in terms of fertilization rates (65.9%), cleavage rates (94.5%), pregnancy rates for both fresh transfers (33.7% overall) and frozen (34.0%), and the spontaneous loss rate (17.2%). Ongoing review of the current malformation rate shows that the observed number of major malformations and minor malformations among all the babies born ($n = 306$) for whom complete birth records are available is 7 (2.29%) and 7 (2.29%), respectively. The exact upper 95% confidence bound for these proportions is 4.25%, indicating that the true major and minor malformation rates for babies born from the use of MicroSort sperm is no greater than 4.25%. This is quite comparable to the 4% rate estimated for all combined major congenital malformations in a general population of newborns *(53)*.

POSTCONCEPTION: PREIMPLANTATION GENETIC DIAGNOSIS

PGD is an extremely accurate sex selection tool. This invasive postfertilization, but pretransfer, method involves testing embryos created by IVF after which embryos with specific genetic traits, e.g., XX or XY sex chromosome complement, are selected for transfer to the uterus. It was first performed in 1990 for patients with known familial hereditary diseases.

PGD testing is typically performed 3 d after egg retrieval, when the embryo has reached the 6 to 8 blastomere stage. There is no evidence to support that the removal of one or two blastomeres at this stage diminishes the ability of the embryo to continue normal fetal development. Because the entire genetic makeup of the embryo can be found in each blastomere, testing for the sex chromosome complement can accurately determine embryo sex at this early stage of development before transfer of embryos to the uterus. Worldwide, more than 5000 PGD procedures have been performed for various indications since the first successful report of PGD by Handyside and colleagues *(54)*, resulting in more than 1000 pregnancies and live births *(55)*.

The ability to identify information regarding the genetic material of embryos when they are only 3 d old allows parents the ability to bear a child with an almost perfect chance of it being the desired gender. Without the option of PGD, parents who are carriers of X-linked diseases or who desire to balance the gender distribution of their children face the choice of natural reproduction, prenatal testing, and possible termination of unwanted pregnancies or foregoing having children.

PGD requires numerous steps prior to the diagnosis of the embryo that include: initial consultations with a reproductive specialist, medical geneticist, or a genetic counselor, an IVF cycle with oocyte retrieval and fertilization, culture of the embryos in the laboratory, biopsy of the embryo to recover one or two blastomeres, and laboratory analysis of these individual cells using either polymerase chain reaction (PCR) or FISH. PCR was the first technique used to diagnose embryos and is still used today for single-gene defects. FISH is used to diagnose embryos with heritable chromosome rearrangements or to screen embryos for the most common aneuploidies found in early embryos and spontaneous miscarriages. Both PCR and FISH can be used to determine the sex of an embryo.

With PCR testing, each recovered blastomere is placed in a lysis solution from which nuclear DNA is captured. Small sections of the captured DNA are amplified so that the laboratory can determine whether a genetic mutation is present or whether the embryo is male or female. PCR is a very sensitive test; thus, care must be taken to ensure no contaminating DNA enters the tube in which amplification takes place, or a misdiagnosis could occur. As an additional precaution against DNA contamination, ICSI may be used as the fertilization method for IVF-PGD cycles in which PCR is the analytic methodology.

For FISH testing, each blastomere removed from the embryo is placed on a microscope slide and observed until lysis occurs. After blastomere lysis, the cytoplasm should float away, leaving the nucleus on the slide. The nuclear material is then fixed on the slide using formalin and dehydrated with ethanol. A final check of the location and appearance of each nucleus is noted before the slides are processed for FISH.

FISH has replaced PCR testing for embryonic sex determination because FISH offers two advantages. (1) Although PCR amplifies small DNA segments on the X and Y chromosome, it does not indicate how many copies of each of these segments are present. In other words, PCR can identify the presence of X or Y chromosome-specific DNA, but does not enable the differentiation between a normal female (XX) and a Turner Syndrome female (XO). Similarly, a Klinefelter male (XXY) would appear to be a normal male (XY) by PCR testing. (2) With FISH, common chromosome anomalies, such as trisomy 21, 18, and 13, can also be screened at the same time as the gender determination. Currently, a panel of eight chromosomes (13, 15, 16, 18, 21, 22, X, and Y) is routinely tested in aneuploidy or sex selection screening cases.

The expected ratio of male:female embryos seen following any PGD cycle should be 50:50. A study at GIVF *(56)* was undertaken to determine if the gender ratio of embryos could be skewed toward the desired gender by using MicroSort®-separated sperm with nonsorted sperm cycles used as a control. In this study, 2005 embryos were biopsied, and gender was determined by PGD using either PCR ($n = 1746$ embryos) or FISH ($n = 259$ embryos). Gender was determined in 1841 (91.8 %) of the embryos. During the time that this study took place (June 1994 and September 2003), the mean postsort purity as measured by FISH for X- and Y-bearing sorted sperm was 88.8% for XSort® and 71.7% for YSort®. For both YSort® and XSort®, the sex ratio of embryos was significantly different from that obtained when unsorted sperm were used (66.0% vs 45.0% and 86.5% vs 55.0%, respectively). These results show that enriching a sample of sperm with either X- or Y-bearing sperm using MicroSort® prefertilization, either for genetic disease avoidance or sex selection indications, will skew the sex ratio among embryos in a cohort so that more embryos of the desired sex are present. This skewing is important in an IVF cycle where all embryos from the cycle may not advance to the proper stage for transfer. In addition, by skewing the ratio of X:Y-bearing sperm prior to the PGD cycle, the physician and patient are likely to have more embryos of good quality and desired sex to choose for transfer.

SUMMARY

The value of a procedure is based on its efficacy and safety. For sex selection methods, these factors can be addressed by determining whether they have a meaningful effect on the sex ratio of babies born as a result of their application and if the babies are healthy. The natural and physical separation methods (density gradients and swim-up) of sex selection are preconception methods that are generally considered safe, but the effectiveness has not been clearly demonstrated. Verifiable data is lacking, particularly for the natural methods, and has not been shown to be independently repeatable or able to withstand peer review. Most claims made by promoters of these methods are unsubstantiated, often confusing and misleading to both the patient and physician. Early data supporting the veracity of the physical separation methods has since been repudiated with the advent of modern molecular testing methods. Although the natural and the physical separation methods are unlikely to harm the sperm, parent, or baby, the effects of the nutritional supplements merchandized by some promoters have not been tested. The cost of these methods is relatively low but their chance of producing a baby of the desired sex appears no different than if the method had not been applied at all (i.e., 50:50).

By comparison, flow cytometric sex selection with MicroSort® results in a verifiable and biologically meaningful shift in the ratio of X- and Y-bearing sperm, which retain their functional competence and lead to an increased likelihood of conceiving and delivering a healthy baby of the desired sex. This preconception method creates a shift in the ratio of X- and Y-bearing sperm from the expected 50:50 to 87.6% for XSort® and 69.3% for YSort®, as validated by FISH analysis of the sorted sperm. PGD results and fetal sex results are consistent with the shift in X- and Y-bearing sperm incidence, showing that MicroSort® does have a significant positive impact on the potential to concieve a baby of the desired sex. The malformation rate for babies born from the use of MicroSort® sperm is consistent with that of the general population.

PGD has been shown to be an extremely accurate postfertilization/preimplantation sex selection method. Although it is invasive, and is necessarily used in conjunction with IVF, it is nearly 100% accurate in determining the sex of an embryo. This accuracy stems from probes that are specific to the X and Y chromosome. When PGD is used in conjunction with MicroSort®, there is a greater percentage of embryos of the desired sex from a given cohort of eggs.

Along with prenatal testing during early pregnancy, the advent of MicroSort® flow cytometric sperm separation and preimplantation genetic diagnosis allows couples to now have additional scientifically verifiable options for gender selection.

ACKNOWLEDGMENTS

The authors would like to gratefully acknowledge Gary Harton, Harvey Stern, MD, PhD, Lawrence A. Johnson, PhD, and MicroSort® Laboratory staff members, Danny Kozink, and Michelle Ballard for their contributions to this chapter.

REFERENCES

1. Shettles LB, Rorvik D. How to Choose the Sex of Your Baby. Broadway Books, New York, NY, 1984.
2. Wilcox AJ, Weinberg CR, Baird DD. Timing of sexual intercourse in relation to ovulation. Effect on the probability of conception, survival of the pregnancy, and sex of the baby. N Engl J Med 1995;333:1517–1521.
3. Chesterman-Phillips H. Boy or Girl: You Choose. Thorsons Publications Ltd, Northamptonshire, UK, 1985.
4. Hilsenrath RE, Swarup M, Bischoff FZ, et al. Effect of sexual abstinence on the proportion of X-bearing sperm as assessed by multicolor fluorescent in situ hybridization. Fertil Steril 1997;68:510–513.
5. Papa F, Henrion R, Breart G. Preconceptional selection of sex using the ionic method. Dietary regime. Results of a 2 years' prospective clinical study. J Gynecol Obstet Biol Reprod (Paris) 1983;12:415–422.
6. Seguy B. Methods of natural and voluntary sex selection. Value for the prevention of sex-linked malformations and of certain recurrent abortions. J Gynecol Obstet Biol Reprod (Paris) 1975;4:145–149.
7. Abbasi K. The spin on sperm. BMJ 1997;315:1386.
8. Ericsson RJ, Langevin CN, Nishino M. Isolation of fractions rich in human Y sperm. Nature 1973;246:421–424.
9. Ericsson RJ. X and Y spermatozoa. Contracept Fertil Sex (Paris) 1976;4:655–668.
10. Quinlivan WLG, Preciado K, Long TL, Sullivan H. Separation of human X and Y spermatozoa by albumin gradients and Sephadex chromatography. Fertil Steril 1982;37:104–107.
11. Beernink FJ, Dmwoski WP, Ericsson RJ. Sex preselection through albumin separation of sperm. Fertil Steril 1993;59(2):382–386.
12. Corson, SL, Batzer FR, Alexander NJ, et al. Sex selection by sperm separation and insemination. Fertil Steril 1984;42:756–760.
13. Jaffe S, Jewelewicz R, Wahl E, Khatamee, MA. A controlled study for gender selection. Fertil Steril 1991;56:254–258.
14. Rose GA, Wong A. Experiences in Hong Kong with the theory and practice of the albumin column method of sperm separation for sex selection. Hum Reprod 1998;13:146–149. Erratum in Hum Reprod 1998;13:1414.
15. van Kooij RJ, van Oost BA. Determination of sex ratio of spermatozoa with deoxyribonucleic acid-probe and quinacrine staining: a comparison. Fertil Steril 1992;58(2):384–386.

16. Wang HX, Flaherty SP, Swann NJ, Matthews CD. Discontinuous Percoll gradients enrich X-bearing human spermatozoa: a study using double-labeled fluorescence in-situ hybridization. Hum Reprod 1994;9:1265–1270.
17. Aribarg A, Ngeamvijawat J, Chanprasit Y, Sukcharoen N. Determination of the ratio of X and Y bearing spermatozoa after albumin gradient method using double-labeled fluorescence in situ hybridization (FISH). J Med Assoc Thai 1996;79(Suppl 1):S88–S95.
18. Flaherty SP, Matthews CD. Application of modern molecular techniques to evaluate sperm sex selection methods. Mol Hum Reprod 1997;2:937–942.
19. Chen Mj, Guu HF, Ho ES. Efficiency of sex pre-selection of spermatozoa by albumin method evaluated by double-labeled fluorescence in situ hybridization. Hum Reprod 1997;12:1920–1926.
20. Lin SP, Lee RK, Tsai YJ, et al. Separating X-bearing human spermatozoa through a discontinuous density gradient proved to be inefficient by double-label fluorescent in situ hybridization. J Assist Reprod Genet 1998;15:565–569.
21. Check ML, Bollendorf A, Check JH, et al. Separation of sperm through a 12-layer percoll column decreases the percentage of sperm staining with crinacrine. Arch Androl 2000; 44:47–50.
22. Kaneko S, Yamaguchi J, Kobayashi T, Iizuka R. Separation of human X- and Y-bearing sperm using percoll density gradient centrifugation. Fertil Steril 1983;40(5):661–665.
23. Corson SL, Batzer FR, Schlaff S. Preconceptual female gender selection. Fertil Steril 1983;40:384,385.
24. Beckett TA, Martin RH, Hoar DI. Assessment of the sephadex technique for selection of X-bearing human sperm by analysis of sperm chromosomes, deoxyribonucleic acid, and Y-bodies. Fertil Steril 1989;52:829–835.
25. Vidal F, Moragas M, Catala V, et al. Sephadex filtration and human serum albumin gradients do not select spermatozoa by sex chromosome: a fluorescent in situ hybridization study. Hum Reprod 1993;8:1740–1743.
26. Check JH, Katsoff D. A Prospective study to evaluate the efficacy of modified swim-up preparation for male sex selection. Hum Reprod1993;8:211–214.
27. Khatamee MA, Horn SR, Weseley A, et al. A controlled study for gender selection using swim-up separation. Gynecol Obstet Invest 1999;48:7–13.
28. De Jonge CJ, Flaherty SP, Barnes AM, et al. Failure of multitube sperm swim-up for sex preselection. Fertil Steril 1997;67:1109–1114.
29. Flaherty SP, Michalowska J, Swann NJ, et al. Albumin gradients do not enrich Y-bearing spermatozoa. Hum Reprod 1997;12:938–942.
30. Reubinoff BE, Schenker JG. New advances in sex preselection. Fertil Steril 1996;66:343–350.
31. American College of Obstetricians and Gynecologists Committee on Ethics. Ethics in Obstetrics and Gynecology: Sex Selection. Committee Opinion 177, AGOG, Washington D.C., 1996.
32. Ethics Committee of the American Society of Reproductive Medicine. Preconception gender selection for nonmedical reasons. Fertil Steril 2001;75:861–864.
33. Human Fertilisation and Embryology Authority. Sex Selection: Report Summary. Available at: www.hfea.gov.uk/AboutHFEA/Consultations/final sex selection summary.pdf. Accessed 2003.
34. Human Fertilisation and Embryology Authority. Sex Selection: Options for Regulation. Available at: www/hfea.gov.uk./AboutHFEA/Consultations/final sex selection main report.pdf. Accessed 2003.
35. Moruzzi JF. Selecting a mamalian species for the separation of X- and Y-chromosome-bearing spermatozoa. J Reprod Fertil 1979;57:319–323.

36. Pinkel D, Gledhill BL, Van Dilla MA, et al. High resolution DNA measurements of mammalian sperm. Cytometry 1982;3:1–9.
37. Johnson LA, Flook JP, Look MV, et al. Flow sorting of X and Y chromosome-bearing spermatozoa into two populations. Gamete Res 1987;16:1–9.
38. Johnson LA, Flook JP, Hawk HW. Sex preselection in rabbits: live births from X and Y sperm separated by DNA and cell sorting. Biol Reprod 1989;41:199–203.
39. Johnson LA. Sex preselection in swine: altered sex ratios in offspring following surgical insemination of flow sorted X- and Y-bearing sperm. Reprod Domest Anim 1991;26:309–314.
40. Cran DG, Johnson LA, Miller NGA, et al. Production of bovine calves following separation of X- and Y-chromosome bearing sperm and in vitro fertilization. Vet Rec 1993;132:40–41.
41. Cran DG, Cochrane DJ, Johnson LA, et al. Separation of X- and Y-chromosome bearing bovine sperm by flow cytometry for use in IVF. Theriogenology 1994;41:183.
42. Johnson LA, Welch GR, Keyvanfar K, et al. Gender preselection in humans? Flow cytometric separation of X and Y spermatozoa for the prevention of X-linked diseases. Hum Reprod 1993;8:1733–1739.
43. Sumner AT, Robinson JA. A difference in dry mass between the heads of X- and Y-bearing human spermatozoa. J Reprod Fert 1976;48:9–15.
44. Levinson G, Keyvanfar K, Wu JC, et al. DNA-based X-enriched sperm separation as an adjunct to preimplantation genetic testing for the prevention of X-linked disease. Hum Reprod 1995;10:979–982.
45. Fugger EF, Black SH, Keyvanfar K, Schulman JD. Births of normal daughters after MicroSort sperm separation and intrauterine insemination, in-vitro fertilization, or intracytoplasmic sperm injection. Hum Reprod 1998;30:2367–2370.
46. Schlaff WD. New ways to prepare semen for IUI. Contemp Ob Gyn 1987;29:79–86.
47. Johnson LA, Pinkel D. Modification of a laser-based flow cytometer for high resolution DNA analysis of mammalian spermatozoa. Cytometry 1986;7:268–273
48. Johnson, LA, Welch GR. Sex preselection: high speed flow cytometric sorting of X- and Y-sperm for maximum efficiency. Theriogenology 1999;52:1323–1341.
49. Johnson LA. Sexing mammalian sperm for production of offspring: the state-of-the-art. Animal Reprod Sci 2000;60,61:93–107.
50. Seidel GE, Garner DL. Current status of sexing mammalian spermatozoa. Reproduction 2002;124:733–743.
51. Ventura SJ, Mosher WD, Curtin SC. Centers for Disease Control and Prevention. Trends in Pregnancy Rates for the United States, 1976–97: An Update. National Vital Statistics Reports 2001;49(4):1–12.
52. Centers for Disease Control and Prevention. 2001 Assisted Reproductive Technology Success Rates. National Summary and Fertility Clinic Reports. US Department of Health and Human Services, National Center for Chronic Disease and Health Promotion, Division of Reproductive Health. Atlanta, GA. Available at: www.cdc.gov/reproductivehealth/ART01/index.htm. Accessed 2003.
53. Marden PM, Smith DW, McDonald MJ. Congenital malformations in the infant, including minor variations. J Pediatrics 1964;64:357–371.
54. Handyside AH, Kontogianni EH, Hardy K, Winston RML. Pregnancies from biopsied human preimplantation embryos sexed by Y-specific DNA-amplification. Nature 1990;344:768–770.
55. Kuliev A, Verlinsky Y. Thirteen years' experience of preimplantation genetic diagnosis: report of the Fifth International Symposium on Preimplantation Genetics. RBM Online 2004; 8:no. 2.

56. Harton GL, Karabinus D, Fallon LA, et al. Embryo outcome as determined by preimplantation genetic diagnosis after fertilization utilizing unsorted sperm vs. MicroSort® sorted sperm. Fertil Steril 2003;80(Suppl 3):S199.

Index